Advanc

MW00454606

PLAY
FOREVER

PLAY
FOREVER

How to Recover from
Injury and *Thrive*

KEVIN R. STONE, M.D.

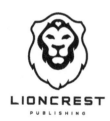

LIONCREST
PUBLISHING

PLAY FOREVER

How to Recover From Injury and Thrive

ISBN 978-1-5445-2678-2 *Hardcover*
      978-1-5445-2676-8 *Paperback*
      978-1-5445-2677-5 *Ebook*

This book is dedicated to

the thousands of patients who have

taught me how to be their doctor and joined

with me in the journey to push

the science forward.

CONTENTS

FOREWORD

Christine Mason

Businessperson, author, and futurist board member,
Stone Research Foundation

I'm standing on the beach watching my friend (who is well into his sixties and has recently rebounded from knee surgery) hydrofoil above the surf on the great Pacific. He is attentive, strong, and graceful in the sunshine. On Monday morning, he will ride his bike to work—and let me say, this isn't your ordinary commute: it's ten miles over steep mountain terrain. A typical winter weekend with his family often includes skiing all day and dancing the night away. In short, Dr. Kevin Stone is the embodiment of playing forever.

What Dr. Stone communicates in this book reflects what he's learned from thousands of patients and from clinical research, *and it is also how he lives.* As a tireless innovator, in orthopaedics and in other fields, he has a commitment to excellence in all things. After witnessing him at work for more than a decade, I believe his innovation comes from a combination of mental habits. These include a willingness to seek feedback and improved outcomes on any procedure he's involved in; to be curious and solution-oriented whenever he thinks things can be better; to listen deeply and between the lines to find out what's really going on; and to look across domains to cross-pollinate ideas. These are rare qualities in life and especially in medicine.

As he lays out in this book, the mental game is also one of the things that distinguishes someone who heals and becomes better from someone who merely recovers. Dr. Stone's life mission is to help people stay active and joyful in their bodies, doing the sports and activities they love for their whole life long. This volume is an extension of that mission.

Play Forever is a treasure trove of useful information, memorable anecdotes, and the collected wisdom of a groundbreaking surgeon with a heart toward healing for all. Whether you're an elite athlete, a passionate amateur, or just someone who wants to bounce back from an injury with full capacity, you're guaranteed to walk away with some new information or insight to lift you up. Dr. Stone, whether in person or through his writing, is that little voice inside of you that says you can do it, and invites you to show up in the best way you can, shining and willing to play.

INTRODUCTION

*P*lay forever—this is what I want for you. It is my wish for each person I have the privilege to work with. I am a physician, surgeon, and scientist, and in each of these roles I have a repository of knowledge, skills, and curiosity to offer each person who seeks me out. I work with world-class athletes, with people confronting arthritis and the effects of aging, with those who lead active and sport-filled lives, and with those who have just begun their fitness journey. I am driven to inquire scientifically about the healing process and technically how to bring better skills to that healing. Fundamentally, I sense that much of what we know in medicine today is only part of the whole human biologic story, and it can be frustratingly insufficient. Thus, I have a compelling urge to combine research and development with clinical treatment. In each case—and no matter what the case—my ability to deliver is based on my belief that my patients can become better than they were before they were injured or afflicted with arthritis.

The key to this is passionate care. Everyone gets injured—even great athletes. The best of them use the injury to come back to their sport better—faster, fitter, and stronger. But to do this, they need information on how to do so, what can help them, and how they can motivate themselves. They need to recognize the recovery process as long, entwined with their habits and mindset, and affected by a large variety of factors. I believe it's the duty of us doctors to provide that guidance. Most of us in medicine have been trained to fix a person and send them on their way, but I see the first encounter with a patient as an opportunity to build a lifelong relationship. The first doctor-patient encounter establishes a level of trust: that I can repair the immediate problem, and that we can embark on a lifelong fitness program with semiannual fitness tests, preseason education about training programs, in-season tune-ups, and outcome studies on treatments and implants placed in their bodies. My team and I become the patient's go-to musculoskeletal health and fitness source forever.

"Forever" here is the important word. My patients and I embark on the journey of excellence together and that cannot be done in short time frames. In part, this desire to become the patient's go-to musculoskeletal health and fitness source comes from my belief that every doctor should know the outcome of any treatment they give, any substance they inject or prescribe, or any device they put into a patient. Thus, if I am going to replace a part of someone's knee, I believe I should study them annually (with X-ray or patient question-naire) for life. Otherwise, how do I know that the implant or surgical technique worked? Secondly, if I am going to repair someone's knee, how about the rest of the body that it is attached to? If my surgery is going to help them return to a sport that led to the injury in the first place, shouldn't I have an interest in how they are returning and in what physical state? Third, if I have a patient with a major injury that is potentially devastating to their livelihood, and I am helping them through the process of healing, shouldn't I offer them tools to deal with or avoid the predictable post-injury depression? Shouldn't I coach them on the mindset they need to triumph over their injury and become physically and mentally stronger?

These are the principles underlying my practice and our treatment at The Stone Clinic, and they are the principles that allow us to reach excellence. Helping people excel is fun. It's always gratifying to hang a poster in my clinic showing a star athlete-patient, post-treatment, wearing a first-place medal—not just from the satisfaction of celebrating that achievement, but also because it represents our shared journey from injury to excellence. I feel that fulfillment with *every* kind of patient—from the high school soccer player to the middle-aged weekend warrior to the octogenarian Masters champion. Creating new ways to accelerate healing, exceeding known limitations, and pushing forward the boundaries of human medical and surgical science are the goals that stimulate me every day.

WHAT IS THIS BOOK ABOUT?

Play Forever is a book about all of these concepts and more. It's about empowering you to reach your level of excellence—mentally and physically, before injury and after—so that you're still playing and enjoying life to the fullest when you're one hundred years old. And by "play," I don't only mean competitive sports. There are many ways to enjoy life to the fullest, and I hope to show you how.

We'll begin our journey with what it means to be "fit." In the spirit of "play forever" and passionate care, Part I will explore what mental qualities you need to excel at sports and life, what general principles are important to staying physically fit—or starting your fitness journey—and how you can keep yourself injury free. Since many of my patients are active and love their sports, I've also included a sports-specific chapter to talk you through the most common injuries you need to avoid with each sport, and best practices in terms of equipment and playing principles. For those just beginning their fitness journey or trying to figure out how, there's plenty in this chapter about different sports and activities you can try, their benefits—and joys—and the impact on your body.

Part II will deep dive into injuries. We'll cover the role of perspective in injury recovery and the common joint injuries, after which we'll explore the landscape of surgical care and novel ways of treatment, including anabolic therapies. As a surgeon, I am honored, humbled, and empowered by repairing injured people. But much of what surgeons do today is based on knowledge that we may discover is wrong tomorrow. I feel the persistent imperative to challenge each assumption and to simplify each technical step to seek out every improvement. I am always thinking about how to improve everything I see and touch. While asking, Why do it this way? is often annoying to others, asking, Could it be improved this way? stimulates a conversation—in my own mind and with my colleagues. My hope is that by empowering you with the knowledge of what is possible, and how we can improve what is currently practiced, you will be encouraged to ask this question of your own physician and create the best treatment plan for you.

In Part III, we'll expand the field a little more to look at the context in which fitness and injury recovery takes place. So we'll explore the current state of medical practice and doctor training, including its flaws and possibilities. Our last chapter looks to the future: what will medical practice look like in ten years, twenty, or thirty? What are the possibilities and the heady potential? As we are striving for excellence today, we know that somewhere in that future is yet another level we and our patients want to achieve.

WHO IS THIS BOOK FOR?

As you might have guessed by now, this book is for a range of people. In these pages, I'm talking to athletes, sportspeople, high schoolers and the elderly, those who have played some kind of sport all their lives, and those who have never kicked a ball before. I'm talking to patients, to doctors, to my juniors in the medical field, and to my peers. This book is for you.

There are two reasons for this. First, the people who come into The Stone Clinic looking for treatment vary in type and profession, so how could I write a book on what I encounter in my practice of orthopaedic surgery—and, sometimes, life in general—for a specific type of person? Fitness and healing relate to everyone. Arthritis can come for you whether you've spent your career shooting hoops or working at the desk.

Second, labels are not always useful. If you look at life as a sports event—and I encourage you to—then you'll see that a label we wear in one part of our lives doesn't apply to all parts. Those who are athletes in one sport are beginners in others. Surgeons and doctors are also regular people who play sports and keep fit in their downtime. Those who are just starting on their fitness journey may already have experimented with a few of these sports and so will be familiar with them, while many who have been playing sports for years may not know the basics of physical health (like standing up straight and working on balance). When you read this book, I encourage you to look beyond the thought of "this section or chapter is not for me." Instead, I hope you will read these pages and see the many selves you are and can become. If you don't ski, don't dismiss the sport-specific advice. Instead, see if you could pick it up. If you've never suffered an injury, don't ignore the advice on how to tune your mindset to recover properly. Instead, see if you can apply that mindset now, before you're injured. (Try it, and you'll see how it impacts so much of what you do.) Everything here is valuable for a sports approach to yourself: mind, body, recovery, and living. Everything here is focused on helping you play forever.

Efficient, effective surgery that repairs, regenerates, and replaces injured tissues is the elegant goal of human surgical restoration. If I can combine these skills with motivating people to become fitter, faster, and stronger than they were before they were injured, I have contributed to their lives in a truly meaningful way. I hope you enjoy sharing this journey with me and—most important—that it motivates you to think of new ways to *play forever.*

PART I

OPTIMIZING PERFORMANCE

CHAPTER 1

MENTAL FITNESS

Almost every professional athlete we see at The Stone Clinic has a solid fitness program involving CrossFit-like extreme training and cross-training in the off-season. They know all about how to get strong, and have access to trainers and coaches who aim to eliminate specific physical weaknesses that can lead to injury.

The pros also know about nutrition. They know that protein is necessary for muscle building and that a balanced diet is more important than the huge carb-laden training tables of the past. All, especially long-distance athletes, know about fueling during sports. Hydration has become a commonplace science with access to electrolyte replenishment everywhere—even poured over the heads of successful coaches.

In addition, the pros know about massage and soft-tissue mobilization as practiced by superb physical therapists. They use the latest in yoga and Pilates along with novel stretching techniques to help them remain flexible. The "wimp" fears of the old days—i.e., an aversion to spending time in Lycra-filled stretching classes—has given way to a useful realization: it is better to spend time in Lycra than in hospital gowns.

And the pros know about coaching—who is good for them and who is not. They know enough to seek out individual coaches if the team coach is not a good fit. They use the resources of the web to find out about the latest strategies that other teams and athletes are employing.

All the pros use technology on both a personal and a team level to monitor performance and strategize about moves, feints, forms, and styles: the choreography of winning performances. These interconnected athletes represent not just local wisdom but the global skillset of the world's best.

And yet, even with all of these components in place, professional athletes can implode. When Serena Williams was penalized during the 2018 US Open, she turned her anger against the umpire rather than remaining focused on her opponent. She lost. At the same event, when Roger Federer suffered from high heat and humidity, he couldn't wait to get out of Arthur Ashe tennis stadium. He lost.

The obvious lesson? We defeat ourselves far more often than our opponents defeat us. Unforced errors in tennis are not just the problems of novices; they pervade sports. Despite the best coaching, phenomenal physical training, fitness, vast sums of money, and even decades of experience, we often remain our own worst enemies.

The patterns that serve or obstruct even great athletes are often learned on children's playgrounds, on youth teams, and through parenting. The phenomenal successes of players, such as Roger Federer,

Tiger Woods, and Serena Williams are brought to a stop by psychological weaknesses—distractions that cause them to lose their swing, their temper, or their confidence, despite seeming at the top of their game. Federer, Woods, and Williams were coached to stunning physical success—but left mentally exposed.

Consistently, the one weakness that is most difficult to fix in athletes lies in the mind itself. Mental conditioning, the approach to an injury and its recovery, the overcoming of psychological blocks that prevent a physical superstar from being a winner—these are so ingrained that they remain the most difficult weaknesses to fix.

Yet it is not impossible to change. We can work on these issues, and many doctors and mental empowerment coaches are successful at it. The first step—a simple but crucial one—is to understand that the body and mind are irrevocably linked. This doesn't only apply to competitive athletes, but to everyone, whether they're dealing with a changing body, playing amateur sports, or simply living. A brain is attached to each body I repair. This is obvious, but in treating the whole patient, I am cognizant of the importance of mental processes as they relate to treatment. The mental health of an injured patient brings another dimension both to their healing and their ability to excel. In short, our daily mental health defines what our body is able to achieve. Naomi Osaka poignantly brought this to light in her refusal to undergo the ritual press conference drilling in the 2021 French Open. Over decades of practicing medicine, I have identified particular mental qualities that enable people to shine—not just athletically, but in all they do. This is a good place to start this book: in the unseen and often underappreciated aspect of fitness and health that can ensure you play forever and play well. These eight mental fitness objectives are:

- Competitiveness
- Grit
- Attention
- Fantasy
- Patience
- Acceptance
- Grace
- Kindness and competency

While these qualities are what take supreme athletes to the top, they are applicable to all aspects of your life. So pay attention to your own mental game—on the court or the playfield or the racecourse, and in day-to-day interactions at work and home. Strengthening each of these qualities is the cornerstone of fitness.

Mindfulness from Day One

I f you knew that your child was going to be on the world stage, performing before millions of people, and that their success depended on their response to adversity, how would you start training them? My advice is to start early.

I believe that the mental fitness required for success as a top competitor is largely formed in childhood. As children, our errors of both judgment and action are met with a wide range of responses. Our teachers and parents may exhibit love or disdain for our actions. They may respond with a teaching moment or with severe discipline. What may be needed, instead, is training in the skillsets that enable young people to control their emotions and their thoughts—skillsets that empower them to become tactical when faced with adversity, to become calculating when surprised by unanticipated events, to become cunning when attacked, and to be mindful at all times.

This is possible. We enroll our children in all kinds of after-school activities, from religious schooling to arts and crafts, from sports camps to computer programming sessions. But where do they go to get the type of mental training that allows them to respond skillfully? Apparently not from team sports, which are often filled with violence and exhortations to hit harder and get "psyched up." Coaching in individual sports certainly addresses the mental game, but it often comes too late.

The mature athlete brings to the game his or her life story of success and failure, which often needs to be accommodated rather than built upon. What is needed is the recognition early on that developing mindfulness—often expressed as the ability to put a pause between the brain and the tongue—may determine our overall success in life. Mindfulness deserves formal early training, which should continue throughout one's life.

The lesson I take from observation of professional athletes' equanimity (or lack of it) is the importance of sophisticated, intuitive, and careful coaching of children. Their approach to sport will be imprinted in their psyches forever. When done well in the beginning, all else is coachable.

COMPETITIVENESS

Competitive. That's how the vast majority of four hundred female corporate executives, the subjects of a recent research report,[1] see themselves. They consider competitiveness an asset to their leadership skills. The study revealed that executive women are more likely to have played competitive sports and are more likely to hire candidates who have also participated in sports. Almost all of the respondents (94 percent) said they participated in at least one sport, and close to three-quarters agreed that an athletic background can help accelerate a woman's leadership and career potential. Approximately two-thirds said that past sporting involvement contributed to their current career

---

[1] EY Women Athletes Business Network and espnW, "Making the Connection: Women, Sport, and Leadership" (2014), https://espnpressroom.com/us/press-releases/2014/10/female-executives-say-participation-in-sport-helps-accelerate-leadership-and-career-potential/.

success, and that a background in sport was a positive influence on hiring decisions. For girls, it seems, the race to the top of the corporate ladder begins well before their first job. It starts with competitive sports. Yet if you ask parents to describe the traits they are trying to teach their children, they typically mention compassion, teamwork, politeness, and diligence—but never competitiveness. Why is this quality not mentioned?

The skillsets needed by executives, civic leaders, entrepreneurs, doctors, and other professionals—both female and male—overlap with those that make great athletes. Determination, grit, focus, teamwork skills, and the ability to drive oneself and overcome adversity come to mind as the most obvious traits. These are often learned while playing team sports. Fortunately, competitiveness is a skill that also can be honed and encouraged.

How can competitiveness be learned? I can think of seven ways.

1. Remind yourself that success is admirable, that it is within reach, and that it is the pinnacle of achievement.
2. Study what competitiveness means and how it can be utilized.
3. Reward competitive skills. (For children, this means eliminating some of the "participation" trophies and making winning important. It matters. Teaching children to win helps them understand their potential and helps them to find their strengths.) Encourage competitiveness by bringing more age-appropriate awards to sports and academics.
4. Develop mental skills required to be a great athlete and/or executive, including the ability to find the mental flow that characterizes the supremely successful person.

5. Learn how to put yourself in a position to execute your best work, while at the same time developing the skills required to manage failure.

6. Measure your potential. Through competition, we reveal our true abilities. We can gather data on our own potential as well as performance, which may lead to identification of sport-specific skills.

7. Adopt a sustainable approach to athletic or academic performance. The message: the best competitors never get too high or too low but focus on getting a little bit better every day.

When you learn to embrace healthy competition, you can find your spheres of success. Often the last-place athlete in one sport is the star of the next. Being rejected by the volleyball team may put the shorter athlete into the gymnastics world. The too-tall ballet dancer may become the rower. It is your competitive fiber that will drive you to win somewhere. That skill is what creates successful people at all ages.

It's okay to want to win. So compete. Teach kids how to compete. Foster competition. Embrace the outcome.

GRIT

Swimmer Katie Ledecky doesn't just win. She crushes the competition. She crushes her own records and then world records. Everyone asks, "How does she do it?" She has nearly perfect form (despite an imperfect body for swimming). She has great coaching. But the secret sauce is grit.

The world-class athletes I have worked with all have slightly different approaches to success. Some pace themselves so as to peak at the right times. Others seem to glide effortlessly in their sport with an elegance and style that raises them above their peers, giving them the efficiency to excel. Many of the best reached the top by putting in longer hours, getting to that ten-thousand-hour number so commonly mentioned as the threshold to superior performance. All these approaches can lead to winning. Without grit, it's possible to win, but it's impossible to crush the competition.

Grit is what makes an athlete push as hard during the last hour of practice as in the first hour. Grit is coming to practice sessions with the determination to push harder than ever before. Grit doesn't give in. Ledecky's goal is not just to win, but also to swim faster than anyone ever has—and possibly ever will.

At the end of the day, among great athletes, grit is a common denominator. Superiority in anything almost always involves sacrifice. Sacrifice of time, distractions, and pleasure are required to rise above your challengers—who want the prize as much as you do. And grit is what permits the sacrifice to continue, even when the goal is far away.

Grit cannot really be taught, but it can be inspired. With sufficient motivation, you can make a decision to flip a switch, to envelop the sacrifice, and to endure the pain. Ask yourself what really motivates you. If you don't know, think it through with the best coaches you can find. Without an overarching purpose, it is tough to win because sacrifice for yourself has little leverage. Only you (and possibly your friends and family) care.

Being part of something bigger than yourself is a strong motivator. When the goal is shared and the sacrifice distributed, the team effect pushes you. The sacrifices seem less painful and the ambition more lofty. When Michael Phelps got out of the pool after the 2016 4x100 relay, his comment was not about how great it was to win, but about how determined he was to bring the gold home to the US. He realized that yet another gold medal just for himself had little significance.

Bode Miller took a different route. As a loner in his youth, he developed a unique, nearly out-of-control skiing style that led to a string of victories on the World Cup tour. He proclaimed his love of the perfect turn, rather than the victory. He eschewed the team training, team bus, and team hotel on the international ski tour. Yet when the Turin Olympics rolled around in 2006, he was overwhelmed by the distractions of the global stage. Isolated and left to his own proclivities, he failed to make a single podium.

The real message? Grit comes a lot easier when the goal is bigger than the athlete.

ATTENTION

Watching any of the Grand Slam tennis tournaments often makes me wonder why the most elite athletes in tennis still have concentration lapses. Why do they miss so many shots, make so many unforced errors, have to psych themselves up between each shot?

Do we not train people from a young enough age to be able to focus for long periods of time? Are we really only capable of brief periods of intensity? Are the unforced errors in tennis similar to the unforced errors in surgery or in driving a car? The world would undoubtedly be better off if we all could focus intensely for hours, performing at our highest levels, and without the errors that occur due to lapse of focus.

Most sports injuries I see in my orthopaedic practice are the result of loss of focus. The world-class skier momentarily loses edge control, the recreational skier gets going too fast, the skater "slips," the dancer lands poorly. These "mistakes" occur in the midst of sequences repeated a million times, yet they can happen easily when the athlete is slightly distracted.

To me, intense focus for long periods of time seems like a trainable skill. If monks can sit over documents and transcribe them faithfully for hours on end, could we focus equally in our daily lives or in our most important sports events? What if we started focus training at a young age? Error-free activities could be practiced in writing, drawing, sports, and more. Successful focus for minutes and then hours could be rewarded. Errors from loss of focus could be penalized. For example, two points lost for an unforced error in tennis. What if we institute penalties for adults' self-inflicted mistakes to incentivize a safer world, diminishing "accidents" that so often result from distraction rather than intention?

The cost of loss of focus is enormous. From self-inflicted harm to damage to others, the range of destruction is breathtaking. Yet the tools for training this skill seem weak.

But back to the psyched-up tennis players on the pro tennis circuit: swearing, grunting, talking to themselves between points, jumping up and down at the baseline, admonishing themselves to do better…This is the best we can do? Time for a crowd-sourced global conversation on human performance and mental fitness. How can we teach ourselves to focus, clearly, for long stretches of time? It's time to blockbust the conventional belief that to err is human.

Psyched Up, Let Down: The Harvey Moment

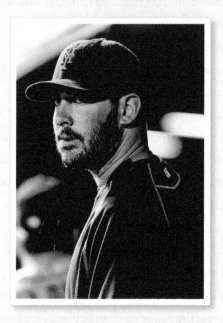

I f you watched the last game of the 2015 World Series, you saw a classic and avoidable mistake. Matt Harvey was pitching a no-hitter. He threw a full complement of pitches through the eighth inning; he was in "The Zone" and ecstatic. Then his manager informed him that he would not pitch the ninth inning. He protested, the manager gave in, the crowd roared, and disaster happened.

If you watched Harvey exit the dugout, you could have easily predicted the outcome. Harvey ran to the mound, psyched up and ready to decimate the opposing batters. The fans chanted his name. The atmosphere was electric.

Pitchers *walk* to the mound. They are focused, not distracted. The ability to throw a ninety-mile-an-hour fastball with accuracy, and mix in two or three other pitches, is what beats batters. Tuning out distractions, lowering the heartbeat, breathing slowly, and delivering powerful pitches takes rhythmic coordination.

Harvey threw high, outside, and almost wildly. The train wreck was just waiting to happen. Whether or not he deserved to be on the mound, he did deserve masterful coaching.

Harvey's mistake was his failure to reclaim the Zen-like focus required of him in that moment. He needed the help of his coach to do this, a coach who could take him aside, get into his head, focus his vision inward, slow his breathing, and create the calm mindset that allows a superstar to deliver in the intensity of a big moment. Psyched up with his adrenaline running, Harvey's pitch control was lost—and so were the Mets' hopes for a World Series ring.

The ability to "center down" in a clutch moment, whether it's exhilarating or life-threatening, determines the outcome of many critical decisions in life. It is a wonder that mental control is not taught as a major life lesson for all of us. We can learn it, we can practice it, and we can use it to improve. And when the forces of enthusiasm are greater than our skills, we should be able to rely on our coaches to bring us to that focus. Harvey was let down by his coach. Don't be let down by yours.

It's incredibly valuable to have a life coach, a confidant, and a trusted friend in your life and to rely on their perspective when yours is about to fail you. But knowing when that moment is at hand, and being able to ask for help, is the hardest part.

FANTASY

Meditation has become the prescription of choice for much of what ails us. Designed to put space between the thoughts and the tongue, or between thoughts and ill-advised actions, meditation invites a state of "mindfulness." It calms our anxieties and permits many stressed individuals to survive their days with less angst.

But what about the many who have tried meditation and failed? Is it because they can't filter out all the noise—the flood of contradictory or stress-filled thoughts—or is it because meditation is hard? Meditation requires diligent practice and time out from "productive activities." Meditation's benefits are often seen only after considerable time has passed, and they may be subtle.

Without diminishing the power and positivity of meditation, may I suggest another mental activity that might be useful for both meditation practitioners and the rest of us? Fantasy.

Fantasy is available to all. It is universal in all cultures and unique to individuals. Fantasy can be goal-oriented or simply pleasurable. Fantasy requires no practice, and the benefits can be enormous.

An example: While bending my knee after my own knee surgery, the therapist asked if I knew how to meditate. Could I quiet my mind and ignore the pain? "No" was my answer. How about fantasizing about being a surfer, kneeling on my board, and paddling through perfect waves? "Ah, yes," I replied. The waves, the kneeling, the flexion of the knee…With fantasy, you can take yourself anywhere—happy, blissful, sensual, or athletic brain spaces—as the therapist cranks the reluctant joint a little harder.

Fantasizing is not the same as visualization. The difference between them is a matter of imagination. Visualization is mentally practicing what you could do; fantasy is creating what you dream to do. Visualization alone can lead to stress: the fear of not performing. An athlete who visualizes will memorize the course, go through it in their mind, and try to repeat the vision during competition. Sometimes that works, but too often the reality of the event doesn't match the practice runs.

The champion athlete is one who dreams of the big win and wills it to happen. Uninhibited fantasy leads to exhilaration and frees the muscle memory to do its thing. Remarkably, the same effect happens for patients dealing with serious injuries or diseases. Surprising results often seem to happen for those who set big goals and have the unbroken willpower to get the results.

There are many situations in which this strategy can be effective. If you're preparing to give a presentation, envision Martin Luther King's "I Have a Dream" speech. Fantasize about letting your oratory soar and empower the audience. Before launching yourself down a mountain onto a ski course, don't just visualize each turn; fantasize about arcing the perfect turn and executing the perfect run. Even in yoga, where meditation is supposed to reign supreme, fantasizing about having the flexibility of a circus contortionist may permit postures you never dreamed possible.

Back pain is another place where fantasy can be useful. The worst part is the fear that it won't go away, and that one's life will be permanently compromised. While there is no all-encompassing solution to back pain, almost every therapy involves strengthening the trunk and core. Fantasizing about this muscle building can promote a new body image in which you stand tall, shoulders back, and belly button sucked in while radiating inner power and grace.

Fantasy is available to us all; it is a form of useful and simple magical thinking. By creating and living temporarily within the images we create in our brains, we can return to our earthbound lives with a smile—and the knowledge that we can indeed create a space where we are gloriously successful and happy.

If Horses Could Dream

t just does not seem logical that an elite athlete—in this case, a pampered, well-fed, carefully vetted, meticulously exercised horse—could be tired after running only three times in four weeks, and only two minutes at a time. The excuses given for why the racehorse California Chrome did not win the third leg of the Triple Crown might have sounded reasonable to some, but not to many of us involved in sports medicine.

In 2014, California Chrome was vying to be the first horse in thirty-six years to win the Triple Crown. But in the Belmont Stakes, he finished fourth, behind Tonalist and two others. It wasn't even close. With the race now long over, we are left with the following question: what makes an athlete—animal or human—perform at peak ability repeatedly and then suddenly, inexplicably, turn in a subpar performance? The answer may lie more in the mind than in the body, which is why the best training money can buy may not ever be enough.

From a physical point of view, the energy output required of a thoroughbred horse in a race is extreme, but very short. Tonalist finished the 1.5-mile race in 2:28.52 minutes. Over the course of a typical race, a horse will utilize a little more than two calories per pound. As an example, a 1,000-pound horse carrying 126 pounds of weight (jockey and saddle) will burn nearly fifteen thousand calories during a race. (That's five days' worth of calories for the average healthy, active human male in his twenties to mid-thirties.) As long as the animal remains uninjured, physical recovery from all of that effort is typically measured in days as the stored glucose (primarily from the liver and fat) is rapidly replaced by hay and feed. Muscle soreness from lactic acid buildup reduces quickly. Top racehorses have massages, walking times, rest times, and feed times all calibrated to aid in this recovery. There would have been every reason for the horse to have recovered from the first two races and be raring to go for the third—but something went wrong.

What is unknowable, although possibly predictable, is the state of a horse's mind when entering the starting gate. Many announcers commented on the serene appearance of California Chrome in the paddock and on the way to the track. The horse's calmness in the gates paralleled his unfortunate lack of spirit on the track.

For humans, similar flat performances can happen at the most inopportune times as a result of conditions known as unexplained underperformance syndrome or overtraining syndrome. However, humans have the capacity to psych up for the event, to imagine the victory, to fantasize about the outcome. An ability to fantasize differentiates successful athletes from equally talented but less imaginative competitors.

California Chrome may have had all the horsepower in the world, but without the mindset to win at all costs on that day, his race was lost before it began.

PATIENCE

Patience is a virtue, for both athletes and patients. Successful older athletes tend to have more of it. While my younger patients set fitness and performance goals and go after them, my older patients set goals and proceed in a stepwise, cautious fashion. My younger patients are often injured. My older patients—especially those recovering from an injury or surgery—avoid repeat injuries by building solid foundations for their workouts and sports.

Nothing demonstrates the difference between the old and the young more than CrossFit. At CrossFit, the young set personal bests every time they can. Their volume of weight training, the amount of weight they lift, and their intensity increase steadily. And their injuries from overuse and technique errors fill orthopaedic surgeons' offices worldwide.

My older fitness-addicted patients learn their lessons. They return to fitness training after an injury with an appreciation for the time and effort it takes to heal—and so they cautiously increase their weights without hurry. Their return rate for repeat injuries is a fraction of that of my younger patients. Even my nationally competitive older CrossFit patients turn their addictive personalities to physical therapy and rehab. They are in my clinic every day after surgery and sometimes twice a day. They follow the therapist's recommendations and gain range of motion before they focus on gaining strength.

My middle-aged patients pose a problem. They believe they are young bucks and reinjure themselves with weekend-warrior workouts and games. They heal more slowly than they want to believe. They see their physical therapists once or twice a week. They get compensation injuries, such as back pain, when they are recovering from a knee surgery. I know. I am that patient.

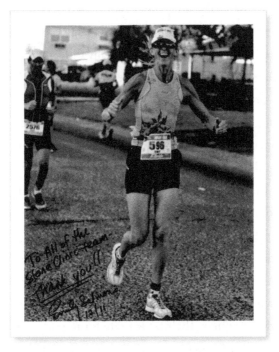

*Emily S • Triathlete and heli-skier, completing her first of six
Ironman races after BioKnee reconstruction in 2010*

Patience may be a virtue, but from what I see, it is also very much an art form. It takes training. Delaying the gratification of intense exercise means regulating the adrenaline, the endorphins, and the testosterone-driven forces within us. On that score, gender matters too. My female patients overwhelmingly outperform my male patients in patience at every age. Many top women runners and triathletes don't even start their sports until after age thirty. After an injury, they quickly reset their priorities by introducing more balance into their workouts. Maybe that's why they excel at older ages, more than their male peers.

Patience is not innate. It is acquired by recognizing that more victories are won with strategy than with impulse and emotion. Patience grows from experience with failure and by learning to excel from that experience rather than being diminished by it. Patience comes from accumulating skills and technique, and refining them. Patience is the art form that expresses the wisdom of the long view. Patience keeps you out of my office.

ACCEPTANCE

"Failure is not an option," people sometimes say. Really? Why not? I believe that failure can be a useful option—if you know how to accept it, learn from it, and move on.

I certainly have failed far more often than I have succeeded when creating new products and pursuing novel, risky business adventures. Without failure, I would never have learned the business and life lessons necessary to succeed in these spaces. As a physician and surgeon, I can assure you that failure is part of advancing the field. Much of medicine is a science in constant development, so it is never static. When I hear a doctor say, "I only do what is approved and permitted," I hear a doctor stuck in the middle of the field. When I learn about a new insurance company regulation stating that they will only pay for "proven" medicines or procedures, I recognize an insurance business that does not understand that most of the practice of medicine has not been proven by high-quality, Level-1 studies, and those procedures that have been proven may have evolved since that study was completed. In fact, less than 5 percent of all papers submitted to one major sports medicine journal, *Arthroscopy*, were graded as Level-1 studies.

Failure is the fuel of smart innovation. Taking risks means accepting that a certain percentage of the efforts won't work, especially in surgery and patient care. Data published by our research group demonstrated that 79 percent of 120 osteoarthritic patients who had their meniscus replaced were still enjoying all the benefits of their meniscus replacement up to twelve years from surgery. That's a high success rate. Yet almost a quarter of these patients did not achieve the level of success we were aiming for. In that sense, failure was part of the risk for both physician and patient.

The surgical procedures we perform remain in continuous development. Outcomes are continually improving, most recently with the additions of growth factors and stem cells. They don't always work, however. Some knees and some patients will fail our best efforts. (We counsel our patients about this before surgery.) Fortunately, we have developed salvage procedures in the event the first try fails, and failure is always our teacher.

So push the envelope. Accept that things might not work out. Acceptance of failure is a great option because it permits the success of novel solutions that otherwise would not occur.

There's another aspect to our acceptance of failure: not wasting energy on regret. Watching football over many seasons, you can't help but notice that the special quarterbacks, the great ones like Tom Brady of the Patriots, Russell Wilson of the Seahawks, or Peyton Manning of the Broncos, don't get hung up on errors. Teams led by superstar quarterbacks get into a rhythm of winning. The quarterbacks enter the zone, feel the flow of the game, and lead their teammates to excellence. But equally important, when errors occur—the interception, the dropped pass, the sack—the quarterback moves on as if it never happened. The great ones don't look back.

Not looking back is key both in sports and in health. My patients who come in with stories of woe, focused on what one doctor did or did not do for them, have a much harder time than the patients who seek advice on where to go from here and how to recover quickly. Some patients are burdened by blame. They focus, for example, on the store that had the wet floor causing them to slip, and they listen for sympathy rather than solutions. Letting go and moving on is sometimes hard to do.

So how do you do what the great ones do? You accept, on a contingency basis. That is, you learn when to look back and recognize what to look for when you do.

We do this in medicine and surgery all the time. We aim for an accurate diagnosis and successful treatment, and when all goes according to plan, we feel proud of our patients and ourselves. When it doesn't, however, we examine every decision, find a new approach, and move on. The ability to park the regret over an unsuccessful outcome, to store it for examination later, and focus on a new solution characterizes the successful physician. The operative word is "later." It is essential to go back *later* and examine what happened, learn from the failure, and use it to improve the next decision.

This ability to park the frustration that arises from failure comes from the absolute confidence that examining it later will be more fruitful, and that any conclusions made in the moment will be incomplete and interfere with the job at hand. Steely assurance of that fact is the magic behind the unperturbed face of the intercepted quarterback. Practice being a Monday morning quarterback. Review your good and bad decisions. Become expert at the analysis and the design of the new action plan. Be creative in your thought process in order to avoid thinking in the same patterns that led to the first error. Speed up your pattern recognition so you can see and then reject a losing play in a set of circumstances. But do it later.

This is what the great ones do. They accept their failure—storing it away for analysis later—and let their acceptance keep them in their state of magical flow, where they can see new possibilities and create novel ones. So let it go and learn.

Recipe for a Hat Trick: Flow

Hat tricks—three goals in a game, like soccer player Carli Lloyd's feat at the 2016 Women's World Cup—occur because the athlete and the team are in the flow. Flow is the stream of consciousness, the momentum of physical activity, the confluence of events that produce success. And success follows success. In surgery, clinical care, work, and sports, flow is both the tool and the goal. The question is: can it be predicted?

At least four criteria are present when flow occurs.

Happiness. A wise advisor once told me that I should never go in to work unless I was 100 percent happy. "Impossible," I replied. His retort was that people make good decisions when they are happy and poor ones when they are not. If I am happy only 75 percent of the time while working as a surgeon, can I really afford to make one poor decision out of every four? Neither my patients nor I would accept it. So happiness is a base criterion for the solid decision-making of flow.

Preparedness. "Chance favors the prepared mind," as Louis Pasteur once commented. Great discoveries are made standing on the shoulders of giants, knowing what came before you, building on data, and laying the groundwork for the eureka moment. Great sports accomplishments are achieved by athletes who have honed their skills with endless practice. Super-prepared people are more likely to succeed.

Creativity. The ability, the desire, the *need* to look at what is and imagine what isn't is the heart of creativity. It often arises from

curiosity based on skepticism, and irreverence born of dissatisfac-
tion. Creativity feeds flow, and flow feeds creativity.

Talent. The skillset that permits you to seize the moment, score
the goals, and realize your dreams.

While seemingly unpredictable, the odds of a hat trick go up
dramatically when these forces are working in unison. It seems
poetic that hat tricks all start and end with happiness. Without
happiness, the score is just a score.

GRACE

While watching the world premiere of a dance program by Amy
Seiwert, I was captivated by a smile.

The program was designed to highlight two independently choreographed interpretations of the same music with the same group of
dancers. In each piece, the gorgeous fitness of the dancers, the beauty
of the expressions, and the stunning movements wowed the audience.
Yet rather than focus on the differences in the creative interpretations
of the music, I was most moved by one dancer's small but beautiful
smile. It radiated warmth and made me smile in response as her head
turned toward me with each spin. What is it about a smile that can
determine the greatness of a performance?

The smile touches the hearts and spirits of both the performer
and the observer. The smile is her gift.

I have provided medical support for dancers since the 1980s. Back
then, the female dancers were rail-thin, smoked cigarettes between
rehearsals, and had no nutrition guidance. They were revered for their

grace, beauty, and ethereal qualities. The male dancers could leap to great heights with elongated—rather than muscular—bodies. The strict style of Balanchine choreography ruled the ballet universe. Ballet was not that healthy and, as far as I could see, not that much fun.

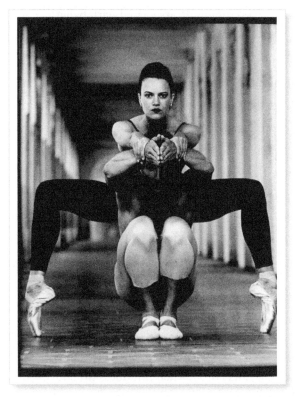

Ballet dancers and Stone Clinic patients Wendy V., Larry P., and Pascal L.,
Photo credit: Mark Estes

Although dancers were paid as artists, they were asked to perform as athletes. Consequently, injuries to their frail bodies were common. Gradually, the ballet masters and choreographers recognized this mismatch and permitted those of us in sports medicine to bring a focus on cardiovascular and muscular fitness training, nutrition, and healthy lifestyles to the ballet world. Today's dancers are both strong and lithe. They are extremely fit and very much aware of their health. It is a joy to watch them perform, and they radiate a degree of happiness not commonly associated with ballet.

Still, when pushed to extremes, their bodies become injured. Dancers' injuries reflect the athletic risks they take—ACL tears, ankle ligament ruptures, back muscle strains, and meniscus and cartilage damage. Yet their response to injuries is now much more consistent with other professional athletes who benefit from early repair of cartilage and ligament injuries and immediate high-quality manual physical therapy. The result is prolonged careers and healthy retirements.

A dancer's performance is up close and personal. It's not only their seemingly effortless technique but also their attitude that determines their success. Their expression reflects this. Dancers who grace their performances—and injury recoveries—with a smile that mirrors their joy do the best.

KINDNESS AND COMPETENCY

Of all the behaviors I discuss here, kindness would seem like the easiest to cultivate. Like patience, it is a virtue, commonly hammered into us by our parents. Perhaps for this reason, it is often overlooked by those striving for success. What does kindness have to do with being a winner? A lot, it turns out, when kindness is matched by competency.

Surgery is a form of collaboration, as is participation in a team sport. Successful surgeries, and probably most complex team interactions, are determined in part by where the collaborators live on the kindness/competency curve. Extremely competent individuals who are also always extremely kind are as rare as unicorns. They are role models, showing us the people we should strive to be, when we think about it. The problem is, we don't think about it often enough. We perform with dexterity, but not with enough kindness—or with kindness, but without studying or working hard enough to perfect our skills.

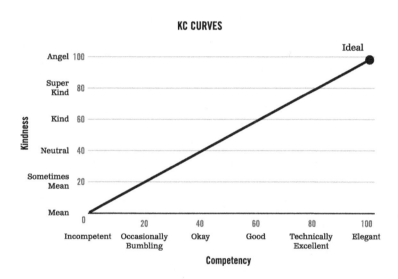

KC CURVES

Look closely at the diagram. Where do you fit when you are intensely focused on your job? Not just when you are relaxed, but when the stress is intense, the outcome critical, or your teammates are relying on you? Unicorns—people at the upper right tip of the graph—are rare not because they are endangered, but because they seldom receive the right encouragement and training. Often, our emphasis in life is to be kind or to be competent. But, how often are we taught how to be both, especially when the stakes are high?

It's true in sports as well. Focus, flow, performance, and aggression are qualities that define the best athletes of our day. The skill of raising a teammate's performance through vocal expressions and acts of kindness—while under our own stress to perform—isn't given much attention on our playing fields, or in our increasingly competitive workplaces. If it were, team performance would improve, and job satisfaction would soar. Outcomes in every facet of life would be optimized.

Good communication can help you become kinder and more competent. The way to get to this place is by publicizing the possibilities of such cooperation, understanding the potential for benefit, and studying the graph itself. Grade yourself and your teams. Ask yourself why you aren't at a higher point, and what it will take to get you there. Because who wants to be a super competent jerk? Or work with one? And who wants to be the patient of an incredibly kind but bumbling surgeon?

It is not okay to be, in the current vernacular, just "a nice person." Let's raise the bar of success and cultivate the superstars we wish our children to be: fantastically competent, kind, and part of a blessing of unicorns.

WHEN THE TRAIN DERAILS

We are all prey to the disappointments that life dishes out. We don't always have the mental bandwidth to brush off or bounce back from disillusionments, frustrations, regrets, and defeats. Often, rallying our internal mental forces is enough, but other times, professional help is needed.

With some of life's blows, it is easy to give in. Whether it is an injury, disease, age, or loneliness, the affliction overwhelms our potential. In such cases, the Latin expression *Illigitimi non carborundum* —"Don't let the bastards get you down"—is a good one to remember.

- Injury is an opportunity to rehab yourself back to a place better than you were before you were hurt. I use this expression twenty times a day with patients, designing a unique path for each one. The idea is not just to overcome their specific injury, but to change their life by treating themselves the way a pro athlete would. The patients who learn how to train around their injury, keep up daily exercise, hire trainers, use physical therapists, consult nutritionists, carve out time to work on their bodies, and have professionals work on their injured parts return to their lives fitter, faster, and stronger than ever before. I know that I have contributed to these peoples' lives for a lifetime. They have learned not to give in.

- Diseases are the same and different in various ways. Some are transient, some debilitating, and some permanent. The psychology of the disease response is often more complicated, and sometimes includes accepting lifelong disabilities. Confronting one's own mortality often comes as a surprise. While sometimes the remedy for a disease can be the same as that for a specific injury, at other times, the response requires a restructuring of daily activities and expectations. Setting new goals is part of the solution, as is working to defy the odds. Willing yourself back to health marshals one's internal systems in a way that no amount of training can provide.

- Similarly, a strong perspective can help you cope with aging. Aging gracefully is an art form. While singer Toby Keith's "not letting the old man in" phrase (from the song in the film *The Mule*) is part of the picture, holding on to a child's sense of wonder and curiosity may be equally important. Giving in to aging is often associated with quitting early: resting when you might be active, riding when you could be walking, letting others do for you what you can do for yourself. But it is also a process of losing vigor, determination, drive, and lust. The testosterone, adrenaline, and pheromones associated with an active life are somehow withdrawn from the aged, just when they would appreciate them the most.

- Loneliness is the accumulation of all these internal processes and behaviors—places where we are succumbing to our perceived fates. We are lonely when we succumb to events and infirmities that seem outside of our control. While being satisfied that our eyes open again in the morning is wonderful, being aggressive about pushing the envelope of activities and sensory inputs is exciting. Giving these activities up leads to decrepitude. We are aged and alone when we leave our senses behind and let the bastards get us down.

And then there is depression—a mental condition that afflicts almost all of us at some point. It may be the more difficult, internal, life-changing kind or the post-injury, temporary loss of performance kind. It is deflating, demoralizing, and debilitating, yet the cause is often invisible.

The effectiveness of drugs prescribed to combat depression have been so remarkably unsuccessful that their record is roughly equal to that of most talk therapies. Most of these drugs try to balance the neurotransmitters in the brain, but often at the expense of other brain chemistry—meaning that balancing one chemical may lead to a suppression of other chemicals, causing such side effects as sleeplessness or impotence. And all these drugs potentially require a lifetime of use as none are meant to be curative.

Other anti-depression therapies, such as electroshock (ECT), were meant to be curative, but were initially so destructive to other parts of the brain that long-term negative personality traits were produced. Refinement of ECT has made it much less invasive and more effective at treating depression, though still with significant risks—so many still see it as a solution of last resort.

Today, other drugs and therapies are being studied. Recent successes with psychedelics—including psilocybin, ketamine, MDMA, and LSD are encouraging. These substances fundamentally work by providing a new perspective and permitting a person to see themselves freed from the psychological chains that have held them captive. A person's ability to see himself or herself as a happy, independent, successful person gives them permission to actually *be* that person, even when the primary effects of the transformative drugs have worn off. The dramatic successes frequently reported with these drugs as part of guided therapies (as opposed to recreational use) to address PTSD and addiction make us wonder if we could free ourselves from our mental entrapments without the use of pharmaceuticals. (Some of this work has been popularized in the recent bestseller by Michel Pollan, *How to Change Your Mind* and *Your Brain on Plants*.)

The question is, why can't we *will* ourselves to relative health and happiness? The answer is, maybe we can. Sometimes we may just need a little help to do so.

Common, usually transient depressions—such as after knee surgery (ACL depression syndrome) or post-partum—respond remarkably well to exercise therapy. The testosterone, pheromones, and
adrenaline released by a sweat-producing workout do wonders to
elevate one's mood. It makes us wonder what other naturally circulating hormones can be induced to rise to the required occasions, and
which activities can target those endogenous chemicals.

Chocolate, the "food of love," is known to contain specific compounds that slow the breakdown of anandamides called "bliss compounds" from the receptors in the brain. What if a concentrated
chocolate compound, formulated without fat or sugar, could be
optimized for brain therapy?

Meditation and massage therapy lower blood pressure and the
levels of stress hormones through different pathways. While both
require skilled teachers and practitioners to help a person relax, the
skills of meditation can be learned and used by individuals to reduce
the depressive states caused by stress.

Now that we know there is a path toward actually curing depression, our job is to expand the ways to help people free themselves
from the depression trap. While not all depressions are the same—
and some may not be amenable to any curative process—we don't
actually know how many can, in fact, be cured. Using the insights
gained from experiments with the psychedelic experience, and those
from a variety of internal hormone manipulations, we now have the
opportunity to explore exciting new pathways that allow us to see
ourselves from different perspectives—since all of us may, at some
time, feel the oppressive weight of seemingly intractable mental stress.

The Lessons of Tiger Woods

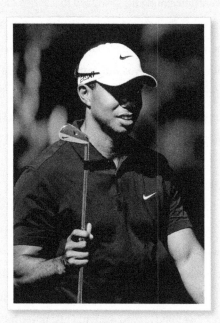

Superstars crash. This happens commonly enough, in fact, that we only hear about the ones who do so spectacularly—like Tiger Woods. Between 1997 and 2011, Woods broke nearly every golf record until his life unraveled with divorce, personal injury, and self-destructive behavior. Without any inside knowledge of his particular issues during this low point in his life, here are a few lessons I believe we can all take away.

Natural swings are just that: natural. For youthful athletes with phenomenal skills, coaching should focus on preserving those skills and focusing the mind to avoid the distractions that destroy them. After his dad, Tiger had one great early coach who guided him through his entry into professional golf. Ditching that coach and repetitively reinventing his swing led to a series of failed efforts to get "better." That's partially because he was already the best. The enemy of good is better, but the enemy of best is a fanatical competitive drive that lives within many top athletes.

Bulking up is good for weightlifting, but not for a golfer's rhythm. Tiger led the way out of the fat, out-of-shape, sloppy golf land of mixed plaids and baggy pants. He also brought a new level of fitness to a game that had little perception of the need for muscles to create power. But he went too far astray when he bulked up—possibly with the help of anabolic steroids and weightlifting coaches. Tiger's physique changed as clearly as Barry Bonds's changed, from lean to huge. He excelled in power but lost the grace we so admired. Whether or not his later injuries were a result of that transformation, no one knows, but we can't help but wonder. If only Tiger had stayed lean and just powerful enough to swing the club with the beauty of the youthful god of golf that he was.

Tigers's back surgeries, which began in March of 2014, didn't help either. That's because back surgery often doesn't work for athletes. Yes, there are many successful back operations that relieve pain and provide stability to millions of people. Yet very, very few athletes return to sports that require high torque, powerful twisting motions, and the ballistic striking of balls, racquets, people, or other objects.

Once the anatomy of the back is changed by injury or surgery, healing is rarely completely normal. While surgery may fix one level of the spine, if a fusion is performed, the levels above and below take more of the force and degenerate. If tissue is taken out, the target vertebrae often collapse. Because of this, new anabolic therapies using growth factors and stem cells are exploding in popularity. The future is hopeful—but for Tiger, his career took a dive once the back-surgery cycle started.

The mind controls the game. Happy people have happy careers. If their personal lives fall apart due to divorce, drugs, or alcohol, few top athletes stay on top of their game. When you see the first public displays of personal dysfunction—such as the crashed car on the house lawn after a marriage fight—both the support team around the athlete and the public need to come together and support the rehabilitation of the athlete's personal life.

When personal lives come tumbling down, athletic careers rarely continue to be as successful. The personal stability that got the athlete to the pinnacle of success is usually what keeps them there. Losing that support, often by looking for greener pastures, is likely to cause so much mental turmoil that the athlete's professional performance is at risk. If athletes were stocks, they would be shorted upon the first disclosure of such difficulties. Tiger failed to correct, to reconcile, and to use his counselors to rebuild trust and relationships. His golden future seemed doomed.

Yet not all collapses are permanent. Tiger made a comeback. As he played his way to winning the 2019 Masters Tournament at Augusta National Golf Club, commentators frequently mentioned his poise and his determination. He was playing with the brain of a thoughtful, strategic golfer. He had the "look" of a winner, and a "stare" on the twelfth hole that left his competitors no doubt that they were holding up the march of a champion.

It is easy to point out life's lessons in retrospect. We are surrounded by thousands of examples of downfalls, displayed in every supermarket tabloid. Still, we continue to cheer on our failing superstars, hoping they have some mental superpower that helps them defy the odds. We all know why we do this. We are hoping that when and if the time comes, we have that power too.

THE EYES HAVE IT

"Look 'em in the eye." This advice—whether in a Western shoot-out, a poker game, or most sports—has served competitors well. Yet few people do it. Why?

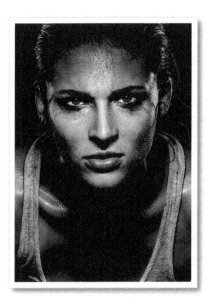

The eyes receive and give away information. They communicate in a language we have yet to define. We know they are windows to the soul, portals into the mind, and transmitters of emotions, intentions, and desires. Because we don't always control their transmissions, we fear their exposure. Shouldn't we start to train our visual communication skills?

When you talk to your family members, do you look them in the eye? Really look at them? We learned from Proust how little we all actually see. We glance briefly, and our mind fills in the rest of the details. Whether this is an evolutionary strategy to save on neurological horsepower or just a bad habit is unknown. In either case, we see what we expect to see. So, when our family members say that we are not listening to them, are they also saying we are not seeing them?

In sports, the eyes often betray the plans of the athlete. Which way is the opponent looking? Are they scared? Did they see the open man? Most of the time, looking a competitor in the eye provides you with information and intimidates them. Yet few athletes actually look hard at their opponent.

Sometimes it is a bad idea to look. If you look at a tree while skiing through the woods, you often hit the tree. It is the open space you want to see. In soccer, if you look at the goalie when shooting a penalty kick, you are far more likely to hit it directly to him.

In cycling, skiing, and race car driving, the body goes where the eyes are looking. Cornering at speed and arcing smooth turns all require "looking" around the corner. On a bicycle or motorcycle, one must "trust the rubber," and tilt the bikes nearly onto their sides to hold the inner line on a tight turn. Looking away from that line can cause a loss of connection with the road and a wipeout. The eyes lead the way.

In hockey, as Wayne Gretzky famously said, "I pass to the open space." He saw where his teammates were and sent the puck to where they would be. He would look his opponent in the eyes, yet that is not all that he saw. He saw the future by seeing where his competitors weren't. When was the last time you trained yourself to use peripheral vision while locking on your competitor's eyes? We can usually see more than we think we can—mostly because we don't think about it.

So look. And see. Communicate tactically. Practice looking. It is a very quiet, and remarkably effective, strategy. There is nothing digital about it that can be usurped by a device. It may be our last human skill that is fully independent of the internet. Seeing isn't believing; it is thinking.

In this chapter, we have highlighted focus, flow, mindfulness, attitude, and how the ability to see is so tied to success. Each skill is fully under the control of the athlete until it isn't, and then injury and failure arise. Whether in sport or medicine, as an athlete or a patient, controlling those facets of your own personality are often more important than the skills you bring to the table. Reflect on what resources you have to refine your ability to be fully present in each endeavor and learn from every athlete we see not just in victory but even more so in defeat.

CHAPTER 2

PHYSICAL FITNESS AND INJURY PREVENTION

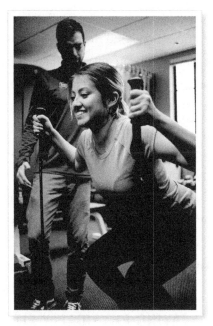

*StoneFit rehab team's ski season preparation and
injury prevention training program*

Fitness is life. The physical ability to do what you want to do, when you want to do it, and to do it well contribute to a life full of purpose and happiness. Yet being fit is not a given. We are all dying, and after we hit maturity, our bodies degrade with time. The only antidote is a keen understanding of our bodies and healthy exercise—constantly building all the key components of fitness and improving both the mental and physical attributes our parents gave us.

Part of staying fit is staying injury free. Injuries from sports or exercise interrupt our routines, throw us off-kilter, and affect both our physical fitness and our mental health. Injuries can be prevented, as so many I see are due to mental errors combined with fitness deficits. The mind wasn't in the game, and the body was not flexible enough to reach for that errant shot. I'm not just talking about injuries from sport. I'm talking about injuries from bad habits like terrible posture, and from the wear and tear that comes with aging.

In this chapter, we'll explore what it means to be fit—both physically and mentally—and what it takes to stay that way, no matter what sport you play or age you are. My goal is to convey to you the inspiration I feel every day—in keeping fit, exercising, and playing, in helping others avoid injuries in the first place, or recovering rapidly from injuries faster than dreamed possible, and by pushing forward the boundaries of medical science.

STAYING PHYSICALLY FIT

Imagine presenting yourself to a fitness venture capitalist as an investment. If you could, the investor would want to know what your "personal fitness business plan" is. You are your own best investment—so why not lay out a plan and execute it?

Components of Physical Fitness

Every business plan follows a fairly traditional format: here is the problem; here is our solution; here is how our team will accomplish it; this is the competition; here's why this is a "must have" rather than a "nice to have"; this is the amount of money it will take to get there; and here's why there is a fantastic return to the investor.

Begin by taking stock of who you are and where you are, both in your fitness program and athletic career. If fitness can be defined as your combined abilities in the following ten areas popularized by CrossFit, how fit are you? Score yourself.

- **Cardiovascular/respiratory endurance.** The ability of body systems to gather, process, and deliver oxygen.
- **Stamina.** The ability of body systems to process, deliver, store, and utilize energy.
- **Strength.** The ability of a muscular unit, or combination of muscular units, to apply force.
- **Power.** The ability of a muscular unit, or combination of muscular units, to apply maximum force in minimum time.
- **Speed.** The ability to minimize the time cycle of a repeated movement.
- **Coordination.** The ability to combine several distinct movement patterns into a singular distinct movement.
- **Agility.** The ability to minimize transition time from one movement pattern to another.

- **Flexibility.** The ability to maximize the range of motion at a given joint.
- **Balance.** The ability to control the placement of the body's center of gravity in relation to its support base.
- **Accuracy.** The ability to control movement in a given direction and at a given intensity.

We'll go through each of these metrics in detail in this chapter, but for now, write down how you think you score in each category from one to ten, with one being the lowest score and ten being the highest. Is your final score a fantasy of your fitness, or is it an objective assessment of you? Now is the time to do an audit. A great trainer and/or physical therapist can lay out a series of tests and measures. At our clinic, we quantify these areas in a program called StoneFit, in which we identify your weaknesses and design programs to address them.

Next, what are your specific goals? How long will it take to get there, and what is your schedule for doing so? If you are muscularly weak but lean, there is a range of options to solve that problem. If you are overweight and cardiovascularly deconditioned—if you find yourself out of breath after even small efforts—there are other specific pathways to follow. Honestly defining your problems is the first step to crafting the successful business plan of "You, Inc."

Once the problem (or set of problems) you are trying to solve is defined, the investor wants to know *why* an investment in you is likely to succeed. Do you exercise every day? Are you willing to adjust your life to do so? Do you have a fitness schedule? Are you on a team that relies on you? Do you have a coach for your skills and for your training regimen? Do you treat yourself as a top athlete would? Do you optimize your diet, tuning it to your output needs and muscle-building goals?

Act as if you were taking over a company and the company's fitness performance was critical. How, in that light, would you assess "You, Inc.?" What would you require to meet those fitness goals? A plan likely to succeed will demonstrate an honest assessment of your performance today, the critical goals you need to achieve, and the team most likely to encourage and enforce the new business plan. Drafting a new and exciting plan takes enthusiasm. The passion of the founder infects everyone around them with the mission, bringing a single-minded commitment to the goal.

The obstacles to achieving this goal often take the form of other obligations of life: time with family, work responsibilities, friendships, the need for sleep, and many more. Here, the best business models are those that turn those forces into allies. Exercising with your family and friends, creating work environments that partner with gyms (and have work exercise betting pools rather than fantasy teams), and strictly shutting off the lights early in the evening and waking at sunrise are common models of fitness success. There are, of course, a wide variety of other models too.

Last, we can't overlook the funding requirements. Once enough time is invested, the other resources available are limited only by one's creativity. At the low-cost end, simple exercises like sit-ups, push-ups, planks, box steps, squats, and running—combined with the unlimited free coaching resources available on the web—are universally available. But it is those people who combine varied fitness programs with personal coaching, nutrition optimization, goal setting, and quantification of accomplishments who are most likely to achieve success and maintain it for a lifetime.

"You, Inc." is not a flash in the pan. It's not the hot company of the moment or a highflier. "You, Inc." is a sure bet to produce fantastic returns, but only with passionate commitment. Got a better investment?

Endurance and Stamina

Endurance is determined by cardiovascular and respiratory health. The ability to raise your heart rate and oxygenate your blood to meet the exercise demands you are placing upon yourself determines, in part, how far, how high, and how deep you can go. If your heart is healthy, with more training, it will maintain lower rates and therefore use less energy and recover to an even lower base rate. A healthy heart conserves energy and supplies muscles with needed blood. With practice, your lungs will inflate and deflate to capacity and more efficiently deliver oxygen to the brain, muscles, and tissues required for an active life. Without practice, you simply won't deliver the goods. Think of the heart and lungs as the fuel pumps for your engine. Fill them up with high performance fuels and tune them constantly.

How far can you go? How long can you last? How painful is it getting there? Stamina is the ability to maintain a level of performance over a period of time. Think of the length of time as your life, and decide the minimum and maximum performance you want to achieve.

Strength, Power, and Speed

Strength is how tough you are combined with how much you can resist, and the maximum force you can apply. How *fast* can you provide your maximum force? This is what power is: speed times force applied. A power hitter swings the bat hard and fast and delivers a maximum amount of force to the ball, determined by his strength, bat speed, and skillset. Like strength, power is trained, and it can be lost without training. It is a key metric of your athletic skill in many sports, yet often ignored by many fitness programs. (You can do Pilates and yoga all day long and never develop substantial power.) For most activities, you want to be strong and powerful and have confidence in your toughness.

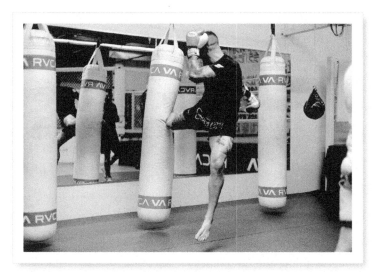

Ray G. • Muay Thai martial artist & kickboxer,
six months after knee surgery by Dr. Stone

Speed is related to response. "I didn't react in time" is not just the complaint of the athlete who couldn't dodge the oncoming linebacker. It is also the comment of the elderly man who didn't lift his hand in time to stop the revolving door. The speed with which you respond to an event is trainable, yet often not practiced in everyday exercise efforts. Try it. Instead of just spinning on a bike, accelerate in interval training. Instead of swinging a kettlebell weight, throw a weighted ball, faster and faster. Speed exercises are fun but have to be built up to in order to avoid overstretching injuries.

The Abs Have It

If you could focus on only one part of your body to change and strengthen, consider investing in your abdominal muscles. Here is why you should—and a simple exercise for getting the abs you deserve.

The abdominal muscles, from the rib cage down to the pelvis, control how you move as much as how you look. When they are weak, the belly protrudes, hanging over the belt and jiggling its way along almost as an appendage. The distended belly acts like a seesaw, with the weight providing strain on the muscles of the back to prevent you from falling over. Back pain, so common in adults, is often caused by weak abdominal muscles and can be cured by strengthening them. Yet many of us ignore our abs.

Until recently, we were taught to do the classic sit-up for abdominal strength. Yet "crunches" can cause neck and back pain for many, and arthritis can make this exercise impossible for some older people. Also, it is difficult to develop a sustainable rhythm that permits enough of the exercises to be performed.

An exercise ball provides the easiest pathway to rock-hard abs. Lie on a large ball centered in the middle of your back with your feet resting against a wall. Lean back far enough to see the ceiling, and rest your hands on your belly. Slowly bend forward to an upright position. This is the motion that works. Suck in your belly button while doing this exercise and it will engage the entire range of upper and lower abdominal muscles.

Don't count. The number of reps you do is not as important

as doing them mindfully. Close your eyes, relax, and feel the rhythm of the motion and the gradual training of the muscles. Find the pace that permits your mind to wander and the exercise to continue forever. Set your phone timer to five minutes, and slowly progress to fifteen minutes over the course of three months.

To gradually make the exercise more difficult, hold a weight of five to twenty pounds. Swing the weight behind your head as you lean back, and bring it forward as you sit up. Be sure to hold your belly button in.

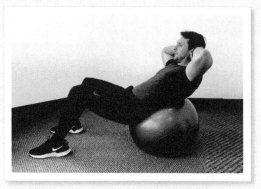

Rehab expert performing an abdominal crunch

The mesmerizing rhythm of this exercise makes it addictive and remarkably effective. Do it daily and notice the effects on your body, your self-image, and your ability to move without as much pain. When walking or sitting, hold your abdomen in, set your shoulders behind your hips, hold your head high, and smile. The key to molding our bodies to fit the image we want for ourselves lies in adopting everyday behaviors that walk the talk—even if the conversation is only inside our heads.

Top Six Dumbest Exercises

Just as important as doing the right exercises is *not* doing the wrong exercises. "Wrong" means exercises that are useless or potentially injury-generating. Here are some doozies that should not be on your list.

- **Wall squats.** At no time in life does anyone sit stationary against a wall. This exercise overloads the kneecap by holding a stationary load on one area of the cartilage. This load depletes the cartilage of its lubricating fluid or—if the joint is already damaged—increases the breakdown of the exposed collagen fibers.
- **Knee extension exercises.** No athlete kicks a ball solely from a knee extension. The kick is generated as the hip rotates the powerful trunk, and then the leg muscles, into the ball. A seated, repetitive leg extension overloads both the kneecap and the trochlea (the groove in the femur in which the kneecap tracks). Repetitive leg extensions can lead to patellar arthritis and patellar tendonitis—and the damage is much worse with the added weight of one's ankle or leg. A simple squat exercise is highly preferred as it exercises all the muscles from the foot and ankle up through the leg, hip, and trunk. Squats are what athletes do in almost all sports.
- **Isolated machine single-muscle exercises.** Exercises like bench presses make your chest look good, but not much else. The time you spend doing a bench press or a biceps curl could be much more beneficially spent doing a dynamic

exercise—such as a hammer curl to overhead press—that utilizes much more of the upper extremity musculature (biceps, triceps, and shoulders).

- **Anything too complicated.** Exercises that require too much setup to perform correctly can result in improper performance, overcompensation, or injury. Doing exercises with proper form, appropriate pace, and resistance is most effective. Don't waste your time on complicated exercises that you can't remember how to set up properly.

- **Highly loaded leg presses.** This means you are pushing against two hundred, three hundred, and in some cases four hundred pounds of weight. If you are looking for lower extremity strength, you should be attempting to squat standing up, double or single leg, with or without resistance (i.e., using a kettlebell, hand weights, or bar), depending on your ability and form. These types of standing exercises will more effectively improve your movements for daily living and will challenge your core more usefully. A step exercise using a box, for instance, will build thigh muscle strength quickly, challenge your balance, and improve your ability to ascend and descend stairs.

- **Multitasking.** Do you spin on a bike or walk on a treadmill while reading or watching TV? If so, you're distracted. To gain the most benefit from exercise, you must feel your heart rate, your breathing, and your muscles as they hit their limits and begin to tire. It is awareness of your body's responses to exercise stress that help you push past today's barriers and become fitter, faster, and stronger. You lose much of the psychological training benefit, as well as the skill improvements, by dissociating your mind from your exercise. Learn how to filter out all other distractions and become mindful during training. Then, enjoy the post-workout bliss. Exercise is the ultimate meditation and a direct connection to the god within you.

Coordination and Agility

The best of all the sports definitions of "coordination" comes from the Merriam-Webster dictionary, which defines coordination as the harmonious functioning of parts for effective results. Often thought of as two different parts of the body—eye-hand for example—coordination can also be of the fingers on a keyboard. Fundamentally, it is the brain-body connection that defines your coordination. Coordination can be optimized for so many activities, but if in the moment you are not thinking, then all the training in the world may not save you from an uncoordinated athletic move. Mental errors beat physical training so often that much of our rehabilitation time with athletes in the rehab clinic concentrates on developing focus, not just skill.

Flexibility

The ability to completely bend or extend our joints determines their health. Any loss of motion signals a gradual decline in joint performance and lifespan. This fact is often overlooked, yet it may be the single most important factor in physical health after injury and arthritis.

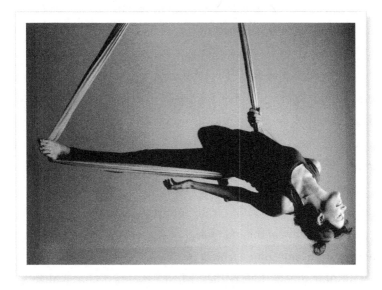

Amy C. • After five ankle surgeries elsewhere and debilitating chronic pain, Amy was on the path to amputation of her right foot. This is Amy aerial dancing after a BioAnkle repair from Dr. Stone.

All joints are covered by a bearing surface called articular cartilage. This white, shiny material (crack open a chicken wing, and you will see its smooth surface) is made up of a long protein called collagen, plus a grout-like matrix with a few cells interspersed called chondrocytes. These cells continually replenish the extracellular matrix and collagen, keeping the cartilage healthy over a lifetime. When articular cartilage is injured it fails to heal on its own. Injured cartilage loses its slickness and gradually wears away to expose the bone underneath, which causes deformity and pain.

Joints are like your car's tires. When out of alignment, they wear unevenly. When motion is limited by scar tissue or bone spurs, weight-bearing forces are concentrated in a smaller area of the joint surface, and the rotation-flexion motion pattern of the joint is constricted. So, like a misaligned tire, it wears faster.

All joints that lose flexibility produce abnormal motions and not just in the joint itself. The joints above and below are forced to compensate. When the knee joint fails to extend fully, the kneecap (patella), which normally moves up and out of the groove of the femur, is trapped against the femur. It is constantly loaded and wears down prematurely. Additionally, the hip above the limited knee needs to compensate to get the foot to land on the ground properly for walking. This compensation leads to hip and back pain.

Unfortunately, in this era of declining reimbursement for physical therapy after joint injuries, most people don't realize how much the lost motion affects their bodies. Most patients do not realize how small losses of motion lead to subsequent large problems.

Each of us takes two to three million steps each year in normal walking. Can you really afford to have two to three million abnormal cycles on each joint of the body over the rest of your lifetime? Focus on range of motion. Regain and maintain it as much as you focus on strength exercises or cardiovascular fitness conditioning. Your body is as finely tuned as a Ferrari. Don't drive it out of alignment.

Balance

It seems so simple: balance is what we do every day when we walk. We put one foot in front of the other. So, why are there so many sports injuries from landing badly? Why does tripping cause so many ankle sprains? Why do so many elderly people die from falling?

Estimates say that ankle sprains occur some 640,000 times per year.[2] While these injuries are not always due to a loss of balance, the common report that a patient tripped or landed poorly from a jump suggests a coordination failure often related to balance. Over three hundred thousand Americans who are sixty-five years and older fall and break a hip each year.[3] Under normal care, the mortality in the first year after a hip fracture has been reported as high as 58 percent.[4] These days, devices and apps can monitor elderly and frail people and send alerts when falls occur, but they don't prevent the fall in the first place.

Balance, simply defined, is the ability to maintain your vertical alignment. This is stunningly easy to lose after an injury. And, though it's easy to train your balance skills, most people never bother. Balance can be trained by standing on one foot with your arms outstretched; eyes open at first, and then closed as you get better. The challenge can be increased by standing on a pillow or on any uneven surface. Balance equipment such as Bosu boards or small trampolines, commonly available at gyms, add yet another level of difficulty. Walking on a balance beam (or better still, a "slack line" stretched between two trees) pushes you to the next level, on par with a gymnast. These exercises are fun and important—yet almost no one in your local gym is focusing on balance.

---

[2] Incidence rate reported in article, 2.15/1,000. Multiplied by 2006 US population of 298.4 million, from US census bureau, to get final figure. Brian R. Waterman et al., "The epidemiology of ankle sprains in the United States," *Journal of Bone and Joint Surgery* 92 no. 13 (October 2010): 2279–84, DOI: 10.2106/JBJS.I.01537.

[3] "Healthcare Cost and Utilization Project," Agency for Healthcare Research and Quality, accessed August 5 2016, http://hcupnet.ahrq.gov.

[4] Scott Schnell, et al., "The 1-year mortality of patients treated in a hip fracture program for elders," *Geriatric Orthopaedic Surgery & Rehabilitation* 1 no. 1 (2010): 6–14, DOI: 10.1177/21 51458510378105.

Balance is crucial for much more than injury prevention. Every sport has balance as a fitness characteristic. If you are training for the upcoming ski season, adding balance to your regimen increases your confidence on each ski, in each turn, and with every landing. Balance determines if a skier can edge with confidence, recover from a caught edge, or arc a smooth turn.

Landing from a jump, in any sport, requires a full repertoire of physical skills from muscle power to flexibility. But without good balance, all the training in the world won't prevent an awkward fall when the unanticipated occurs: an uneven surface, a slick floor, or a slight error in timing. Where is the disconnect? Why spend hours lifting weights but barely seconds training your balance?

I believe it is because we take balance for granted and don't realize how poor at it we actually are. Measure yourself. Time how long you can stand on one foot with your eyes closed. After you realize how brief it is, set a goal to increase that time by a few seconds every week. This is a cheap, easy, and always available training tool. And while you may never compete with Simone Biles on the balance beam, you will likely avoid unnecessary trips to my office, excel at your sport, and live a longer life.

Getting low is a big part of the balance equation. In most sports, when you're upright and locked, you're begging for a fall. I'll always remember a valuable ski lesson I received years ago in the Austrian alps. "Bend ze knees!" my instructor shouted at me. "Pretend like you are making love, ja!" This memorable guidance holds true today for all sports. Watch a great surfer. The back leg is bent so far that the thigh is parallel to the board. A soccer player with power bends his planted leg in order to generate enough force with the striking foot to fire the ball into the net. The best linemen in the NFL bend low despite their massive sizes.

Bending your knees sufficiently is a challenge, and it only gets harder as you age. Golfers progressively stand up more, losing that ideal position for addressing the ball. Tennis players fail to get low enough to generate core rotation power. Bowlers don't plant with enough knee bend, and the ball hits the alley hard, losing spin.

Knowing this, you might think that people train to bend their knees. Oddly, as with balance training, no. Many believe that regular gym workouts provide what it takes to get low, but watch these "cross-trainers" at the gym. Most use an elliptical machine or ride a stationary bike, perhaps lift some weights, and maybe even take a yoga class—believing that variety is the key to maintaining the bent-knee position.

The reality is that most sports demand power in knee bending. Generating power to strike a ball, to hold a position while rotating the hips and the back, to get low enough to apply pressure to the back of a surfboard or ski, takes concentric and eccentric power in the muscles, meaning the ability to generate force while bending and extending. You can only develop that coordinated power by repeating the motion with progressively higher weights and volume of repetitions.

So, if you are going to train to become a better athlete, the ideal method is the simple squat exercise. The squat, when done properly, perfectly trains all the muscles of the lower extremity and the core, the gluteal (butt) muscles, the abdominal muscles, and the paraspinal muscles in a coordinated fashion. Done with body weight alone, it can be performed anywhere. When adding weights to a bar or making the squat more complicated, such as adding an overhead thrust of a bar with weights, more of the body is engaged and the goals of coordinated fitness are achieved earlier. Proper squat form means the head is in a neutral position, the chest is upright, facing forward, the knees are bent over—but not beyond—the toes, the hips are lowered as far as they can go, the weight is on the heels, the abdomen muscles are sucked in, and the butt is pushed backwards. There you have it: the cheapest, most available, and most effective exercise for nearly every sport.

Accuracy

Accuracy is the ability to control movement in a given direction and at a given intensity.

Though accuracy comes last in this list, it is the foundation for many of the other measures. If you are inaccurate, you trip, jump, and land poorly; you lift weights (or a ballet partner) with poor technique; and frequently, you miss the target in other activities. Accuracy is such a part of our daily activities that we forget to train specifically for it. There are no Fitbit measures, no stopwatch pressures, and no reminders except the failure to achieve some of our goals. We spend hours spinning, lifting, running, and stretching, but precious few minutes targeting.

The consequences of inaccuracy are the falls we see in the elderly, the sprained ankles we see in all athletes, torn ligaments from landing a ski jump a little off target, and a multitude of "minor" injuries that can result from even slight errant placement of our body parts.

Think about practicing accuracy, and remember that the tools we use to train our muscles can also be applied to train our skills. Place a weight down in exactly the same spot, ten times in a row. Press against a Pilates footplate with exactly the same knee and foot position every time. Throw a ball at a precise position on a backboard. Kick a soccer ball—or putt a golf ball—repeatedly into a small target. You can even practice accuracy by placing your pen or cell phone down on your desk in exactly the same position each time (you can use a piece of tape to mark the position, and if you are teased, challenge your colleagues or housemates to an accuracy competition). Focus on being accurate in all the physical motions of your life. See how far off you are on the first few tries, and take it from there. Correct and practice, time and again. The phenomenally simple mental and physical game of practicing accuracy is sport's version of mindfulness.

Pace Yourself

"Go full out, give it everything you've got, push harder than ever, all the time, full bore, full on, never stop, full power, 100 percent!" These are the exhortations of today's coaches, teachers, and advisors. We are inferior if we aren't at the bleeding edge of our performance abilities. We are slacking off if we're not redlining. But guess what. I'm an 80-percenter. And I'll be a happy one for the rest of my life.

Pacing yourself is key to fitness. You get to a stage of life when you realize that "good enough" is truly good enough. That exerting yourself on your skis at 80 percent of your maximum speed, taking 80 percent of the risk, on 80 percent of the runs you could have taken, is a gift. Eighty percent of sleep is just fine. Eighty percent of the time for sex still satisfies. You learn that in training for the sports you love, 80-percent effort is sustainable, saves energy for later, diminishes injuries, and actually feels good. You push yourself at a more than moderate pace, dipping into extremes if desired or needed, but not as a baseline. You push others at rates that demand they perform, but at paces they can sustain. Your expectations are high, but not unachievable.

You learn that 100 percent is short term, shortsighted, and sometimes dangerous. Maximum exertion predisposes you to injury. It impresses, but it drains your tank. You mentally compare options: a consistent 80 percent, or intermittent 100-percent periods broken up by zero-percenters due to injuries.

For competitive athletes, success favors those who are willing to own the 100-percent territory. Their willingness to sacrifice their bodies for a gold medal is what sets them apart. But for athletes who are looking beyond that finish line, 100-percent exertion, 100 percent of the time, with 100 percent of the risks, is just not worth it.

For those of you who push yourself to the outer boundaries, relinquishing your addiction to giving your all is difficult. Reprogramming a body that's satisfied only when operating at its upper limit takes willpower. Scaling down to 80 percent can feel like defeat. It can make you question whether another run, bike ride, or full day of skiing even makes sense.

But after the readjustment, you'll find that a life at 100 percent has prepared your 80 percent to be pretty damn good. You'll find that your eighty can best other people's hundred. You will still sweat, your heart will still thump, and your muscles will still ache. You'll still summit the mountain, you'll still finish the race, and you'll still feel like an athlete. You might even gain a few additional friends who find your 80 percent to be welcoming—while your 100 percent was threatening.

The Sleep Dilemma

The data is now overwhelming. Eight hours of sleep each night is what humans need for optimal health and performance. Yet most of us don't get it. What is the fix?

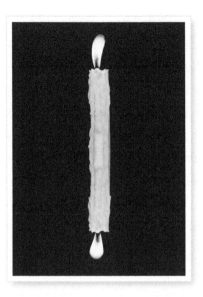

It turns out that eight hours of sleep does a host of beneficial things. Our DNA repair system works diligently during sleep, repairing the damage done by our exposure to toxins, sunlight, bad food, and worse behavior. The learning mechanisms for storing new data and transferring that data from short-term memory to long-term storage occur during sleep and are interrupted when we sleep less than eight hours.

Shockingly, in data presented by Dr. Matthew Walker from the Sleep Lab in Berkeley, testosterone is reduced significantly in people with less than eight hours of sleep. This makes them function as a person a decade older. In experiments with animals as well, inadequate sleep means dramatically increased aging. Mood, blood pressure, cognitive performance, and a host of other critical processes are optimized with the magic eight. The research by Walker and others has crystallized these findings so well that apprehension is now pervading our nightshift-enabled world—a world where students, ER physicians, nurses, and night foremen are all expected to perform superbly while sleeping poorly.

If workers are required to alternate between night shifts and day shifts without sufficient adjustment time, and if pilots are expected to fly airplanes in and out of shifting time zones with reduced sleep hours, and if students are expected to be at school at 7:00 a.m. after finishing their homework at 11:00 p.m.—all behaviors now proven to be harmful to their health—is this not a form of abuse? If so, it's an abuse that hurts both the abuser (now deprived of the best performance results) and the victim (e.g., the employee, pilot, trainee, physician, or student).

What can we do about it? Drugs to induce or improve sleep actually inhibit the high-quality REM sleep known to be most effective for human optimization. Meditation may address a few of the sleep deprivation symptoms but not solve the problem. Melatonin and supplements may help regulate the sleep clock, but they do not compensate for the missing time.

Exercising to optimize your weight improves nighttime breathing, exhausts the muscles, and improves the quality of sleep. Avoiding alcohol and caffeine also removes impediments that interfere with your sleep cycles. Eliminating electronic screen time a few hours before sleep diminishes conflicting brain and body rhythms. Adjusting the time you take certain medications can also help you avoid systemic interference with sleep.

It will require a fundamental remodeling of our educational systems and workforce to truly make a difference in the population's ability to raise its personal and professional performance through better sleep. Educational institutions are the first and easiest place to start. They should clearly understand the science and see the benefits of teaching when students are alert and retention is highest. Students and parents must reject early morning classes. Stand up and protest now!

Medical training programs should hire scribes and support staff with regular shifts to reduce the workload for key medical staff, many of whom are up at night. Safety records will improve. Otherwise, the dreaded lawyers may soon figure out that these institutions are exposing patients to unnecessary risk—and exposing the programs to liability.

Employers must design shifts so that employees stay on a single time schedule for long periods, with sufficient time between shifts. Do this now—the quality of your products and services will improve. Labor laws and OSHA guidelines may soon be enforced to reflect this health and safety reality.

Sleep is the new health food. It is organic, biodegradable, recyclable, and allergen free—and crucial to our fitness. Free-range humans are the ethical choice. Well-rested humans are happy—and happy humans make happiness universal.

Keep It Simple When It Comes to Food

Maintaining a healthy weight—as any doctor, health column, or nutrition scientist will shout at you—is an important component of fitness. Yet *how* to do this can be baffling. Many people are overwhelmed by the food choices and diet trends that make the news. Low fat or low carb, vegetarian or paleo, food pyramid or keto…What should you eat and not eat, and how much of each? What should you feed your kids? How do you teach kids about food and health, food and sports?

In a nutshell, my advice to my kids and my patients is: Eat simple foods, the fresher the better. Eat only what you need and only fill up to three-quarters full. Drink water.

Let me dive a little deeper. Assuming you have not been diagnosed with some specific reason why you cannot eat a certain food, then food is fuel. (Notice I did not use the term "food allergy," since I believe that the field of immunology and its understanding of what allergic reactions really are, and whether or not they are temporary, is in a state of flux.) Food is not for pleasure, yet should be pleasurable. The difference is important. Food is fuel needed for specific output needs. The better you come to understand your energy requirements, the better you will manage your food intake and choices, and the more pleasurable your meals will be.

Here is how. Eat when you are hungry. Start with a protein-centric diet and use carbohydrates and fats as condiments. Protein fuels your muscles and your brain. Foods that are lean and protein-rich (i.e., low in fat, high in protein) are fish, lean meats, and quinoa. Make protein the main ingredient of each meal. It takes effort to get protein—but if it is consumed in the morning, protein carries most people through the day's activities longer than the other choices. It is protein that builds muscle, provides the longest-lasting energy supply, and helps the immune system resist infection. Protein allows bones to build mass and helps tissues repair injuries.

Most of the efforts to measure how much protein you should or should not eat have failed. Nobody measures for a long time or has a clue how many grams of protein are in each portion of food. Our experience is that if you make protein—especially lean protein—a central part of your diet, you will have adopted the right approach. (By lean protein, we mean the type without excess fat: lean meats, pork, chicken without the skin, fish, and some beans.) Surround that protein with enough carbohydrate and fat to fill you up to three-quarters full and you have a meal. Since we do not judge ourselves to be full until we have overeaten, we are much better off stopping when we know we could eat more but choose not to—thus, the three-quarters-full recommendation.

The hard part is what to reach for when you are hungry between meals. The world is full of fatty fast foods and, worse, sugary ones. The brief high from an immediate sugar fix is both addictive and destructive. Every disease known to man—from tooth decay to fat deposition—has been linked to poor dietary choices. In addition, the gut microbiome adjusts itself to our dietary intake. Eating fatty foods induces fat deposition, while consuming sugar promotes the overgrowth of destructive bacteria—bacteria that communicate to the brain the desire for more sugar. But if you can reach for protein instead, the snack will fuel your efforts—both muscle and brain power. And a high-protein snack will carry you to your next meal without the rollercoaster of the sugar high and crashing low.

If you are growing a lot or exercising heavily, follow the same rules but eat more frequently. If you want to lose weight, drop the carbohydrates significantly. Focus on protein and vegetables, with water as your primary beverage. Excellent new studies demonstrate that carbohydrates in the diet increase cholesterol, drive blood sugars abnormally, and increase fat deposition. Eliminating unneeded carbs leads to weight loss, especially when combined with daily exercise that raises the heart rate for an hour a day. This approach will help you reach your ideal body weight more rapidly than any specific diet program.

Choose foods that have been minimally processed. Farm-to-table or wild, sustainably harvested sea-to-table foods means there has been no intermediary manipulation of naturally nutritious ingredients. Avoid packaged or processed foods whenever possible. Cook food lightly and present it beautifully. Inhale the pleasurable aromas that evoke emotional sensations. The pleasure in the eating is matched by the pleasure in knowing you have tuned your intake to your needs.

Drink a lot of water. All of the tissues in our bodies work better when well hydrated. When your tongue and lips are dry, your body is diverting precious fluid to your brain and other key organs to maintain life. And most people are dry much of the day. They sleep and often mouth breathe, losing water at night. They drink coffee without other fluids, and the caffeine further dehydrates. They drink alcoholic beverages, which increases urination without compensating hydration.

Water is the ideal beverage. No calories, no sugar, pure taste, and an optimal source of hydration. Try drinking water as a pre-beverage drink—a full glass of water before a beer or a cocktail. A glass before each meal reduces caloric intake. A glass before bed reduces nighttime dehydration. There are very few athletes who need to replace electrolytes, despite what the advertisements say. Yet there are millions of people who, if they drank water more often, would save untold dollars while improving their performance. Think of washing your insides as frequently during the day as you wash your hands. Make plain water your key beverage, and always have a glass before you lift a fork and between any alcoholic drinks. Finish the glass of water whenever you lift it.

Simple as that.

Mind, Body, Gut

Gluten-free, vegan, dairy-free…all of these diet variations designed to address irritable bowels are exploding—apparently, because people's bowels are now explosive. Celiac, diverticulitis, irritable bowel syndrome, and their relatives are being diagnosed more frequently than ever. As a society, Americans are becoming more stressed. Could these be linked through the gut?

We now know that a healthy gut is critical to overall well-being and fitness. An unhappy gut not only affects us physically, but its effects ripple out mentally—you only have to ask someone suffering from irritable bowel syndrome how deeply it can contribute to stress. But keeping the gut happy is not straightforward. It is a complex system colonized by trillions of bacteria and other organisms, only a small percentage of which we have identified. We know that when we take an antibiotic to kill bacteria in one part of our body, it acts as a nuclear bomb in the gut, wiping out populations of organisms living in precarious balance with other organisms. When one group is wiped out, other populations of bacteria—and possibly viruses, fungi, and prions that were previously suppressed—are free to grow. Some of these populations may not process gluten as well as others, leading to the shocking surge of gluten sensitivities. For some people, the newly dominant life forms create widespread havoc.

Havoc in the bowel produces a variety of disabling disorders, from prolific gas production to diarrhea to weight loss. The bowel becomes inflamed—either due directly to the new organisms, to their overactivity, or to the immune system's response to the now-dominant bacteria colonies. Thus, inflammatory bowel diseases are labeled, possibly often incorrectly, as autoimmune diseases—illness caused by the body rejecting itself. The far more likely explanation is that we simply have not yet identified the primary inflammatory agents. Newer DNA bowel diagnostic testing should help clarify these invaders. At present, we have not yet identified possibly 60 percent of the DNA in the gut codes for organisms. There is a long way to go.

And it is not just the bowel that gets disordered. When we cannot process foods correctly, we naturally become stressed, hungry, and irritable. Stress alone causes the release of cortisol and other hormones that increase bowel activity. In many cases, in fact, the initial insult to the bowel is stress from the mind. This stress-induced excess bowel activity leads to poor food processing and an inflamed bowel lining—leading to the selection of organisms that thrive in the newly swollen tissue.

In this circle game of our bowel's life, the common denominators are stress and inflammation. The unknowns are the specific organisms that respond to stress and induce inflammation, and the therapies needed to reduce them.

The most novel approach to date involves reintroducing an overwhelming dose of the healthy microbiome that exists within a person's family population. If four members of a family have normal bowels and one is afflicted with an inflammatory syndrome, it's possible that introducing the fecal matter of a digestively healthy family member into the ill person may destroy the nasty bacteria and recolonize the bowel with a healthier population. This common-sense approach called fecal therapy is gaining acceptance as evidence of its success grows.

So, when combined with a program that includes stress reduction, mindfulness, visualization, and exercise, an overpowering dose of normal gut bacteria may reverse the bowel disorder tsunami.

My grandmother once said that the definition of serendipity is falling in poop and coming out smelling like a rose. If the gut does control the mind, and the mind controls the gut, may we all experience serendipity when we need it the most.

Stress: Make the Most of It

We all experience it. Sometimes, we can use it to our advantage. But more often than not, stress is a disease, rotting our insides. Let's look at performance, relationships, and sleep. Each is affected by stress in a different way, and each has a variety of useful and useless responses.

Performance stress drives us to deliver our best. We push ourselves out of pride and fear, desperately wanting to deliver the best outcome, and we're frightened of failing. We use stress to work harder, to show up early and leave late, to double-check our work, and go the extra mile to get the job done. We use stress to train harder, to lift more weights, ride more miles, hit the gym with more vigor, and enjoy the pain of exertion. Yet the fear of failing ourselves or others raises our blood pressure to unhealthy levels. It causes us to do unhealthy things to hit unrealistic marks and to miss our targets due to performance anxiety.

Relationship stress makes us work harder at being better spouses, parents, and friends. We struggle to maintain our multitude of friendships, sometimes at the expense of work responsibilities. We try hard to be great lovers. We add worry where bliss should be and arguments where conversation should take place. Jealousy enters our minds when welcoming would be more effective.

Sleep more than seven hours? We all know that sleep is extremely healthy and restorative. Yet life's stresses interfere, whether in the form of bad dreams or bad habits. Too much alcohol, too little water, excessive caffeine, and outside forces disrupt the best of relaxing plans. All conspire to disturb that most effective of all health remedies. And then, of course, we stress about not getting enough sleep.

What is the common thread here? Everyone's life is inconsistent. Some days are better than others, for a dozen reasons. Our relationships have ups and downs. We have hot streaks in our work, but they don't last forever. Stress is how we experience these erratic outside forces and internal thoughts.

Stress is a force worth harnessing. It is a ubiquitous, omnipresent energy flowing through the ether—as are love, tranquility, anger, and a host of other human emotions. But stress is one of the few such forces that we can train for, teach our children about, and modify at every stage of life. Watch the athletes who "center down" before a big match. Study the exceptional public speakers who use presentation tools to calm their voice and deliver their message. Talk to military commanders who lead their soldiers into battle. When the chips are down, certain people rise to the challenge. They do so by taking stock of the situation and organizing their responses.

Stress is not a disease that requires a treatment, a vaccine, or a cure. It is a tool that most of us have yet to master. We're not very good at attending practice sessions though. It's time to stop playing hooky.

Travel Fitness

In today's globalized world, travel is an intrinsic part of our lives—it's less a rare disruption to our routine and more a *part* of our routine. So, how do you include it in your exercise regimen and stay fit while travelling? It can be hard. Between airline food, cramped airplane seats, hotels without gyms, and time changes, the home-based fitness glow is dulled. Here are some fitness tips for travelers, for when you're on the plane and at your destination.

- **Book only hotels with good gyms.** Check this out by looking at the photos on the hotel's website. Most importantly, book the hotel gym's trainer into your schedule for a one-hour meeting. Give this the priority of any other important meeting. In a career that requires a lot of travel, missing workouts on the road is the single most destructive obstacle to your fitness program. Regular training is much harder to avoid when the appointment is pre-booked and paid for. The workout can be a gym circuit, a Pilates session, a swim, or running with a partner. Suddenly, being on the road becomes a great way to vary your fitness regimen.
- **Exercise hard before getting on the plane.** Swim, bike, run, lift weights, do whatever you can before you fly. If possible, use the airplane time for rest and recovery from sports, rather than work. The times we have awake and in a cocoon are precious and can be internally private, thoughtful, and restorative.
- **Hydrate before and during the flight.** Water is lost on long flights and in fitful sleep, and brain cells work poorly when dehydrated. So if you want to think well, sleep well, and avoid gaining weight, drink plain, non-carbonated water all day long, a full glass every hour. (Non-carbonated, because when you lift the glass of water, try to finish it before putting it down. This is harder to do with a carbonated beverage.) Increased water intake will lower caloric intake, wash out

the body, and make you feel good. When we're hydrated, everything works better.

- **Avoid alcohol or coffee.** Alcohol dehydrates and debilitates. It is an anesthetic with a long post-infusion tail. It slows metabolism and increases weight gain in three ways: added calories, slowed metabolism, and increased desire to eat while drinking. Coffee and tea with caffeine accelerate heart rate and metabolism but add stress and anxiety and stimulate the bowels to move more often—leading to more hunger.

- **Walk every hour (at least).** Book an aisle seat and get up frequently. This movement decreases blood clot risk, diminishes back pain caused by poor seats, and reminds you to exercise. Set your phone alarm to vibrate every hour. The reminder is the key as it's easy to be lulled into mindlessness by the airplane's drone.

- **Exercise while sitting.** Here are five:
  - » Ankle pumps: Do a set of one hundred every flight.
  - » Posture adjustment: Roll your pelvis forward, suck in your abdominal muscles, and set your shoulders behind your hips. Hold the position for a minute. Do this once every fifteen minutes. You will be shocked by how much time you are slouching; this will help you discipline yourself to sit up straight.
  - » Simple biceps curls: Lift your computer (or your book) from the tray table to your chest. Do this sixty times. Repeat every few hours.
  - » Push-ups on the hand rests: Push down on the hand rests, lifting your body off the seat. Do this fifteen times, every few hours.

» Shoulder muscle strengthening: Squeeze your shoulder blades together and hold them in that position for as long as you can. Suck in your abdominal muscles while you do this exercise. Do this thirty times.

Exercise when standing in the aisle. Here are three simple exercises:

» Calf raises: See how many you can do before the flight attendant tells you to sit down!

» Single stance balance: Stand on one leg, and count the number of rows on the plane. See how long you can go. Repeat each time you get up.

» Hip strength: Stand next to your seat, facing forward, and push your leg firmly against the seat. Hold the position for fifteen seconds. Try ten, then switch legs.

• **Bring your own food.** It's easy to bring healthy fruits, vegetables, and even yogurt. If you prepare a meal the night before, make an extra portion, and put it in a baggy with a plastic fork. You can control what you eat when you travel if you plan ahead. (If it is a multi-leg trip, order an extra-healthy dinner in the restaurant the night before and have them bag it for you.) Cold shrimp, cut-up steak, or lean pork are good protein options.

• **Travel with a friend.** If your schedules include overlapping free time, organize sports and recreation activities together. Work travel should not be twenty-four hours of work.

• **Think.** We tend to fill our hours with conversation, reading, working, and writing, and take too little time to just think. Close your eyes and tap into your most creative self.

- **Sleep.** Sleep without sleeping drugs. Practice meditation and centering down. Use an eye shield and music if it helps you. Use the airplane time to increase your rest time.
- **Stand up frequently.** Stand up on the airplane and at meetings. Meetings without chairs have been shown to be more efficient and clearly more energy consuming. Walk, talk, and stretch whenever possible. Take whomever you are meeting out for a walk, not for a drink or coffee. You will be surprised by the positive reception to this idea and pleased with the flow of conversation. If you must sit, sit forward on the leading edge of the chair: stomach in, pelvis in neutral, shoulders square.
- **Eat well.** Seek out restaurants with healthy menu options. Ignore the hotel's mini bar—nothing in there is good for you.

The Wizard of O2

F ootball players sit on the sidelines sucking oxygen from masks and tanks. Hip millennials lounge in oxygen bars, breathing bubbling oxygen through multicolored water canisters. Pooh-poohed by most experts as a money-wasting (and possibly dangerous) psychological massage, oxygen bars are nonetheless expanding their reach, from dugouts to mountain spas. Why?

The science is simple. We normally breathe 20 percent oxygen from indoor air. At sea level, this saturates our blood cell hemoglobin to 98 percent—leaving little room for more. At altitude, the concentration of oxygen is the same, but the atmospheric air pressure is lower (you are farther away from the center of the earth, so gravity has less pull). Thus, you get less oxygen with each breath, and the saturation of the hemoglobin drops: usually to the low- to mid-90 percentages for healthy people.

Breathing higher concentrations of oxygen (40 percent from most oxygen bars or 100 percent from anesthesia machines during surgery) seems like a good idea but can have serious negative consequences if used for too long. That's because higher concentrations of oxygen liberate free radicals: oxygen molecules with charged sides that can damage lung tissue, affect various inflammatory control systems, and instigate a variety of health problems. Therefore, most medical experts recommend that you avoid increased concentrations of oxygen for prolonged periods of time.

Still, oxygen bars are popular. The concentration of O2 is only 40 percent, not 100 percent, and exposure is usually measured in ten- to twenty-minute increments—not long enough to produce any damage. And people love them. That's because short intervals of oxygen do produce a "high" feeling. This is especially true when the O2 is combined with aromatic scents and definitely when you have a hangover (or an altitude headache). The air smells good, and the act of breathing slowly—closing your eyes and inhaling "purifying" air, with the resulting increase in hemoglobin oxygen saturation—produces a wonderful state of bliss. The endorphins released have not yet been measured in any scientific way, but ask any oxygen bar user why they spend twenty dollars on air and they will tell you: the experience is dreamy.

This observation is not new. In Jules Verne's 1870 novel *Around the Moon*, the author states the following:

> Do you know, my friends, that a curious establishment
> might be founded with rooms of oxygen, where people
> whose system is weakened could for a few hours live
> a more active life. Fancy parties where the room was
> saturated with this heroic fluid, theaters where it should
> be kept at high pressure; what passion in the souls of the
> actors and spectators! What fire, what enthusiasm! And
> if, instead of an assembly only a whole people could be
> saturated, what activity in its functions, what a supplement
> to life it would derive. From an exhausted nation they
> might make a great and strong one, and I know more than
> one state in old Europe which ought to put itself under the
> regime of oxygen for the sake of its health!

So for those at higher altitudes, having danced a little too much and drunk even more, that morning headache can be treated with a lot of hydration and a little extra oxygen. The treatment works. People feel better. The headache goes away. A little extra oxygen actually helps.

For those huffing and puffing on the sidelines of the football field, oxygen slows the breathing and provides confidence that the next round of contact will be answered with full force. The psychological effect is as powerful as the physical force that drives the legs, and it's available instantly.

For those in search of urban refreshment, peering behind the curtain of that long zinc bar reveals the Wizard of O2. That extra shot of oxygen infuses customers with a dose of atmospheric bitters, a temporary shot of rejuvenation.

My advice? Use what nature gives us first, but feel free to have an extra helping sometimes, and radiate well-being. To paraphrase the song in the movie, "If we only had more lungs..."

STAYING INJURY FREE

An essential part of staying fit and healthy is, of course, staying injury free. So let's start this section with a fundamental question. Why—when we know we are the most fit when we are uninjured and we know about injury risk associated with sports—do we keep playing sports?

Injury Prevention

Every day, I hear something like this: "Doc, how soon can I get back to playing soccer?" This can be a question from somebody with significant cartilage damage, torn ligaments, and arthritis at age thirty, after having had six operations for both knees. For this person, returning to soccer means a chance of further bodily injury. Not to mention brain damage.

In soccer, there's the added risk of injury when heading the ball. A sixteen-ounce soccer ball traveling at up to fifty miles per hour smacks the head deliberately and repeatedly. How often? In a range of thirty-two to fifty-four hundred times per player per season, according to a 2013 study of amateur soccer players.[5] The brain changes detected by MRI were not subtle, nor would you expect them to be.

And it's not just soccer. In skiing, an ACL rupture—injuring the key ligament in the knee—permanently changes the biomechanics of the knee (whether or not it is reconstructed) and leads to a high rate of arthritis. In boxing, the goal is to produce a concussion. Knocking someone out impacts their brain so profoundly that the victim loses

---

[5] Michael L. Lipton et al., "Soccer heading is associated with white matter microstructural and cognitive abnormalities," *Radiology* 268 no. 3 (2013): 850–7, https://pubmed.ncbi.nlm.nih .gov/23757503/.

consciousness. Football is a full-body contact sport in which nearly every bone and tissue is affected. When a Super Bowl player gets his bell rung, the chimes may last forever, but sadly, he may not realize it. The brain injury from that concussion can lead to initially subtle and later overt mental acuity loss.[6]

Why is it that the fun and satisfaction of participating in sports impedes recognition that they could significantly harm our bodies, be it our knees or our brains? The answer, I believe, is that as athletes, we just can't comprehend the impact of the damage. We don't understand that sports injuries build up and lead to arthritis or that repetitive brain trauma gradually reduces our cognitive power. Either that or we choose to ignore it because we feel invincible. Simply put, the fun outweighs our belief in the risk, and even if we acknowledge the risk, in many cases, we think it is worth it.

As an orthopaedic surgeon, an athlete, a former soccer player, an avid skier, and a dad, I have multiple dilemmas. I work hard at developing the best methods for repairing my patients' injured joints and at developing new tools so their injuries do not lead to arthritis later in their lives. A goal of sports medicine is to get players back to the sport as soon as possible. However, I know our tools are limited, and the science is just developing to replace meniscus, cartilage, and ligaments in ways that prevent arthritis. The tools for assessing brain injury are even more primitive, and there are no treatments at all for the subtle and not-so-subtle brain injuries.

---

[6] The concussion story came to light in part because of the determined forensic pathologist Dr. Bennet Omalu, portrayed by Will Smith in the movie Concussion. Another reason was the top scientific work done by University of North Carolina Dean Kevin M. Guskiewicz. He looked at how sport-related concussions affected both balance and brain function in young athletes, and the long-term neurological issues related to playing sport. A final factor, of course, was the activism on the part of aggrieved families.

Am I wrong to help these sports warriors back to the fray? Although I warn them that further impact on their repaired cartilage is likely to shorten their active lifestyles, and I tell them that arthritis ruins more lives than cancer kills people, is that enough? And what about our kids? Is encouraging them to play soccer and football simply crazy?

My answer, and I look forward to hearing yours, is that there *is* a little craziness to it all. To live without any risk entirely is both impossible and foolish. "A ship is always safe at the shore," observed Albert Einstein, "but that is not what it is built for." And so we must teach our kids and our patients to do dangerous things safely, to measure the risks, and take the newest knowledge and apply it to the best safety gear and methods. Then we must encourage them to go fully enjoy the thrill of sports and learn the wonderful lessons that only team sports can teach. The alternatives are not palatable.

At the same time as I am enabling these activities, I must commit myself and inspire others to research, develop, and test novel ways to protect the athlete and repair the damage once done. It seems reasonable that in the twenty-first century, we should be able to repair, regenerate, and replace injured tissues, which, while it won't make athletes indestructible, will certainly cut the risk of long-term damage. That is my mission and my obligation.

What is your role in the equation? You can make it *your* mission and obligation to do what you can to minimize your chances for injury. (For most of my patients, all it takes is one bit of serious damage, and they become much more motivated to pay more attention to smart preparation and risk calculation.) When it comes to diminishing self-inflicted injuries, staying confident in your body's remarkable abilities, and lengthening your sports/athletic career, here is my number one, rock-solid, solid-gold piece of advice: *Listen to your body and know when to stop.*

Pain is a sign of injury. Pain in muscles stems from the overuse of the existing muscle fibers. It's a balance. We need just enough overuse to stimulate the body to build stronger muscles but without tearing the muscle past the point of natural repair. Pain in the joints is often due to damage to the weight-bearing surfaces. Since we are often caught up in the excitement of our sport when the body is calling out, we fail to stop in time. We extend past the helpful pain of muscle training into the damage zone.

Think about any past injuries you may have sustained and what led to them. Were there points along the way when you could have stopped and listened? And, having listened, stopped? Think about your current activities. Do your muscles ever tell you that you are overusing them? I have trained myself to listen when my body is trying to have a helpful conversation with me. Here are examples of chats my mind and body regularly have, which lead to activity modification.

- **When I am waterskiing,** I am in a state of bliss—until I notice the front of my knee hurting. This usually happens just as I am getting really tired. If I drop the handle right then, I won't overload the patella cartilage and may avoid suffering irreparable damage. Much anterior knee pain comes from overloading—whether from weak muscles, poor alignment, or previous injuries. Gradually building strength distributes the forces across the knee and may stop the pain.
- **Doing squats while weight lifting** is my single most important gym weight-training maneuver. Almost no other exercise builds muscle power in the legs, trunk, and core

while also improving balance and flexibility as much as a well-executed squat. It is my go-to exercise—yet it's one that, if done poorly, leads quickly to back pain. As soon as I feel an odd tweak in one side of my back or the other, I stop the squat. I then stretch and attempt to return with a lower weight, or call it quits with squats for the day.

- **When I'm riding my bike,** I often notice lower back stiffness. This is a function of being on the bike for several hours in the forward-curled position of the road-bike rider. The stomach muscles are not engaged, the lower back strains unequally with each pedal stroke, and the neck is awkwardly extended, with the weight of the helmet pushing against the paracervical muscles. All of this conspires to produce soreness, stiffness, and pain. I've learned that I have to get off my bike every hour or so to stretch. I also change my hand positions frequently during the ride. Either I respect the not-so-subtle signals of muscle overuse, or I find myself dropped from the group.

- **When I'm standup paddling,** the rhythmic motion of the paddle in the water lulls me into forgetting that if I don't engage my core, bend my back deeply, reach out, and use short strokes, many of my joints will talk to me. My arm complains of a tennis-elbow-like pain if the paddle's not truly straight when entering the water. Standup paddling is all about technique. If I don't listen when pain signals me, my technique leads not to bliss but to injury.

- **Ski season arrives** and tempts all the fates. There are no better sports than skiing and snowboarding to keep you engaged for hours at a time. Your knees are bent and loaded for as many as six hours a day, with your body weight at the mercy of gravity. The bumps on the slopes are just waiting to force rapid bending and extension, while temperatures fluctuate to heat and freeze the blood flow. On the first day out, and throughout the season, I really try to listen— even though all I want to do is keep on skiing.

Listen to your body. Notice the first signs of overuse muscle pain, and change the activity just enough to avoid the second (the cramp), third (muscle strain), and then fatal signs (the tear) of muscle injury. When we position ourselves to stop when we need to, we will achieve our ultimate goal of sliding into the home plate of life well used up.

Perception and Injury Recovery

No matter how careful you are, all athletes get injured, and the odds are that at some point in your life, you will too—the steepness of the odds tied, of course, to the particular sports you engage in. Perception of your injury and of yourself as a fit athlete plays a crucial role in how well you recover from your injury and what happens to your fitness levels. It's not just about repairing yourself physically. Your mind is instrumental to how well you fare on the recovery journey.

The best athletes use injury as an excuse to come back better than they were before they were hurt. Others may not be able to do so, often due in part to an inability to let go of the self-image they are attached to. We tend to become tethered to our own models of ourselves— images we then broadcast to others. Remaining open to multiple visions of our athletic selves, rather than fixing on a static portrait, makes us more resilient and able to bounce back from injury.

The severity of injuries varies. There are injuries that leave people with significant disabilities, and others that just take a long time to heal. Most injuries heal on their own or can be repaired. Surgeons and therapists can control many but not all of the outcomes. While it used to be said that after the initial intervention by the medical and surgical team, the rest was up to the patient, the reality is that the "rest" is actually quite susceptible to intervention by caregivers.

Before you get injured—meaning, now—spend some time thinking about your image of your athletic self. What do you see? Are you fitter than you have ever been? Are you muscular, toned, trim, and powerful? Are you a couch potato? Are you the image of yourself in your youth, or the image of your parents? Of all the things about yourself that you take for granted, what would it be like if you lost just one of these qualities, or even two?

Next, ask several objective people to assess you—a trainer, a physical therapist, or a coach. Really take an honest inventory of your physical attributes and skills. Then, look at all the sports and activities that you don't do, and widen your vision of yourself in the athletic world.

Almost nobody does this unless they are competing to make a team and a coach takes the time to share his or her assessments. You might have been trying out for a quarterback position, but the coach may see your potential as a running back, to use a football analogy. If you do this self-analysis, you may refine your own picture of yourself and your potential. This becomes phenomenally helpful if you get injured, because your options have increased.

After people are injured, I see a wide range of responses. These are often based on the person's flexibility in thinking about themselves —including their ability to absorb the loss, take inventory of what is and isn't available to work with, and how they will engage in a recovery program. Those people for whom a realistic self-imagery is absent, or who stay locked into one vision, are often seriously hampered by their injuries.

Your caregivers play an important role in assisting you in developing your other selves. If they are tethered to an image of you as a patient—an image they may form on first meeting you—they may not bring a commitment to the care that achieves your goals. But the physicians, surgeons, and therapists who treat you as a person with infinite potential will start you down the road of becoming a better athlete—though maybe different—than you were before you were injured. These caregivers will repair your injuries in order to facilitate a return to sports. They focus their words and actions on partnering with you to set new goals, and bring creativity and inventiveness to the science and practice of medicine. This partnership in injury recovery, if directed not just at recovery but at improvement, determines the final outcome for many.

Those who have the flexibility to see themselves as athletes-in-training for the same or a new sport, despite their injury, excel. Those who engage the care team with a shared vision excel even more. Yes, developing a range of new conceptions of ourselves requires insight and imagination. But untethering our self-imagery to allow these new models prepares us for the unexpected. Why wait? You might even try on your other selves *before* you get hurt.

Supplements 2.0

"My vet gave my pet glucosamine, and the animal stopped limping. So I started taking it, and I feel less stiff. But I sure hate those big horse pills!"

In the mid-1990s, patients were coming into my office and telling me that their aging pets—even horses—weren't stiff or limping anymore after veterinarians started them on glucosamine. The patients reported that *they* felt better after taking it as well—though they hated the big pills. Inspired by their remarks, I researched the science behind glucosamine and its relative, chondroitin sulfate. I concluded the data was convincing enough. The supplement could be helpful to counteract the wear and tear and injuries from aging, and it certainly had no health risk. I then created a glucosamine-rich beverage called "Joint Juice" to make it easy to consume.

The science behind glucosamine was thin at the time. In the laboratory, glucosamine had been shown to stimulate joint tissue cells to perform several positive actions. First, the glucosamine was a precursor: a building block of the natural lubricant of the joint called hyaluronic acid. The more lubrication, the better the joint worked and felt. Second, glucosamine was a natural anti-inflammatory. Even low levels of anti-inflammatory agents appeared to have positive effects on multiple diseases, not just joint arthritis. Third, glucosamine was a building block for the matrix of articular cartilage. Articular cartilage, which covers all of the bones in a joint, is the surface that becomes damaged from sports or from the disease osteoarthritis. Last, glucosamine suppressed some of the degradative enzymes produced in the joint after injury—those enzymes that break down cartilage.

Glucosamine appeared to be the ultimate supplement: one that both relieved symptoms and improved the actual underlying disease. And it did no harm. Early fears that people with shellfish allergies could not take the supplement were solved by sourcing it from vegetables.

As with many natural food supplements, however, the pharmaceutical industry saw glucosamine as a threat.

A major NIH-funded, double-blind study, which compared glucosamine and chondroitin sulfate to the leading arthritis drug, Celebrex, demonstrated fewer efficacies when all patients were included. In patients with moderate-to-severe arthritis, the supplements showed similar efficacy to the more expensive drug.[7] Since the lead investigator was an industry consultant, the press release claimed that glucosamine didn't work. Yet those of us who treat patients didn't care if glucosamine wasn't as effective in people with very mild symptoms. We did care that it was as good as Celebrex for people with moderate-to-severe pain. Over the last few decades, basic science has clarified the mechanism of action. The supplements work by increasing the production of charged sugars in the articular cartilage matrix of joints. These sugars attract water, hydrating the cartilage and surrounding tissues. Glucosamine and chondroitin are the key building blocks to produce the normal lubricants of the joint called hyaluronic acid. And glucosamine and chondroitin affect the genes, upregulating specific genetic activity involved in maintaining the health of joint tissues. However, the supplements are not effective enough to stop arthritis or restore damaged cartilage to health, because damaged cartilage leads to inflammation and pain.

Until recently, few other supplements showed adequate benefits. This is about to change, as leading-edge science shows that modifications of inflammation itself may actually permit cartilage regeneration. This is a completely novel concept, as traditional orthopaedic science taught that articular cartilage had no healing potential.

---

[7] Daniel O. Clegg et al., "Glucosamine, chondroitin sulfate, and the two in combination for painful knee osteoarthritis," *New England Journal of Medicine* 354 (2006): 795–808, https://pubmed.ncbi.nlm.nih.gov/16495392/.

There is now emerging evidence that some other supplements affect inflammation in novel ways. Some may clear away dead cells (called senolytic cells). These cells, in the process of dying, release degradative enzymes into the joint tissues. In arthritic tissues, as well as in other diseases, the natural process that allows new cells to build restorative tissues is overwhelmed by these toxins. This causes damage to the surrounding tissue as well as irritation, leading to painful inflammation. Pioneering work, led by Johnny Huard, PhD, is demonstrating that if senolytic cells are cleared away with certain anti-inflammatory supplements, the tissues can rebuild themselves— even the articular cartilage of joints.

Various medications used for blood pressure control, infection, and other problems may also have a role in conditioning the tissues to be receptive to anti-inflammation supplements. Again, this is a novel concept. Who would have thought that a blood pressure medication or an antibiotic could affect musculoskeletal tissues in unexpected and helpful ways?

The confusing part of the puzzle is that inflammation has both good and bad features. Inflammatory cells kill cancer cells, which pop up in our bodies every day. They control harmful bacteria that escape from our gut or mouth into our bloodstream. Inflammation is a normal part of wound healing. It is becoming clear that inflammation has a wide range of features, is far more complex than we thought, and can be viewed as good or bad depending on its specific location and situation.

Overloading ourselves with anti-inflammatory diets, supplements, and drugs is probably not the best strategy for longevity. But selectively targeting specific tissues with just the right combination of supplements and drugs may make our joints happier, lives longer, and surgeons less busy.

Supplements and Sharapova

The amazing Sharapova. How could she blow her doping confession so badly? And why do so many top athletes blow theirs?

"I took a medicine given to me by my doctor for several health issues I was having...I got the flu, I had irregular EKG results, I have a family history of diabetes..." A laundry list of explanations.

Athletes' confessions are bumbling, defensive, confusing, and always disappointing. How come? Given their incredibly expensive retinue of advisors, lawyers, press agents, and coaches, why is it so hard for them to simply talk honestly about their efforts to succeed?

The Sharapova case is educational for athletes across all sports. What she could have said is that for years she used every supplement, every drug, every training technique, and every mental focus technique in existence and optimized them to achieve her stellar performances.

Don't all athletes want to do the same? Isn't the whole point of training and competing to develop all your skillsets and push yourself beyond previously accepted limits of human performance? Top athletes spend their entire lives optimizing their speed, agility, strength, coordination, and coaching to push themselves ahead of everyone else. The best ones also optimize their nutrition, supplements, and legal medications to build muscle, stay healthy, and recover from injury and illness.

The future of sports performance may include more than just supplements and drugs that build muscle and increase blood flow. Tomorrow's athletes will likely use genetic manipulation that stimulates the body to produce higher levels of proteins for muscle building, phosphates for energy use, and brain chemicals for focus and processing speed.

Think this is fantasy? It is already happening, and you, too, may be taking substances to optimize your body's capabilities. For example, when you take glucosamine—the drug we discussed in "Supplements 2.0" that is now sold over the counter to aid arthritic joints—one of its side effects is to stimulate the production of specific sugars in the matrix of cartilage that lubricates and protects our joints. Glucosamine, along with chondroitin sulfate, regulates metalloproteinase activity by decreasing the protein synthesis of the enzymes, decreasing the production of the cell-signaling molecules that up-regulate them, and increasing their natural inhibitors. In short, the supplements affect the genes that affect cartilage health. This genetic stimulus of joint health permits people to perform better whether walking, hiking, or playing a top-level sport.

And it's not just glucosamine. Many of the substances we put in our bodies affect multiple genetic and epigenetic systems, some for the good and some detrimentally. The odd thing is that people get so upset about eating genetically engineered foods, when we genetically manipulate ourselves in other ways daily.

But, back to Sharapova. Her statement might have been, with head held high, "Of course I took the legal supplements and drugs that my team doctors and coaches said would improve my blood flow. Every athlete should investigate healthy options that can help them build better bodies. I erred in not knowing that one drug had just become illegal in January—and for that, I apologize and accept a fine."

Look no further than the Olympic motto: *Citius, Altius, Fortius* —"Swifter, Higher, Stronger." What is so hard about acknowledging the fact that we all want to win? And that we will do whatever it takes, within the rules and spirit of sport, to do so?

Medical Myth Busting

In my twenty-five years of practicing as an orthopaedic surgeon working with people with joint injuries and arthritis, I have learned that much of what we think we know turns out to be only part of the truth. Here are a few commonly held beliefs which I believe may do more harm than good.

Myth 1: Antioxidants Are Good for You

Many people seem to be obsessed with antioxidants. They want to eat antioxidant foods, adhere to an anti-inflammatory diet, and take drugs that act as antioxidants. They consume turmeric and cumin along with vitamins E and C, the powerful antioxidant supplements. Their belief is that these foods and vitamins—which can absorb free radicals formed by oxygen—can improve skin appearance, slow aging, reduce cancer risk, and prolong life.

Well, guess what. Oxidation—the formation of free radicals by oxygen—is exactly what kills cancer cells. Oxidation is your body's response to "micro cancers," which are abnormal cells that occur in our bodies literally millions of times. Your system destroys these cells through the oxidative ability of free radicals. If you take a lot of antioxidants, you may actually be suppressing your body's ability to keep down these micro cancers and abnormal cells.

So are you helping yourself or hurting yourself when you take lots of antioxidants? In fact, there's very little high-quality science that supports any benefit from an increased ingestion of antioxidants over the amount one would get in a normal diet.

Myth 2: Sunlight Is Bad for You

Your dermatologist friends will tell you to stay out of direct sunlight and to use lots of skin care and skin protective products. This will prevent you from getting much UV radiation, which can cause skin cancer. But you absolutely have to have sunlight to produce the active forms of vitamin D.

All of those pale dermatologists that you see—and their patients, who also look pasty white—may have very poor calcium uptake, precisely because they are not activating vitamin D through sunlight. No matter how much vitamin D you take, sunlight is required to convert the vitamin D into the active form the body uses to regulate calcium uptake. That's why people in northern climates experience more osteoporosis (bone loss) than people in southern climes: their sun exposure differs dramatically.

The directive to "Cover up, cover up, cover up!" may be destroying your bones. Thirty minutes of total skin sunlight exposure each day (skinny-dipping may be the most efficient way) is the dose the body needs, rationally followed by skin coverage with high UV-protection zinc or titanium skin products and clothing.

Myth 3: Don't Exercise That Arthritic Knee!

Whether or not you have had an artificial knee replacement, a major cause of disability with aging—as well as the loosening of artificial implants—is bone loss. Resistance exercise is the only strategy shown to build up bone without side effects. Lack of exercise is responsible not only for more rapid bone loss but also for loss of muscle power, range of motion, coordination, loss of balance, and a decline in our sense of well-being.

Furthermore, regular exercise is the antidote to arthritis. The trick is to find the workouts that stimulate those abilities, are fun to do, and can be done daily—*and* to do them. Better yet, do them with a partner. Because one fact that's not a myth is that partners who play together stay together.

Myth 4: Diet Alone Can Lead to Weight Loss

It is well known that shockingly few people who lose weight dieting actually maintain their weight reduction. In our experience at The Stone Clinic, only a fundamental change in lifestyle will do the trick. That includes a combination of athleticism (not just exercise), diet, and attitude work. Athleticism means setting a fitness goal and combining exercises and play to achieve fitness. Fitness is the combination of cardiovascular endurance, stamina, strength, flexibility, power, coordination, agility, and balance. Getting there requires dedication and good coaching. Staying there, and maintaining a healthy weight, means the process must be satisfying—both mentally and physically.

Myth 5: Water Intake Doesn't Matter

While several recent studies have called into question the notion that most people are relatively dehydrated during the day, our experience is that increasing plain water consumption decreases appetite, quells an urge to drink sugary beverages, and improves mood. All the cells in our body depend on water and function better when hydrated than when not hydrated. Almost all of our behavior—including sleeping, drinking coffee, alcohol intake, etc.—pushes us toward dehydration. So increase your water intake substantially, and watch the good things that happen.

Myth 6: Vitamin Supplements Matter

Unfortunately, there is so little regulatory oversight over the vitamin and supplement industry that it is impossible to know what is actually in a vitamin pill. What's more, no clinical study has demonstrated a substantially beneficial effect from vitamin supplements for normal people. Well-balanced diets with substantial amounts of protein, fruits, and vegetables are a far better way to nourish the human body than popping pills of dubious pedigree.

Myth 7: Cartilage Can't Be Regrown or Replaced, Especially in Arthritis

There are two types of cartilage in the knee: the fibrocartilage meniscus tissue and the hyaline cartilage covering the ends of bones in joints. When these tissues are torn or damaged through injury (or removed by surgery), the joint develops arthritis. Arthritis is loss of the normal cartilage, bone, or surrounding tissues in joints. Patients are often told that once cartilage is lost, only artificial joint replacement is possible. But the techniques for meniscus replacement and articular cartilage repair have improved so much that biologic joint replacement is often possible. The trick is to repair or replace the injured tissue as soon as the injury occurs and not wait for the arthritis to set in.

If you consider each of these myths individually, you'll find that the "common sense" answer is almost always the right answer. It is amusing to note, though, that sensible answers are not always common.

Stand Up Straight

Stand up straight, like your mother told you to! Bad posture is a cause of multiple musculoskeletal problems. You age yourself artificially by curling up. The overload on all of your joints and on the disks in your spine, caused by poor posture, leads to arthritis. And weakening your abdominal muscles sets you up for back pain. The image of a bent-over, decrepit you does you no good. So *really* stand up. Inhale. Feel strong.

Training your posture takes practice and discipline. Set your phone, computer, Alexa, and Siri to remind you to do the following simple exercises regularly.

Simple Exercises

Start with your eyes. Look around you. Notice how many people are looking down. Then look at *their* posture. My bet is that their shoulders and backs are curled forward, aging them prematurely. So, start your new image of yourself by looking forward. Look directly into people's eyes, at the horizon, at the world around and above you. We all spend too much time contemplating our navels, literally and figuratively. Lift your chin, not just your eyes. Lead with your chin and notice what it does to your neck. The curve shifts. The weight of your skull, holding your massive brain, now centers over your spine. Your blood flow and cerebrospinal fluid have smoother tracks in and out of your mental computer. This diminishes overheating and burnout and oxygenates the neuronal cells that transmit your prodigious thoughts.

Set your shoulders behind your hips, and keep your shoulders open. When they are curled forward, as you tap away at your phone or computer keyboard, they become stuck in the closed position. The scapular rotator muscles on your back weaken from that biomechanically disadvantageous position. Shoulders rolled forward, your rotator cuffs—the four tendons that guide your shoulder motion—get impinged on the bone of the acromion. This causes pain when you try to lift your arm above your head.

As your shoulders roll back, suck in your abdomen. Stuck out over your belt, your abdominal muscles and the fat that covers them are dead weight, pulling on your spine. Try holding a glass of water out in front of you, and notice how hard this is to do even for a few minutes. Without the benefit of muscle contraction and abdominal strength, your back is holding up your stomach like that all day.

With your abdomen tucked in, take a deep breath. Imagine that your lungs have three compartments to fill with each breath. First, fill the space at the bottom, near your belly button. Next, fill your chest area. Lastly, fill the area above your clavicles. Notice your shoulders rolling back, your lungs lifting, and your stomach sucking in.

Roll your hips forward as your shoulders square back. It is not just soldiers who can stand erect for hours, looking proud—you can too. Now walk squarely into the world. Sit down squarely at your desk, keeping your erect posture. Your mother would be proud, and your joints won't ache so much.

Tom Brady's Mouthguard

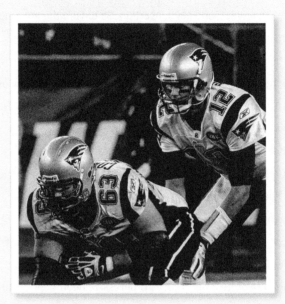

Remaining active and fit isn't just about staying injury free. It is also about staying healthy.

Watch Tom Brady's mouthguard. In and out of his mouth, covered in football sweat and dirt. Hanging in or out of his helmet. And where else has it been? Common places that football players stash their mouthguards between plays are on the face mask, in socks, on the bench, inside skullcaps, or held in the hand. Not surprisingly, studies reveal that mouthguards are typically covered in all kinds of bacteria, fungi, and yeasts associated with disease and infection.

So, why doesn't Brady get sick?

In essence, it's because the microbiome, the organisms that live on that mouthguard, are actually changing with each football field, each helmet, and each insertion. So too are the immune system and the genetic makeup of Tom Brady.

It turns out that we are not mostly human. Of the ten trillion microorganisms that make up the human microbiome, only one in ten is identified as a human cell. What's more, only a fraction of our nine trillion non-human organisms have even been clearly identified as bacteria, virus, or prions, or any other living organisms that we understand. The rest are organisms that we have yet to know.

Let me explain. We've known about bacteria since the 1600s, finally making the link between germs and disease in the 1860s and 1870s. The first virus was discovered in 1892, while the first prion (a protein that causes progressive neurodegenerative conditions) wasn't identified until the 1960s. These discoveries have been enormously helpful in medicine. However, 20 percent of the DNA in your nose and 40 to 50 percent of the DNA in your gut has the genetic code for organisms we have not yet identified, the so-called "biological dark matter." This large amount of unknown genetic coding and "organisms" makes up most of what we consider as us.

In addition, the ecosystem of the human body is constantly invaded. The immune system responds to known and unknown new intruders with varying strength and effectiveness. While a small portion of the response may be preprogrammed by your genetic makeup, the reality is that there are too many new and unknown organisms. Fortunately, instead we have a response system that both modifies itself by recording each new invader (memory cells) and modifies our genes so they can produce a range of proteins and other molecules to defend ourselves in the future.

The average lifespan of cells in our body is estimated to be four thousand seconds. So the Tom Brady you see in the beginning of the Super Bowl is not the Tom Brady raising the trophy or mourning the loss.

Brady doesn't usually get sick, despite the presence of all kinds of nasty things in his mouthguard, because of the flexibility of his response system and the natural turnover of the human cells in a healthy body. You can avoid getting sick too, by maintaining a vigorously healthy body to defend against the blitzing invaders.

The Aging Athlete

In a recent conversation with a sixty-year-old colleague, the subject turned to aging. "My body is like my old sailboat," he said. "Every time it gets taken out for a sail, something breaks. Not something major, like a keel falling off, but a fitting here, a line there. The thing with sailboats is that you have to maintain them constantly. If you don't, big things will go wrong."

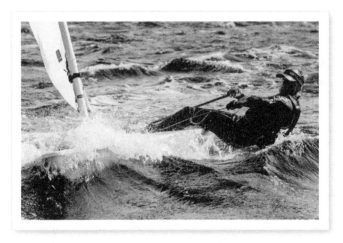

Andrew H • World-class sailor, Melges 32 world champion,
and knee/elbow growth factor injection patient

The body is the same way. Ignore it, and the issues accumulate; then something big typically does go wrong. But pay attention, and you can live well until the day you die. *Drop dead in your 100s—playing a sport and loving life.* This is our goal for our patients. If you can stay fit, recover from illness and injury, and keep your eye on the ball, it's an achievable goal. It starts with regular evaluations of where you are as you age—inventories of strengths and weaknesses, and game plans for making the best of the former and improving the latter. If you want to grow old happily, train your body for the sport of aging. Here's what to do.

Keep up with preventive care. Physical exams are a form of inspection and maintenance. Your doctor offers you wise, personalized guidance, up-to-date information about developments in medicine that may apply to you, and warnings about little things before they become big things. Physicals are also an opportunity for bonding with the person who may save your life.

Don't get injured. Injuries that damage the joints often lead to arthritis if the damaged tissues are not repaired or replaced. Avoiding injuries as you age is not as hard as it was when you were younger. My older athletes pick their sports with care. They lean more toward swimming, cycling, and running, but even those who play soccer try to avoid making the mistakes that can lead to injuries. My golfers and tennis players tend to be more thoughtful about the mechanics of their swings.

All my older athletes seem to choose their times to exercise based on brain power, rather than on rash, adrenaline-infused decisions. They are mindful while they play. Most of my long-distance female runners began running in their thirties and forties, and some as late as their sixties. They don't suffer from the overuse injuries my younger males do, in part because they manage their runs, titrating their efforts to match their health. Not getting injured doesn't mean not playing—it means playing smart.

Repair and replace what does get injured. The old days of taking out torn meniscus cartilages in the knee, living with torn rotator cuffs in the shoulder, injecting cortisone, and toughing it out are over. As soon as key tissues are torn, they should be repaired, regenerated, or replaced. For example, there is overwhelming data that simply repairing rather than resecting a torn meniscus cartilage dramatically decreases the chance of arthritis in the knee. For arthritic knees, resurfacing only the part that is painful is an outpatient procedure that can return people to most sports in two months.

Train for balance. Falling is one of the main killers of older people, and falls often occur as a result of poor balance. Balance and the mind/ body connection, called proprioception, are rapidly lost after an injury and lost slowly with aging—but both are completely trainable.

Standing on one leg with your eyes closed or on a pillow is an easy way to train balance every day. If you live near the water and can swim, the number one best exercise for balance is standup paddling. It can be done at any age. By widening the board to the width of a door, anyone can stand on one. The constant balancing and gentle paddling strengthen the trunk and core muscles. Working on the small muscles of the feet, and the neuro-sensory or proprioceptive feedback system improves balance more than any other activity.

Train for strength. Weak muscles are mostly from disuse and low natural testosterone. Often the advice people are given for their aches and pains is to go home and rest, further weakening all the structures. In China, many old people are in the public parks performing Chinese dances and Tai Chi, while our old people are home watching TV. We can change this. Exercise programs designed to build muscle should be part of everyone's day. An entire field of elderly sports and fitness training would do wonders for our aging population. Progressive, competitive, and creative fitness programs that focus on muscle building work for the elderly but are rarely encouraged. We need CrossFit to mature into AgeFit.

Build bone. Bone responds to stress. More stress stimulates the body to make stronger bones; lack of stress on the bones leads to mineral loss and weakening. Increasing stress by resistance exercises, such as weight lifting, is proven to be the most effective bone-building activity at all ages. Elderly weight lifting gyms and programs should be the norm. Wheelchair-bound elderly people can learn from wheelchair-bound young people to exercise their upper body and trunk muscles. It takes courage, determination, coaching, and education to build bone, and it is worth it.

Join a team. My happiest older athletes don't just hit the gym solo. They play with others. Team sports build the camaraderie that we all remember from high school and college but often lose in our working years. Masters leagues are the easiest sport communities to identify and join. Running partners, rowing clubs, hiking groups, and sailing clubs all inspire the "group think" that leads to long-term sports participation.

Eat like you plan to live forever. Optimizing your weight usually means getting lighter in your fifties through your seventies and getting more muscular in your seventies through your hundreds. Since everyone has unique issues with metabolism, kidney function, and GI tolerance, a smart sports nutritionist can customize your diet to your output. In general, older athletes need more protein. Ingesting protein in the hour just after exercise leads to the best utilization of the nutrient for muscle building. Obtaining a serum albumin level and a testosterone level may help guide the program for men and for women. I don't have any eighty- to one-hundred-year-olds who are too muscular.

Water, water everywhere. Both to drink and to train in. Most people are perpetually dehydrated from sleep, caffeine, alcohol, and mouth breathing. Increasing water intake hydrates all the cells in the body, including the ones in your brain. Have a tall glass of water before even lifting a fork, and place a glass on your desk all day. The need for frequent trips to the bathroom often discourages my older athletes from drinking enough, but the trade-off is worth it, from both a health and a fitness point of view.

But don't just drink water; immerse yourself in it. Everyone, every joint, every injury feels better in a warm pool. You don't have to be a swimmer. Just walking laps in the pool, in waist- to chest-deep water, is a great cardiovascular workout. Try walking twenty laps. Time yourself, and try to walk a little faster each day. Set a goal for your hundredth birthday of walking for ten minutes in the pool, twice a day.

Reframe what you can and can't do. I happen to love skiing moguls, but I don't ski them in the backcountry anymore because if I fall, I may not get up. I ski them on the main slopes and only as a treat. Road biking is the same. I've learned that if I want to take an aggressive bike ride for a number of hours, I'll have to take breaks and stretch out. Each birthday, I like to ride my age in years in miles. Maybe at some point I'll switch to doing it in two days rather than all at once. If so, I'll see it as doubling the pleasure, rather than halving the effort.

Waterskiing keeps my entire body strong. Nothing else tunes the muscles so fast and so enjoyably. Yet making that hard carve on the outside turn isn't as pretty as it used to be and carries more risk than reward. That's really the whole point. Is the risk of the extreme activity worth more than the longer-lasting joys of the moderately extreme activities? At my age, moderately extreme has more longevity and more appeal. Getting older means doing something great, often—and passing up something spectacular, occasionally.

Each little tweak, each warning sign, if ignored, can turn into a chronic pain. I don't have time for chronic pain. So I learn to pay attention sooner, fix the problems, and do the preventive maintenance. That way, I'll get to keep sailing this "old boat" until—one inevitable day—the wind dies.

The Stone Aging Impact Score

Staying fit—and injury free—takes daily commitment. What you do to yourself ages you. The work you do, the activities you engage in, the food you put into your body—these and many other lifestyle factors have impacts on your fitness levels, what you can achieve, and the aging process. Since how well you live each day determines the quality and the length of your life, how about starting to keep score? Here is a scorecard. Rate yourself on a scale of negative ten to plus ten on these ten items.

- **Starting at daybreak, do you feel like you slept well?**
  Sleep is a key criterion of well-being, and its duration and quality affects both your day and your life.
  » *If yes, a full eight hours is worth ten points. Pulling an all-nighter is a negative ten. Somewhere in between? Rate accordingly.*

- **If you normally exercise in the morning before breakfast, did you get your best workout in?** A great Pilates class, a spin, a run, a swim?
  » *If yes, give yourself a ten. Missing a day is not a negative ten, but possibly a negative two—as long as it doesn't keep happening. No exercise during a full week? Negative ten.*

- **Is your breakfast a breakfast of champions?** Data is overwhelming that a breakfast high in lean protein (and lunch, too) provides energy for the whole day. A consistently healthy diet that optimizes your weight and provides fuel to play the sports you want to do is worth more than you can imagine.
  » *A plus ten if what you eat for breakfast carries you to a healthy lunch. A high-fat, high-carb breakfast, powered by extra caffeine, is a negative ten.*

- **Do you commute to and from work?** Is the trip filled with
  wonderful books on tape, podcasts, and music? Or is it
  defined by heavy traffic and the anxiety of running late? Can
  you commute to work on a bike? The new e-bikes are powerful enough to go thirty miles. Those that only assist you
  when you pedal give you a mild workout without the sweat.
  Freedom from the prison of the car or public transportation
  and traffic, combined with that extra exercise, is a bonus.
  » *Plus ten if relaxed; negative ten if you were frenzied or
    late for a meeting. On a bike of any kind: eleven points!*
- **Your work environment.** Is it inspiring, one that you cherish,
  one that motivates you? Do you feel you are contributing to
  the world, are well paid, and appreciated?
  » *If yes, give yourself a plus ten. If you labor in a hostile,
    high-stress environment, give yourself a negative ten.*
- **Healthy friendships and work colleagues, nice waiters,
  and flight attendants.** What your behavior elicits in others,
  and your interactions with others during the day, all add up.
  A smile to everyone you meet starts the relationship at a ten.
  » *Rate yourself from a positive to a negative ten each
    day, depending on your balance of helpful versus
    fraught encounters.*
- **Relationships are important.** Is the love of your life in your
  life? Or are you in a relationship that was once great but is
  now "just average?" If the latter, enlist a pro to help you both
  get back to a state of bliss.
  » *Plus ten if you have a warm, supportive partner. If you
    are in the middle of an acrimonious relationship or a
    bitter divorce, a negative ten.*

- **How about sex?** Sexual satisfaction, orgasms, and communication are correlated with well-being.

  » *A positive ten if there are fireworks between you and your partner! Absence of sexual love may not be a negative, so in this case enter a zero on your score. But if you're in an abusive or deeply unsatisfying physical relationship, score a negative ten.*

- **How much do you partake?** Alcohol, drugs, and ingestibles at levels that impair you get a negative score. A single glass of good Bordeaux, a refreshing beer, or any socially acceptable indulgence may increase your well-being.

  » *Positive ten for balanced imbibing; negative ten for anything that gives you a hangover. (Abstinence equals zero.)*

- **How was dinner?** Did you share it with family and friends, with time to share stories, reflect on world events, counsel the kids on their homework, and generally relax? Did you ditch the devices? Or was it a rushed takeout meal with stress from the day carrying over?

  » *For the former, a huge positive ten; the latter, negative ten. Most electronic device time is either a neutral or a negative. You judge the effect of devices on the quality of your interactions and digestion.*

Your Stone Aging Impact Score may affect not just your aging process but your response to illness, injury, surgery, or other life-challenging events. As we've seen in this chapter, you can't separate physical fitness from good mental fitness. The body is not divorced from the mind. Approach fitness by building it into your routine through exercise, diet, stress management, outlook, and injury pre-vention, and you'll be well on your way to those three contributors of life fulfillment—doing what you want to do, when you want to do it, and doing it well.

CHAPTER 3

SPORTS-SPECIFIC INSIGHTS

T raining and playing. The choice on how to balance these is yours. You can train just to train, and never play a sport. You can play a sport and never get fitter or better. Or you can train for your sport and play it, and become fitter and better. Preferences differ for each person and each activity and sport.

My goal is to enable you to drop dead at the age of one hundred years playing some sport—or at least to have the ability to do so. To get there, you'll need to constantly improve your body and your mind to counter the natural degradation of time and biology. For you to succeed means: 1) that you want to be fit and live a healthy lifestyle; 2) that you find it fun and not drudgery (because otherwise you won't persist at it); and 3) that you avoid the injuries that lurk out there

and can severely reduce your fitness program and/or that you have
the tools to recover from those setbacks.

Here are a few insights on the most common sports and activities
I deal with to help you avoid the usual injuries. Let these activities
inspire you to pick up a sport you may not have tried, and make sure
you're still playing when you're one hundred years young.

SLIDING ON SNOW

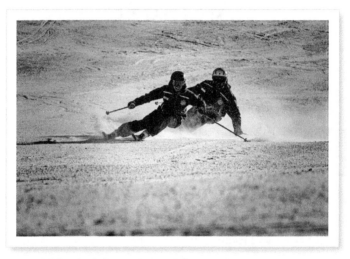

*Mark M. • Avid skier and growth factor study patient, carving on
skis after meniscus replacement, & shoulder reconstruction*

Winter brings the opportunity for you to slide down nature's slopes,
bringing bliss to those of you who plan to enjoy it. The operative
word here is *plan*. If anyone ever truly understood the injury rate
from skiing, they probably would never ski. But we skiers keep skiing
because it is just so much fun, and so addictive, that we choose to
suppress our worries about the risks. As a lifelong skier and a former

physician for the US Ski Team, I see a disproportionate number of skiers each year, and thus think about ski injuries often. While I know that my thoughts will not completely protect me, I share them with you in hopes that we spend more time talking on the chairlift than in the operating room.

Here are the things you can do to limit your skiing injury exposure this year.

- **Fitness matters.** Thanks to high-speed lifts—which are becoming ubiquitous—lift lines have shortened. This has increased our time on the snow, and therefore our exposure to injury. Weakened, tired legs respond to changes in terrain more slowly. Preseason ski fitness classes can be an enormous help. And remember, many people lose fitness during the ski season as they ski only on the weekends. Train daily (focus on flexibility, trunk, core, quad, and hamstring strength), stretch daily, swim, and focus on flexibility.

More specifically:

- **Strength training.** There is no other sport that involves staying in the flexed position, loading the front of your knees for four to six hours at a time—so training for skiing and boarding really does help. Increase your time in the gym doing squats, Pilates machine exercises, and uphill cycling. These are the most efficient training tools.
- **Balance.** Given the current shapes of skis and boards, carving—the act of making a ski turn completely on its edges through the entire arc of the turn—requires balance

more than strength. Train on a balance board or a slack line, or simply stand with one leg on a pillow and close your eyes. Proprioception or balance/awareness/ feedback training is the least practiced exercise and yet the most important for injury prevention. If you don't know where you are in space, or where your limbs are, it is hard to make in-course corrections to land safely. This applies to the racer at seventy miles per hour and to the beginner about to tip over from the slipped ski on a patch of ice.

- **Cardio.** Snow sports are rarely at sea level. Most people do not enjoy their first few days in the mountains due to the low atmospheric pressure of oxygen and dehydration. Increasing your cardio training and upping your water intake at high altitudes makes a huge difference.

- **Flexibility.** Can you lie all the way back on your skis or board and get up? Try it at home. If not, start stretching. Pool workouts, combining cardio and flexibility, are the fastest way to improve both.

- **Equipment matters.** Tune your skis and boots to work with your type of skiing. Boots that fit well may make a difference not just in improving your performance and enjoyment but also in preventing harm to your joints. Sharp edges and well-tuned skis grab snow snakes less often and get you out of trouble when you really need that edge. Go to the ski shop now and tune your gear.

If your gear is well used, or more than a few years old, consider investing in new components. With shaped skis and boards, the effort required to turn is significantly less. In skiing, the mid-stance position is far more comfortable. But radically shaped skis are not safer. The increased tip/tail-to-waist ratio increases the "catching" of the ski and increases torque on the body. Fortunately, skis are now returning to a narrower design with a less radical difference from tip to tail. Most importantly, the tails are getting narrower, which should diminish some of the ACL injuries seen when a skier loads the tails of the skis.

Wide skis are fun in powder, but they increase the injury rate on groomed slopes. If you are skiing mostly on groomers, choose the newest ski designs with longer arcs and softer flex. If you have radically shaped skis from just a few seasons ago, trade them in. The wider the ski, the harder it is to lay them over on their edge, which creates more torque on the knee. No one ski is best. Rent skis for conditions that don't suit the skis you own.

Softer boots have replaced rigid boots for older knees. Fit your boots snugly, as they transfer the forces to and from the ski and to the binding for release. Ski boots are slowly evolving from the "one-shape-fits-all" to more customized designs that will permit the transfer of force through the foot's arch and great toe rather than the boot's rigid cuff. This design change will mimic the way we walk— loading our feet, not our shins, and thereby increasing the feel of the ski and the snow. (Read more about ski boots in Appendix A.)

For poles, consider that the most common injury on the hill is a thumb injury from falling with your hands in the pole straps. Many orthopaedic surgeons won't use pole straps. Do you really need them?

Last: helmets have not been shown to reduce neck or significant head injuries, except in some collisions with tree branches or other objects. Clear visibility of your goggles and headgear probably matters more. For racing, however, there is no doubt: no helmet, no starts.

Binding settings matter; binding brands don't. Surprisingly, there isn't much that's new or more effective on the market when it comes to bindings. And no existing brand has been shown to be safer than another by any high-quality study—neither the KneeBinding binding nor the Brainless binding. Not until there is a computer embedded between the ski and the boot, reading the real-time forces on the skier's body and releasing the ski a split second before a potential injury, will there be a truly safe release mechanism. Bindings that have both toe and heel lateral releases (like those made by Howell design) are probably better, though there is still no clear data that they reduce ACL injuries yet.

The most common error for recreational skiers is having the bindings too tight. Bindings were designed to avoid pre-release for ski racers who didn't want to fall prematurely. Often, their injuries were greater from the pre-release than from the ACL rupture that can occur when the binding doesn't release. Unless you are jumping, racing, or skiing in hard moguls or chutes, set your bindings slightly lower than the recommended DIN settings. You may (or may not) have a few more releases than you planned, but you'll also have fewer ACL tears. We see far fewer pre-release injuries than injuries in which "my binding didn't release." Bottom line: get bindings adjusted to the right release setting for the skier you actually are and not the one you imagine yourself to be. (Read more about bindings in Appendix A.)

Get prepped. Don't hit the slopes cold. Stiff backs, cold feet, and cold muscles lead to an overall reduction in the ability to respond to sudden changes in position. Warm up in the morning with yoga, flexibility exercises, and hot soaks. Don't stretch on a cold floor. If you have poor blood circulation, get boot warmers, heated socks, and heated gloves. (They really work—though they're not durable and don't survive washing.) Upgrade your clothing to the newer materials that are thinner, warmer, and stretchier. Ride the covered lifts. Drink warm fluids. You will be surprised by how much staying warm decreases minor injuries—which lead to major injuries. **What are you here for?** Being mentally compromised includes "distracted skiing" too. Focus, relax, and enjoy the sport by keeping your mind on the hill and off your electronic devices. Our hope is that cell-zone-free mountains are coming to a hill near us all, and soon! Be bold. Leave the phone at home, be in the moment, pay attention, and ski intelligently.

Substances and skiing aren't a safe cocktail. Drugs and alcohol are legal in many ski states, but both truly reduce athletic performance. Alcohol, not surprisingly, plays a significant role in skiing injuries. Skiing and boarding half-baked sounds cool to some, but can be dangerous for most. (Whether or not this will decline in weed-legal states is an interesting potential research study, with data yet to be revealed.) Skiing while mentally altered decreases one's perception of all the wonderful stimuli in the mountains and increases the potential for injury. Since mental errors still account for a large number of injuries, it is best to wait for happy hour to increase your happiness.

Mind your speed. It kills on the highway, and it ruptures ligaments on the slopes. "I got a little out of control," is the most common comment I hear when I see patients with ski injuries.

Read the map. Look at the updated grooming conditions on the mountain. Surprisingly, not many skiers do. There are far fewer injuries on groomed trails than in rough skiing conditions.

Take a guide. Most people do not appreciate how many hidden ski trails there are on every mountain. While skiing is already extraordinarily expensive, local hosts and mountain guides are often relatively cheap compared to ski school instructors. The hidden stashes will put huge grins on everyone's faces.

Mind any injuries. Fix what's broken before the season. If your back, shoulder, knee, or other joints are holding you back, get them repaired. The science of joint repair and rehabilitation has advanced so far that almost all joint injuries and arthritic conditions can be repaired well enough to return you to skiing.

ACL, MCL, and meniscus injuries, shoulder dislocations, and rotator cuff tears—these are the most common major injuries resulting from falls. (Hand injuries happen often as well, but they're not our focus.) Fortunately, the increasing use of donor tissues preloaded with stem cells appears to be speeding recovery after replacement and repair of damaged tissues. While early repair has made injuries less life-interrupting, they can still end your ski season. Research on speeding the recovery is a major focus for those of us in the tissue regeneration space.

Enjoy yourself. If it isn't fun, it isn't snow sports. Quit when it isn't. Ski during the best sun and best snow conditions of the day. Eat lunch when few other people do. Pass on the icy, low-visibility conditions. There's no shame in being smart and quitting early. The goal is to ski for a long time in life, not a long time in one day.

Schiffrin and Sacrifice

M ikaela Shiffrin has brought ski racing to an entirely new level. Her extreme focus, commitment, and ambition dwarf those of other competitors. Is this what it takes to win?

First let's consider Lindsey Vonn. She was on track to be the greatest ski racer of her generation, with eighty-one World Cup races, four overall World Cup titles, and three gold medals. She combined beauty with awesome power, challenging the men in a sport where power and guts often determine the outcome. Yet along the way, she became a very public figure with a social life highlighted in the media: a marriage and divorce, a high-profile relationship with Tiger Woods, and multiple injuries. Despite her often career-threatening injuries, she inspired us with her phenomenal comebacks. Still, one has to wonder: do public distractions lead to irregular performances and—in a sport where mistakes lead to sometimes fatal crashes—avoidable injuries?

Along comes the Shiffrin family, a prodigy skier and her parents. Her mother, a woman willing to dedicate her entire life to her child, becomes Mikaela's coach, confidante, roommate, and guardian against all outside influences. They travel (in name only) with the US Ski Team but with their own physiotherapists, trainers, and hotels. They put a 24/7 laser focus on Mikaela's sports performance. She wears headphones to block out any extraneous distractions. In this virtual bubble, the athlete whose talent starts out at the "gifted" level achieves absolute dominance of her sport. Until she doesn't.

Mikaela set her sights on excelling beyond the range of technical ski events where she had trained most of her life. She turned her attention to the speed ski events, the Super G and Downhill, which she had avoided as a youth. She courageously applied her skills to those races, where a loss of focus lasting even a few milliseconds can lead to a crash at seventy miles per hour (and often a severe injury). While she has won World Cup races, the Olympics presented a whole new level of stress.

Mikaela is intimidating to all who compete in skiing. She and her training style raise disturbing questions. Must an athlete become a robot to dominate? Is there no room for variety of life, especially in a world-touring sport? Must one be insulated so completely that one's mother, coach, roommate, and protector are one and the same? Is the sacrifice of a full, diverse life the price one must pay to reduce the risk of injury? And are such athletes then more vulnerable to unexpected bouts of stress that can cause them to become unglued? The lives of Lindsey Vonn and Tiger Woods—to name just two examples—show how phenomenal talent can be derailed by social misadventures and the stress of public scrutiny.

During any Olympic season, as you watch the nauseatingly up-close-and-personal television interviews and vignettes that punctuate the sports events, look for the telltale signs that distinguish "well-rounded" athletes from high-performance human machines. Try to predict which athletes will succeed. Then ask yourself: How would *you* define success? Is it only through absolute domination? And if so, is it worth the sacrifice?

HIGH ON CLIMBING

Going to high elevations pushes all your cardiovascular systems to respond. With altitude, as the force of gravity declines, the partial pressure or density of oxygen declines progressively. While the percentage of oxygen in each breath stays the same (21 percent), due to the lower pressure, the amount of oxygen available to the lungs at five thousand meters drops by half. The body is unable to access the amount of oxygen normally needed without dramatically increasing breathing, blood flow, and sometimes blood pressure. Relative hypoxia, or lowered oxygen concentration in your blood, occurs when you cannot adapt fast enough to lower oxygen at partial pressure.

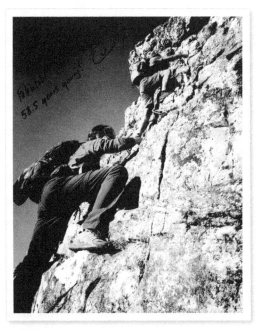

Dianne L. • Sixty-year-old female avid hiker/climber and meniscus transplant & articular cartilage repair patient

Certain behaviors inhibit your adaption mechanisms—smoking chief among them. Smoking brings carbon monoxide into the lungs, binding the hemoglobin that carries oxygen to tissues. Smoking three cigarettes effectively raises you to the equivalent of fifteen hundred meters of elevation. This not only makes you breathe even harder to get enough oxygen, but also, in trying to conserve oxygenated blood for the brain, the cardiovascular system distributes blood away from the peripheral parts of the body. As a result, your muscles don't work as well. And higher levels of carbon monoxide and hypoxia lower visual acuity immediately. You simply don't see as accurately. Alcohol also shifts the dissociation curve of oxygen, making it less available to all tissue.

If you have heart disease or arteries that are calcified or restricted by plaque deposition, your system may not be able to distend and contract effectively enough. If you have lung disease—or simply a cold—your ability to expand your lungs and fill their small alveolar spaces with fresh air may be restricted. Clearing the lungs before going to altitude helps, if possible. Once there, using inhalers, nasal washes, and decongestants all improve your reactivity to altitude stress.

But you have to pay attention to more than just the oxygen concentration. Dry air at altitude dehydrates everyone, and few lowlanders remember to hydrate as much as they need to. All cells in the body are negatively affected by dehydration, and none are more sensitive than the brain. Water consumption of as much as eight glasses a day makes a huge difference in how you think and how you perform at altitude.

Abrupt weather changes at altitude trap many an unsuspecting visitor. Getting wet from light rain (or even from sweating) just before the temperature plummets has led to hypothermia in athletes of all sports. Extra layers of clothing and accurate weather reporting are the best preparation for the arrival of sudden afternoon cold fronts.

Despite all these potential problems, most people excel at altitude. There is something about the clean air and majestic mountains that frees the spirit from the constraints of everyday life. Changes in lighting, the sunrises and sunsets, and the challenge of pushing oneself all merge into an unmatched beauty of spirit, perception, and physicality. It is important to go up—to get high in the best possible way and carry that elevated state home with you.

RUNNING FOR LIFE

I often get this question: "Doc, does running hurt my knee?" The answer is no. Injury hurts your knee.

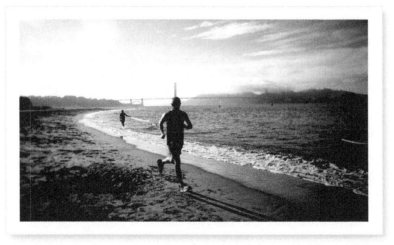

Richard Donovan • Ultra runner and double partial-knee-replacement patient.
Richard completed a Trans America Run, was the first marathoner at the North
& South Pole, and holds the world record for the World Marathon Challenge
(7 marathons on 7 continents in 7 days). He continues to run brilliantly.

Running is safe. No joint is injured solely by running, despite what you may have heard. Running only damages already damaged joints. You can run forever if you have healthy joints and good running mechanics. However, if you have lost your meniscus cartilage, suffer from arthritis, or have lost motion from tight hips, ankles, or a torn ligament that causes your knee joint to move abnormally, running can indeed cause damage to the cartilage in the joints.

Let's consider the knee's components: bone, cartilage, and ligament. Most people have a rough image of the bone configuration, the bulbous lower end of the femur meeting the platform of the tibia—but there's a lot of material between these surfaces. Let's start with cartilage.

Articular cartilage, typically 1.69 to 2.55 millimeters thick, covers the ends of the bones (as in all joints) and provides a smooth, bearing surface. As I have mentioned before, this surface is roughly five to ten times slicker than ice sliding on ice! When you injure the articular cartilage or get arthritis, this smooth surface begins to get rougher. As the surface roughens, there is a dramatic increase in the friction between the surfaces in the joint. This increased friction leads to gradually increasing wear of the joint surfaces. During activities such as running, the damaged surfaces can't absorb and distribute the impact force from your foot hitting the ground as well as normal joint surfaces can. So higher peak forces on an injured knee produce damage.

The normal knee also has two meniscus cartilages, which distribute forces and stabilize the knee. If they are torn or missing due to injury or surgery, the impact forces are concentrated on a smaller area of the knee leading to more rapid wear.

Ligaments stabilize the knee. Unstable knees lead to tearing of the meniscus, and just like a car out of alignment wears out its tires, the abnormal motions of the unstable knee lead to an acceleration of the wear patterns of the joint surfaces.

Running produces peak impact forces on the knee of one to three times your body weight, depending on a host of factors, such as the smoothness of your gait, your running technique, and the surfaces you run on. Heel striking increases peak forces, whereas midfoot landing produces lower peak forces, as long as the running shoe is soft enough to permit compression of the arch tissues of the foot. Interestingly, when running is compared to walking, since you take fewer steps per mile when you run, the total amount of force that the knee sees is often less in smooth running than in walking. So, technique and surfaces really do matter.

We have found that people are able to return to running even after injury by repairing their articular cartilage and replacing damaged meniscus cartilage or ligaments with donor tissue. A long-term outcome study of some of our biologic joint replacement patients found that many were able to run again after fearing they had reached the end of the road.

The following, in no particular order of importance, are specific tips for extending your running life indefinitely.

- **Stretch first.** Pay attention to which joints are tight, and work on loosening them up. Get your mind into the sport you are about to do, while leaving the stresses of work and life behind.
- **Run with short strides.** Most people don't know that whether you walk a mile or run a mile, the same total force or load is placed on the knee joints. But the peak forces

are higher with running—especially if the heel lands first. Running with short strides makes midfoot landing easier and has been shown to reduce the high-peak forces generated when the heel strikes the ground first.

- **Run on soft surfaces.** Reducing peak forces can be achieved by soft landings. Grass, soft tracks, beaches, and trails are preferred over streets.
- **Run with new shoes.** While your running shoes may not look worn out, the midsoles (the layers between the sole and the shoe bed) become stiff with time and use.
- **Add sprinting to your regimen.** Most runners I talk with don't sprint anymore. They did in high school and then forgot about it. Numerous studies have shown that short workouts can have the same (or sometimes more) benefits than long ones. Interspersing sprinting into your running workouts raises both the intensity and the cardiovascular benefit.
- **Fuel and hydrate.** Are you trying to break down your body or build it up? If you want to improve, you must take in nutrients before you run, during your run, and after your run. This way, your body can incorporate these fuels into the new musculature you are trying to build. Many runners run dry and hungry and then wonder why they break down.
- **Get a run-fit assessment.** While most serious cyclists have a bike-fitting session before buying a new bike, few runners ask a pro to look at their gait. Many top physical therapists and running coaches spend hours with patients, helping them recover good walking and running form after injuries.

Book a pre-injury appointment, and hopefully you'll never show up again.

- **Treat injuries aggressively.** Running on an injured joint destroys the joint surfaces and shortens running careers. Get full, accurate diagnoses and repair damaged tissues early. The entire field of sports injury treatment is moving in the direction of accelerated healing with stem cells, growth factors, tissue repair, regeneration, and replacement. The days of removing the torn tissue and returning to the doctor years later for an artificial joint replacement are over. You can run forever if you keep what you have, fix what you break, and use your head in addition to your body.

The assertion that normal knees can run forever is backed by observations of huge animals, such as African elephants. Though weighing more than thirteen thousand pounds, an elephant can run extraordinarily fast and live for sixty years without joint arthritis.

Nothing beats running. Running provides endorphins, pheromones, adrenaline, and testosterone so efficiently that the addiction to running and the bliss from it is difficult to replace. In terms of cost and time, running provides benefits that outdo almost any health-care program. If you have healthy knees, you can run, but make sure you run efficiently with a smooth technique involving short strides, midfoot landing, well-fitting running shoes, and soft surfaces. If you have injured knees, repair them or find your bliss in "simulated running," but don't miss out.

Running Alternatives

I have many patients in their fifties, sixties, and seventies who come into my clinic asking for a new meniscus to act as a shock absorber so they can continue running. Anything to avoid stopping. The depression that settles in when an injury causes a layoff from running can only be cured by a return to running. Running is nirvana to the dedicated runner. So what to do when you can't run? Simulate it.

In my experience, the two closest substitutes to running are using an ElliptiGO machine and pool running. An ElliptiGO is similar to the bicycle-like elliptical machines commonly found in gyms, but it can actually go outside on the road. You ride it in an upright position, like a cross-trainer. Using an ElliptiGO entails many of the same physical mechanics as running, but without the impact. When it is used to climb hills, the core and gluteal workouts of an ElliptiGO are actually better than running. This is because the posture is upright, with significant smooth resistance that engages the trunk musculature more efficiently. The motion, the wind in the hair, and the cycling back and forth of the legs all come very close to the experience of running itself.

Pool running is my next favorite alternative. There are two varieties. The first is performed in shallow to chest-deep water, pushing off the bottom of the pool and running laps. In most pools, where the water gets deeper down the length of the pool, this means running along the shallow ends of the pool. The resistance of the water provides a huge muscular and cardiovascular workout. I try to run twenty laps as fast as possible and improve my time each day. The buoyancy of the water diminishes the joint impact significantly. Pool running can even be performed with a severely arthritic knee. Form is important. Leaning forward or staying upright uses different muscles. Experiment with both.

Deep-water pool running is another, more difficult version of this exercise. Here the hands are cupped, providing vertical stability. The knees are pumped high into the chest, just as a sprinter pumps his or her legs and hands. Forward motion is gained by slightly leaning forward. Time is the measure of this workout. Your heart rate will rapidly climb in deep water as your legs cycle furiously to keep you afloat.

Each of these tools helps bridge my dedicated runners from their injury, through their recovery, to a return to outdoor running. For my patients whose running careers really are over, lifelong substitutions are only limited by one's creativity in finding the best alternatives. And yes, many of them are fun, effective, and even addictive, but as with your first true love, nothing compares to running.

CYCLING:
OUR BICYCLES, OURSELVES

They love to ride. The camaraderie of riding in a peloton, or the solo inspiration of riding and daydreaming, keeps them on their bikes for hours. They find themselves adjusting their diets to get leaner, drinking fluids loaded with carbohydrates, and wearing clothes that diminish wind resistance. Over time, their fanatical addiction to riding increases. They measure their output in every conceivable way. The bikes get more expensive. The materials get lighter. Sucked into the vortex of staying in the saddle, updating their gear, and becoming "real" cyclists, the other activities fall by the wayside. And therein lies the problem.

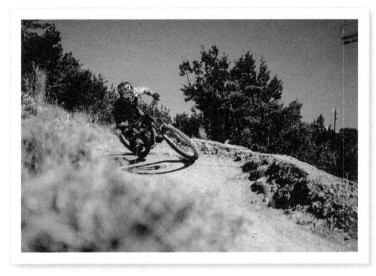

Tony A. • Mountain biker & robotic total knee replacement patient

My cyclist patients are not always fit. Yes, their aerobic capacity is impressive. Their quads are like iron. But watch them when they get off their bikes. For the first minute or two, they can barely stand up. Their backs ache. Their necks are sore. Their hips are tight. They look like the classic picture of abused laborers.

So where is the disconnect? Cycling, while great for some parts of the body, is not so good for others. The abdomen, even if lean, hangs down and does not get stronger. The oblique muscles of the trunk and core experience the same repetitive motion for hours on end and become weak in all other planes of motion. The back is curved on the bike and sees repetitive strain to the lower portion where the pelvis rocks up and down at the lumbosacral interface. When combined with weak abdominal muscles, the strain on the spine and on the musculature of the trunk leaves the cyclist prone to increased back pain and disc degeneration.

Our bones build mass according to the amount of force applied to them. This law of bone physics, called Wolfe's Law, comes into play for cyclists who ride for hours on end. Without the impact of walking or the vertical loads of weight training, the bones weaken. Confirming this observation, a study[8] of twenty-seven older (average age fifty-one) and sixteen younger (average age thirty-one) competitive cyclists shows lowered bone mineral density in long-time cyclists.

And that's not all. While riding, the cyclist's neck is extended, with a helmet increasing the weight that the neck must support. The head acts as a lever arm, straining the neck muscles. Add the force of road bumps, and the discs between the vertebral bodies of the cervical spine suffer repeated sudden loads. Want proof? Take a look at cyclists' tense necks when they get off their superlight, super stiff, carbon fiber, body-abusing machines.

Finally, the knees. The bike is almost always kind to the knees, even arthritic ones. It's hard to injure the knee on the bike unless you fall off. Tendonitis at the patella or the iliotibial band is usually easily fixed with better bike fit.

So what is a cyclist to do? Cross-train. CROSS-TRAIN. Do weight training, Pilates, hiking, and yoga. There is a whole list of fantastic opportunities to increase flexibility, strengthen other muscles, and build bone mass—all key to a cyclist's health. But even more fun than a laser-like focus on cycling is a return to being a multi-sport athlete. Add new sports each year to your activity repertoire. Love the bike, but leave it more often.

---

[8] Jeanne F. Nichols, Jacob E. Palmer, and Susan S. Levy, "Low bone mineral density in highly trained male master cyclists," *Osteoporosis International* 14 no. 8 (2003): 644–649, https://pubmed.ncbi.nlm.nih.gov/12856112/.

Spinway to Heaven

We grew up mastering stairs that went nowhere, eliptical-ing on gym pterodactyls, encouraged by fitness gurus and suburban yogis. Now we spin. Spinning classes have grown to millions of sessions in the US each year. The bikes, too, have progressed—from first recording our pedaling rates, then our heart rates, and finally our soul cycles. The group dynamic pushed us to perform harder than we would do alone in the gym. The hot instructors drew us in. The fad became a craze.

The latest version of spin's evolution is the Peloton, a high-tech carbon fiber bike fitted with a huge iPad-like screen that sits in your garage or living room. The Peloton accesses the best of the crowd-rated instructors: those who have optimized the perfect engagement style and the right encouragement at the right moment. They keep their riders spinning up virtual hills and in and out of Tabata interval training cycles, all the while appealing to the competitive spirit in beginners and pros alike.

Peloton bikes—and those that will follow—have completely changed the fitness game. We no longer have to leave our house, hurry to class, wait in line, use other people's sweaty seats and handlebars, and breathe their dirty air. We don't have to wait for our preferred instructor or class type. We are always in the front row.

And since we have to walk right past our beckoning bike to get out the door in the morning (or to cocktail hour at night), time-based excuses are less valid. We now have the very best instructors, the perfect classes, the most scenic virtual rides, and even the calming cool-down stretch classes on demand, every hour, in our living spaces.

Spinning on a bike is an exercise that almost everyone can do.

Arthritic joints feel better with spinning. Even back pain can be reduced by the increased blood flow, muscle use, and elevated circulating testosterone that spinning produces. Lack of impact, combined with gentle resistance, provides the right amount of muscle stimulation to heal most injuries.

Without a coach, though, it's hard to push yourself past your current fitness level on a spin bike in order to build strength, endurance, and cardiovascular conditioning. The addition of the screen—which shows the metrics of your heart rate, resistance, cadence, and output—provides objective data on which to progressively build a program of improvement. And the live or recorded coach who cajoles and winks at just the right times helps push us onward when we would otherwise pause.

Spinning is not the only exercise required for true overall fitness. To achieve this, we must cross-train. But spinning sure is a fun way to get part of the way there. If heaven on Earth is being fit until the day you drop, spin your way to heaven.

Electric Bikes

Augmented bicycling is about to "hit the hockey stick" on the product adoption curve. Translated into English: we are all about to have a lot of fun.

An electric bike is powered by a small motor, traditionally mounted on the frame, that assists with pedaling. "E-bikes" have been around since the 1890s, but early models were heavy, short on range, slow to recharge, and expensive. During the last few years, they have evolved into lighter, smarter versions. As goes Tesla, so goes the e-bike. Power supplies have gotten lighter, and range has increased. The e-bike market has quickly expanded from a novelty to a credible choice for both road- and mountain-bike fun. E-bikes have become cool.

For sports enthusiasts, the impact of this simple technology is huge. A grueling, three-hour bike ride over steep mountain foothills is out of the realm of possibility for many, including some fit athletes. On an e-bike, the ride can now be done in an hour, with the fun factor increased dramatically. And the whole family can come along, with some using more of the "assist" setting than stronger, younger, and/or fitter members.

If you grimly tolerate a deadening car commute, with traffic, tolls, and parking fees (because the alternative, riding a bike to work, involved sweating, finding a shower, and sometimes being late), you now have a workable option. The questions now are how fast you want to get to work, and how sweaty you can afford to be. Having visited Beijing, where there seem to be a million noisy, polluting motor scooters, one can imagine a government decree insisting they all become electric bikes. The city would be transformed.

Even more remarkable are the new powered "wheel only" devices. Instead of buying a somewhat weighty electric bike, you can now simply purchase an electric wheel that will fit on any bicycle. A wireless connection to your smartphone, mounted on your handlebars, gives you all the feedback you could dream of—from the wattage output of your pedaling to the charge remaining on the enclosed battery. And the price is a fraction of even the most discounted e-bikes. At a TED Conference in Vancouver, a company called Superpedestrian demonstrated a powered wheel that, like a Tesla, has the option of a slight assist for hills or a "ludicrous" setting for bursts of speed.

It may be time to reexamine your need to use a car to get to work. For most people, the commute is reasonably short. What if that commute were fun, as athletic as you wanted it to be, free of gas, tolls, and parking, and made you feel like you were helping the planet? What if your individualistic sport of cycling suddenly became as social as we imagine it could be? *That* is an idea worth sharing.

DANCE LIKE A BUTTERFLY

Dancing recreationally is the perfect merger of play, sport, and fitness. You can't necessarily dance well to every kind of music, but you can always dance, even if various body parts are not working well. You can always improvise and feel the beat. If you're a professional dancer, then you can move your body gracefully to any tempo—until an injury occurs. A joint injury that limits motion can be career threatening.

An ACL tear is often associated with a popping sound, a giving way, and the nauseating feeling that something really bad just happened to your knee. When a ballet dancer's knee is injured—often in a performance when landing from a leap or from twisting in an unplanned way—that dreaded feeling is amplified by career-ending fear. *Will the knee ever be the same again? Can it be fixed so I can dance? Who comes back from this injury? Why did it happen to me?* The sound of the pop can be so loud that it is heard by fellow dancers or theatergoers in the front row. But the scene of the agonized dancer being carried off stage is never choreographed, nor even dreamed of.

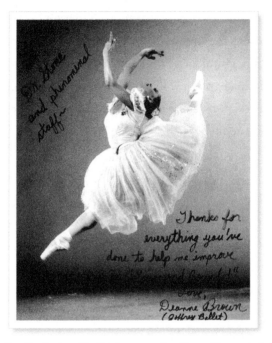

Deanne B. • Professional ballet dancer and ankle cartilage repair patient

Fortunately, those of us who care for such injured performers bring
not only our skills but also our philosophies of rehab and recovery to
these artists—who may be dancers, but are athletes as well. Dance has
evolved from the Balanchine days of whisper-thin ballerinas to the
raw and beautiful athleticism that so many choreographers demand
today. Out are cigarettes, anorexia, and the aversion to muscle bulk
that characterized that bygone era. Today's dancers have adopted
the training and nutrition techniques of Olympian champions. They
have built graceful, powerful bodies required to leap ever higher and
dance more demanding routines. But along with these adaptations
have come the injuries of overuse, the ligament ruptures of soaring
feats, and the cartilage injuries of repetitive impact.

While routine aggressive care of frequent soft-tissue injuries is commonplace, the care of ACL injuries remains controversial. Our success in returning dancers to ballet is based on several approaches and, admittedly, biases.

First, immediate care makes an enormous difference. Minimizing the injured dancer's emotional fallout—the mourning of the injury and anxiety about the future—by treating the problem and initiating rapid return to the studio reduces the likelihood of the injury becoming a career-ending event.

Dancers cannot afford to lose a portion of their patella tendons or their hamstrings. So, when the ACL is completely ruptured, we reconstruct it with something called a "bone-patellar tendon-bone graft," from a donor and preloaded with the patient's own stem cells. During surgery, the graft is placed so as to permit the knee to extend the same extent as the opposite knee—which, for many dancers, actually means hyperextension. Traditional graft placements often did not allow this extra motion. Without it, though, the dancer will never be the same.

Local, long-acting anesthetics allow dancers to watch their knees extending fully in the recovery room. This visualization makes the recovery process significantly better since full range of motion seems harder to achieve once normal post-surgery pain kicks in. The video provides a mental affirmation; just knowing the knee can go there makes all the difference.

For reduction of swelling, we alternate cold compression and soft-tissue massage. Day-one postoperative physical therapy is followed by daily physical therapy sessions. As soon as the dancer is comfortable exercising at the barre, standing on the non-injured leg, and working the injured leg, a return to class and the theater is possible. Full return to dance is judged by strength and agility tests in our clinic. Once the dancer can lift and land with confidence while protecting the leg, their on-stage career can resume.

The more we ask our artists to perform as athletes, the more we must treat them as both. Few populations have better mind/body aware-ness than ballet dancers. It is a thrill to help restore that integration —not only for their benefit but for ours as an audience as well.

THE SPORT OF CROSSFIT

CrossFit became one of the world's largest sports gym chains by moti-vating people to compete with themselves and with others in a variety of fitness tests. While initially focused on Olympic weightlifting and gymnastics, the CrossFit world morphed into a dizzying variety of athletic performance drills. Along the way, it became a sport unto itself.

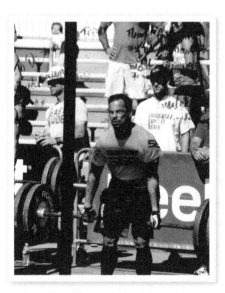

Rich L. • Competitive CrossFit athlete and Achilles tendon repair patient.
Rich has had Dr. Stone repair both shoulders, an ankle ligament,
and a hamstring. Still competing at age sixty-five.

CrossFit's definition of fitness encompasses a conditioning program with ten constantly varying functional movements. The program aims to increase:

1. Cardiovascular/respiratory endurance
2. Stamina
3. Strength
4. Flexibility
5. Power
6. Speed
7. Coordination
8. Agility
9. Balance
10. Accuracy

In the initial model, the complete CrossFit athlete perfected all of the prescribed movements while striving to beat everyone else—first in their gym, then through local, regional, national, and international games (CrossFit called them "sectionals"). I was privileged to see one of my women's ski team athletes, Eva Twardokens, adopt this program more than twenty years ago. She developed her body and athletic ability up to Level I—an achievement I had not before witnessed, from conditioning alone, in female athletes. Eva was amazing, and I recruited her to teach my own family as well as our physical therapy team at the clinic.

My thinking at the time was that the CrossFit program—if carefully supervised and calibrated to a patient's injuries—could accelerate healing and a return to sports after injury and surgery. With this in mind, we hired and trained Kelly Starrett, fresh from physical therapy school, to merge CrossFit with physical therapy in our clinic. He cleverly focused on mobility as well as strength. Starrett eventually brought his methods to the CrossFit world through his own gym, webcasts, and books.

Even though CrossFit tried to incorporate diet and health elements into their program, the popular image of the CrossFit athlete focused more on strength than on health. Unfortunately, along the way, we started seeing a number of injuries at various CrossFit gyms. The box jump became a common referral source for knee injuries. Squatting with heavy weights, without proper technique or hip flexibility, sent us numerous back pain patients. And human shoulders often rebelled at the number of repetitions attempted by competitive CrossFitters. Word got around that CrossFit was somewhat dangerous—even though the data from other training programs may have shown the same rate of injuries.

Simultaneously, the World Wide Web made international competitions viewable by everyone. As the competitions grew, so did the size and power of the most addicted CrossFitters. Now it was no longer about fitness for sport but about the sport of CrossFit itself and the awards it gave. A new wave of obsessively driven athletes with perfectly honed bodies sought to increase their power, speed, and accuracy by any means possible. Their lives became CrossFit driven.

More recently, we are seeing other reactions come in with CrossFit athletes. The conversation has turned more toward health than victory. Merging diet, sleep, and mindfulness into one's workout plan changes its direction. It is no longer about beating the competition. It's about winning the individual game of life. The definition of fitness is evolving as well. Success is defined not only by what you can do but by how well you can live. This direction seems more in line with our own efforts to help people live to be one hundred, while playing the sports and activities they love.

To all those who are taking this activity in more nuanced directions, I say "play on!" But remember: if it is not fun, it is not play, and it is not as healthy as it could be.

CrossFit and the High School Athlete

Year-round single-sport training has been the dogma (and often the reality) for many youthful athletes during the past twenty years. The level of play has increased so much that single-sport athletes dominate the teams, with summer specialty camps and private coaches thrown in when affordable.

Those of us who treat high schoolers—and counsel their worried parents—talk endlessly about the old days of three-sport athletes. Those were days of building well-rounded attitudes, not just bodies, and of decreasing injuries by reducing exposure to repeated impact and developing varied athletic skills.

We have mostly failed. In high school and even elementary school, serious athletes train year-round in their single sport. A kid from a mediocre school with limited financial or parental support often believes their only path to economic and academic freedom is the college sports recruiter. To get his attention, you'd better be big, strong, and a starter. The steroids offered in many gyms, along with single-focus dedication, appear to be the only way forward.

CrossFit (and a few of its imitators) may be changing this. While no training program substitutes the wide-ranging benefits of playing multiple sports, some of the missing attributes can be obtained by these novel, multifaceted training programs.

CrossFit is cheap, available, open to everyone, and cool. Intra-gym competition replaces the missing trainer that many high schools can no longer afford. The fitness variation partly substitutes for the cross-training and skill development available to the three-sport athlete. Metrics posted on the whiteboard at the CrossFit gym quantify the athlete's progress and compare his or her achievements across the entire CrossFit world. And the daily workouts, posted online, make the fitness program so ubiquitous that the barriers of cost, travel, and organizational support have completely disappeared.

Best of all, it works. High school athletes are bringing a soaring level of fitness to the practice field, and the sponsorships are following. Nike, Adidas, and other brands are competing to get on the bandwagon. Simply look at any high school or collegiate golfer. In a sport not previously known for fashion, teens in Under Armour's high-tech sportswear have replaced the plaid-clad, baggy-bellied, fairway strollers of our parents' era.

CrossFit's health effects, while mostly positive, do have some downsides. The platform's extreme competitiveness leads to multiple overuse and even contact injuries. The "box jump" sends more knees into my office than any other training device. Overhead repetitions at high weights have injured many a shoulder.

But, as always, a little caution can go a long way. Despite the conventional wisdom that children should avoid weight lifting, there is little evidence to support that advice—as long as the progression is age and size appropriate, guided, and reasonable. So eliminating the competitive edge of CrossFit, at least until the teenage years, probably makes sense.

In the balance, though, the training benefits are huge. Welcome to the new age of super fitness. It's not just for making the team. It's for building well-rounded athletes of all ages.

STANDUP PADDLING

It used to be "pedal." I would pedal my bike at a wonderful, regular pace, my mind roaming from idea to idea, hot riders male and female blowing past me up the hills and down the valleys. That was just fine. Riding provided the free-thought time that when combined with exercise, led to a productive day, and sometimes to a bounty of new ideas.

Today it's "paddle." Standup paddling has rocketed to the top of the water sports world with sales of new boards growing rapidly. Surfing has been around on the US mainland since 1912, so what took so long for someone to stand up on the board with a paddle? Canoeists used paddles while standing for hundreds of years, and a few surfers in Hawaii in the 1940s stood on their boards to patrol the beaches. The sport itself took off in the 1990s with the first competitions in the early 2000s. Novel board shapes and improved paddle design opened the sport up to the masses—so much so that it became the fastest growing water sport in 2013.

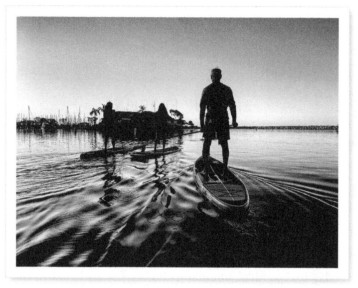

Dr. Stone standup paddling at sunset in the waters of Dana Point, CA

I began with a long version of a surfboard designed by Donald Takayama. As I paddled rhythmically, letting my mind wander, I found new levels of fitness. Standup paddleboards can be so wide that an elephant won't fall in, yet the sport develops balance, coordination, and power through the trunk, core, and shoulder muscles as no other sport does, and with almost no injuries. The boards are so wide, you can even use them as platforms for Pilates and yoga.

But like cycling, some enthusiasts of the sport have succumbed to newer board and paddle designs and a "modern" style of paddling. Short, powerful strokes with high stroke rates beat out the longer, deeper paddle strokes. The sport is becoming a frenetic, high-velocity competition waged on high, fat longboards that keep the paddler's toes out of the waves. Weeknight races and downwind multi-hour events are now staged at every port.

The injuries are piling up too. I see shoulders with inflammation from overloading and rotator cuff tears from pushing through the pain. Back injuries roll in from torquing the spine. Crash injuries show up with lacerations and torn tissues caused by paddling down rivers and into huge waves that are unforgiving to fat boards with stiff paddles. The exhilaration of taking a new sport to unexplored territory still thrills water-sports fanatics, but the pressure to compete is not for everyone. When thrill replaces serenity in a sport, physical creativity may go up, but mental creativity is put on pause.

My old, thin, surfboard-like paddleboard, which responds to my metronomic paddling and carries me through the ocean chop to the local surf spot, still works just fine. My mind is unencumbered by the need for speed. My breathing is regular, and my uninhibited, productive thoughts continue to flow. I never paddle faster than I can daydream.

Downwinders

Downwind standup paddling, a hybrid of standup paddling and surfing, is solid fun. All you need is a windy place with rolling waves. Rivers, bays, large lakes, and the ocean can all provide great conditions. The equipment you need is a paddle and a special board. Use a board twelve to fourteen feet long and twenty-six to thirty inches wide, with a bottom rocker that permits it to ride up and over waves (though it is too big for surfing in the current style).

Once getting upwind, either by land or boat, one paddles out into the middle of the waterway and points the board downwind. While you can stand still and glide, or paddle continuously and glide even faster, the skill of the sport involves accelerating at just the right time.

You do this by paddling quickly, catching the motion of the wave, and then surfing it downwind.

Unlike in normal surfing—where the wave you catch is the one behind you—the standup paddling (SUP) downwinding board goes faster than the waves, so the wave you want to catch is the one in front of you. This means riding up the back of the wave by paddling, cresting the top, and then surfing down the face over and over again. The windier and wavier, the more fun, the more exhilarating, and the more addicting.

So why my fascination? There are few sports that provide speed, excitement, athletic power, balance, and a little fear (from being out in the ocean and/or the speed of the waves)—all without injury. Unless you fall onto your board, it's pretty hard to get hurt downwinding. Increasing your sports fun factor while not getting hurt becomes more important as you age.

I love taking risks, pushing the limits in sports with physical challenges, and competing with myself to achieve new goals. But I detest downtime from injuries associated with almost all other high-thrill sports.

We teach our children to do dangerous things safely. For a sports injury doctor like me, nirvana is experiencing dramatic excitement with little danger of injury. If you're the same, and you want to be one hundred years old and still playing, SUP downwinding may be for you. I am actively searching for other sports like downwinding—for both me and my patients.

GET WET!

Water, water everywhere—so get in it! There are more than ten million swimming pools in the US. (The greatest per capita concentration, surprisingly, is in the Cleveland area.) Pools are not just in the backyards of the rich; they are everywhere. Most people have access to a pool, though they may not know it. Here is why you should notice pools and get wet.

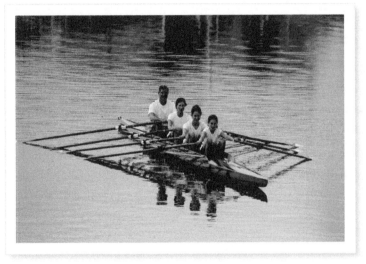

Dr. Stone rowing with his family

Almost every sports injury, arthritis, muscle pain, and surgical recovery program is helped by water exercise. Back pain from pregnancy is one of the most common complaints relieved by water sports. Injury rates from exercising in water are stunningly low, except for occasional shoulder overuse injuries in competitive swimmers. Every training program for physical fitness is enhanced by the use of water, yet few people use their private or local public pools regularly.

When I ask patients if they have access to a pool, most say yes but provide an excuse for why they don't use it: it isn't heated, or they haven't renewed their membership, or it didn't occur to them. Heat it, renew it, sign up for a class or a membership!

You don't have to be a swimmer to use a pool. Stretch in the pool. Do jumping jacks using the water as resistance. Walking or running from side to side in the pool, in chest-deep water is my favorite exercise. Try running twenty laps, and do them a little faster every day.

Finding a good pool exercise instructor is just a web search away in most communities. Call one and have them guide you through a workout. Take your Pilates, spin, CrossFit, yoga, and weight room exercises straight into the pool. The water provides a level of resistance that the air does not, along with a cooling effect on the muscles. All of your joints will feel less stressed, more flexible, and more comfortable.

And there are many other ways to include water in your exercise routine. It doesn't have to be a pool. Do ocean runs along the beach in shallow water; perform jumping jacks in the lake. Use water as a training tool. Here are more ways to stay wet, and don't forget to hydrate while you're at it.

- **Resist.** Hire a water exercise instructor to give you a water workout routine. You will be surprised to find that weight lifting in the water is far superior to weight lifting on dry land.
- **Get foiled.** It now seems that every boat and board known to water sports is being lifted by foils. Surfboards foil, kiteboards foil, and windsurfers foil. These days, the technology is being applied to monohulls for foiling in the next America's Cup. Just wing it.

- **Row, row, row your boat.** There are community-accessible rowing clubs in many locations—yet few people actually access them. Everyone can row, as long as the boat is stable enough. Once you start, you can progress to narrower, faster vessels. Or just paddle along and use muscles you haven't recognized in years. Take your family and friends. Make rowing a new group sport.

- **Hand fins.** Got waves but don't surf? Hand fins were traditionally used by swimmers trying to increase water resistance in their pool-training workouts. Now the fins (and wider handboards) are available for beach wave riding. After just a little practice, anyone can bodysurf with them and look like a pro.

- **Remember windsurfing.** It was supercool a decade ago; now kiteboarding and kitesurfing have taken over. I still love my windsurf board, but I admit, the kiters seem to be having more fun. This water sport definitely needs lessons and supervision as the dangers can be serious or fatal. But the fun factor and accessibility to great windsurfing spots trumps the danger for a growing legion of wind enthusiasts.

- **Swim with the fishes.** Take snorkel gear with you on vacation or rent it. Most of the pretty fish live in shallow water, where the sunshine illuminates their colors. Snorkeling is inexpensive and can be a serious workout—especially against a current.

- **Go deeper.** Scuba diving involves more gear and expense than snorkeling but offers views of another world. You can't help but feel small, yet part of an extraordinary planet, when

you go deep into the sea. After only four or five lessons—
first in a pool, then in the ocean—you can become safely
competent. Taking an instructor along on every dive greatly
improves the experience and safety, at least for me.

- **Stream in streams.** Leave the devices at home and get
  into the local streams. Fish, paddle, kayak, or canoe. There
  is something magical about running water in nature that
  washes out the brain, clears the stress, and puts you in tune
  with Mother Nature. She's waiting for you.

Get wet, as often as possible with others when available, and enjoy
the benefits of the water in a place surprisingly near you.

Natural Gyms

An eighty-year-old came in to see me for his knee pain. He was having trouble with a longstanding knee injury and had finally sought care. What struck me immediately was his appearance. He had the physique of a fit thirty-year-old: not overly muscled, but well-shaped and toned. He moved with grace and with a spring in his step.

"What do you do to keep fit?" I asked with a bit of jealousy.

His story was this. As a middle-aged executive for an international pharmaceutical company, he had accepted a post in Monaco. A friend owned a motorboat, and each morning they would waterski before work. As the man aged, he kept up the activity. In his seventies, he gave up waterskiing on a single ski and followed behind the boat for at least twenty minutes a day on two skis. When the water was calm, he would go even longer. Every muscle in his body benefited from waterskiing, and it showed. The man simply radiated fitness.

Though access to a boat and flat water to ski on is available only to a small number of people, the environment around us provides natural gymnasiums everywhere. Finding that hill to climb, that body of water to swim, or that sports field to use is often as simple as looking out the window. Setting a routine to take those opportunities, and doing it every day, creates lifelong fitness. There is something extra special about exercising outdoors that expands the mind and the perception of freedom and health that the indoor gym just never achieves.

Gym workouts should be the grout between the tiles of our sport-focused lives. The equipment encourages us to use ever larger weights, and the combination of exercises can lead to total body fitness when we're coached well. The efficiency of just hitting the weights, of straining each muscle, of timing and counting each rep allows these workouts to be inserted between work, family, and the other demands of life. The benefits of these exercises make people better athletes in their other sports. But games that are played outdoors, without the metronomic repetitions or endless counting, are the ones that touch the fun chord of the human instrument. The notes played are music to the athletic spirit. Don't let the grout become the cement.

Likewise, spinning indoors on a bike can be fabulous. There are amazing instructors and calibrated pedals, and there is inspiring music. Many of my patients use stationary bikes for rehab and spin bikes for exercise. Whether at home on a Peloton or at Soul Cycle surrounded by a scrum of sweating, Lycra-clad peers, they cycle their legs and turn off their minds. But my patients who ride outdoors—individually or with friends—experience the sounds, smells, and changes of nature that touch a different part of the psyche. The daydreams we have while going somewhere lead to ideas that take us elsewhere.

Pilates reformers and barre classes isolate individual muscles. You focus on the perfect form, executing the repetition with precision. Form matters more than power. Stretching is intertwined with strengthening. Progressively harder exercises lead to a degree of bodily self-awareness that only a nearby mirror can reflect. These exercises are inextricably tied to form and our success to the instructor's commentary. But have you ever watched people doing Tai Chi in the park? You see all of the same motions: beautiful body strokes and carefully placed legs with arms curling and extending. Yet the participants' eyes are often closed, their minds floating on the overhead clouds.

Pools are wonderful places for extending your cardiovascular endurance. With your head down, arms and legs swinging, your lungs expand and contract, inflating your chest and keeping you level. Laps in lanes are the required metric for water exercise accounting. Each stroke is a little different, but each outcome is the same. In a lake or in the ocean, though, the constraints are lifted. The joy is in survival: up and down in the waves, wind and sun on your head, sand and mud between your toes. Blood pressure declines outdoors. The spirit rises.

Yoga classes in hot or cold studios may be the ultimate contemplation of the navel. Contorted beyond its usual limits, the body aches gently while the mind centers down. In this spiral of self-absorption, we often find calmness: either recognition and acceptance of ourselves and our limits, or frustration with these discoveries. Yet you can also find yourself on a long hike, on a run, on a rhythmic cross-country ski, or just sitting outside a swell on a surfboard. And what you find you may enjoy sharing.

Life has turned inward. The smartphone, the personal computer, streaming platforms, and even our counseling sessions have turned our view inward. If you really want to see what's inside, get outside. In all weather conditions. For every sport. There is nothing comparable to experiencing nature while playing a sport or enjoying an exercise. When you get out, you get more deeply in.

GO WIDE AND GO LONG

Exercise, working out, and play are three components of fitness programs that when combined, provide the ultimate physical and mental health benefits. Exercise is doing an activity often without a specific goal. Working out is a training event where the goal is to increase your fitness, and the path to get there is often calibrated, quantified, and recorded. Play is what we do primarily for fun—usually with other people and hopefully with laughter. In this chapter, we've explored the many sports that combine two or three of these components and what you need to watch out for to ensure you stay injury free. Incorporate these sports in your lifestyle, and you're looking at a wealth of fulfillment and joy.

The key here is to *do*. If you're one of those people who believe that exercise is difficult or impossible to fit into your life, or that it's a chore, then you're simply not considering all the alternatives. It is true that exercise programs—either in a gym or recorded on a fitness app—are often designed to help you improve yourself. That means to be successful, you must exceed your normal limits, break down muscle, get short of breath, and sweat. If not, your musculoskeletal system is not going to be better tomorrow than it is today.

But is that entirely true? We used to think so. Now we know there are other ways to strengthen and renew our systems. I am talking about "sustainable exercise"—that is, exercise that you will actually consistently *do*.

You are not in homeostasis. The body is not balanced perfectly with just the right proportion of muscle breakdown balanced by muscle building. The fact is, you are dying. We all are. Life is a fatal disease. Left at rest, the body declines more rapidly. The pumping systems of the heart and lungs, the muscles supporting the bones, and the bones themselves need resistance exercise to build more tissue. They respond effectively to force. This is why the only successful treatment for the bone loss associated with aging is resistance exercise.

Despite this, efforts by the healthcare community to motivate people to go to the gym and lift weights failed miserably. Yes, the number of gyms proliferated, but the population got fatter, which is the key metric for whether or not the exercise-to-consumption ratio is in the healthy zone. Pushing people to lift weights in gyms doesn't work.

There are other solutions. It turns out that you can tip the balance of your musculoskeletal fitness in your favor by mindful extensions of your limbs, sustained muscle poses, prolonged lower-level activities, or even with hyper short, intense ones. The activities and sports of yoga, Pilates, barre methods, and their relatives have filled the streets with stretch-clad men and women displaying incredible fitness and physiques. The high intensity, short-interval programs on stationary bikes, in pools, and with stretch cords have been shown to build fitness with exquisitely short workouts. Lovely, long walks on trails and country roads can be effective at balancing caloric intake. These exercises and activities, in one form or another, are available to everyone and are often free. For the body to stay ahead of its natural degradation through time, increasing all the systems' energy use to a level above baseline improves their resilience.

Simply put, there are a wide variety of activities that can be added to everyone's day that are doable, not just aspirational. So the next time you think about recycling your trash, choosing a sustainable fish, or conserving energy for the environment, look inside. Apply the metrics of sustainability to yourself. Recognize that it is often not what you do that kills you, but what you don't do.

And don't tie yourself down to a single activity. Among all my patients, regardless of age, those who are happiest seem to share a secret: they each add a new sport or activity once or twice a year. For the young, regularly taking up a new sport counters the professionalization of youth sports. When I was young, all kids played three sports a year and took the summer off. The multi-sport kids learned agility, power, and sportsmanship from a variety of angles and coaches. The well-rounded athlete entered college and professional sports with skills that brought new dimensions to every sport.

The benefits of multi-sports are not only for high schoolers. Among my twenty- to thirty-year-old athletes in college or early in their work careers, single-sport athletes are out of luck in the off-season, or when weather doesn't permit their sport in season, or when work hours start early or finish late. Multi-sport athletes, on the other hand, always have an arrow in the exercise quiver and a variety of friends to play with. More importantly, by regularly adding a new sport or activity, they broaden their horizons and expand career and happiness options.

Many thirty- to sixty-year-olds consider themselves too busy to think about new sports, yet they are the ones who need them the most. By adding something new every six months, they could bring spice to their life, now likely dominated by work, and add new challenges for their children and spouses to admire and join in on. Those who do this tend to push their midlife bodies to experience what we in sports medicine call healthy stresses and strains. The aging diseases of bone loss and sloping posture are counteracted with muscle strengthening and cross-training. The malaise of midlife is challenged by the healthy anxiety of being a beginner in a new sport and then mastering it.

My sixty- to ninety-year-old athletes tend to have hit the comfort zone in their sports activities and have an increasing fear of injury.

Yet these people often benefit the most by the new friends made in a new gym or group sport. Choosing sports that stress but don't hurt the body determines their enthusiasm for new challenges.

So no matter what your age, every six months, add a new sport, make new friends, and smile all the way to life's finish line.

PART II

FOCUS ON
YOUR JOINTS

CHAPTER 4

INJURIES

I n Part I, we talked about how you can be fit, be healthy, stay injury free, and enjoy sports and activities that allow you to play forever. But what happens if you do get injured? How do you recover from it, both medically and mentally?

Injuries are no fun, no doubt about it. They drag you down into a parallel universe of frailty. But if mindset is destiny, I encourage you to see that injury is an opportunity to become fitter, faster, and stronger than you have been in years. In Part II, we will deal with how you can recover from injury and thrive. A variety of factors play a role in this: a good understanding of how your body works so that you know how to identify warning signs of an injury and seek intervention early; various medical and surgical interventions—new and old—to repair the injury; a post-surgical or post-intervention recovery plan that includes fitness training, physical therapy, and good diet; and, of course, through it all, your attitude and perspective on the healing process.

Chapter 4 will tackle mindset and the more common injuries usually located at the joints. Chapter 5 will focus exclusively on the knee since it is such a delicate and complex joint. We'll explore the different parts of the knee that can get injured, the many types of injuries, and how medical practices in knee repair and surgery are progressing in leaps and bounds. Chapter 6 talks about the bright landscape of what I call "anabolic therapies," which is the use of stem cells and growth factors to repair tissue. Lastly, Chapter 7 will deal with surgery itself: how the field has progressed, what you can do to actively aid your healing, and the elements of a well-thought-out post-surgical plan.

So let's begin, as always, with the mind.

FINDING THE RIGHT
PERSPECTIVE

Perspective is everything.

You fall off your bike and land on your shoulder. The history and physical exam are consistent with a torn rotator cuff. The MRI shows the tear. The surgeon repairs it. Off you go, yet still with all the problems you had before your accident.

True, you fell. True, you tore your rotator cuff. But also true for years is you've held your phone between your chin and your shoulder. Your range of motion was never great. You are relatively weaker on that side. You had some night pain before you fell. The new injury is, in reality, the icing on top of the two-day-old cake.

You tweak your knee skiing, tearing the ACL. The knee is unstable.

The meniscus is also torn. The surgeon replaces the ligament and repairs the meniscus, but unless also treated, the underlying articular cartilage damage will progressively lead to arthritis. It is true that your injury tore the key tissues in the knee, but it is also true that the surfaces of the knee are now abnormal and could lead to painful arthritis if not addressed. Newer treatments, including stem cell paste grafts, can restore durable surfaces with biologic tissues (if in the repertoire of the treating surgeon).

You twisted your ankle as a college athlete years ago, suffering a torn ligament. Immobilized in a walking boot, the ligament healed but with ankle stiffness. Your gait has been off for years due to the lack of motion in the ankle, leading to hip and back pain. It is true that the ligament was torn leading to potential instability, but it is also true that the treatment may have led to a worse outcome. A stiff joint is always worse than a loose one. Early protected motion of the injured tissues may have avoided the scar formation and stiffness, but afterward, you needed careful guidance on how and when to move.

I see each of these injuries as opportunities to highlight other issues people have that make them prone to more injury and less likely to have a full recovery. So often, the injury and the diagnosis are properly identified and treated, but the consequences of the treatment are not considered fully, or the patient as a whole is ignored. Injury is not this setback you must overcome to return to the same fitness level you were at. Injury can be seen as an opportunity. For the doctor or surgeon, that opportunity is better understanding how to improve surgical practices and medical care. For you, it is an opportunity to become fitter, faster, and stronger than you were before.

What you need is an attitude shift. How often do you say to yourself when you see someone with an obvious injury, *I'm grateful to not be that guy.* That same gratitude is what you need to feel when it's you who is hurt.

I have never met a *para*plegic person who did not, at some point, mention how lucky they were not to be a *quadri*plegic. I have often met quadriplegic people who are grateful to still be alive and able to enjoy their families and their work. We have all met injured people who, despite their disabilities, astound us with their optimism and good humor.

Yet we also tend to feel depressed when a relatively minor injury has ended our sports season or interfered with our performance. The contrast in the severity of an injury with the range of emotions people feel toward them is both striking and useful.

All athletes get injured at some point in their careers. The best ones use their injuries as an excuse to train other parts of their bodies. The very best train their minds to focus on new skills instead of dwelling on the lost season, and they park their depression in their mental storage containers. There it stays, accessed only as a reminder of how detrimental such self-defeating emotions can be.

An injured person becomes disabled when they cannot overcome the physical or mental setbacks they encounter. Many people with an apparent disability are not disabled very much at all and appropriately resent the label. Yet many people with relatively minor injuries have tremendous difficulty moving past the temporary interruption in their lives.

What prepares us to be injured and to overcome? Early childhood experiences ingrain behavior patterns, yet surprise injuries later in life often create disappointments that children didn't face. Fear that you won't recover (very common with back pain), concern that you will let down your teammates, and worry over the cost of medical care and rehabilitation—these negative emotions magnify the potential depression.

Prepare for future injury now by looking at your life and truly appreciating what you have: your physical and mental skills, the beauty of the environment you live in, and your potential to improve the world with your contributions. Constantly remind yourself of your emotional and physical strengths. That way, when the snow snake reaches out and grabs your ski and you come to the sudden end of your winter ski sports season, you can instantly shift to finding other, equally exhilarating activities while developing new gym skills.

Disability is only as bad as you perceive it to be and only as disabling as you let it be. Empowering your mind and your body to be a multidimensional, multi-specialty athlete is your best insurance plan.

Why You Should Google
Your Symptoms

My friend is a hypochondriac. Every ache or pain is dramatized into a mortal illness, possibly even contagious. She should not Google her symptoms—but perhaps you should. Here's why: the internet offers helpful resources for differentiating between inconvenient symptoms and fatal ones. These resources are improving due to search engines' expanded use of artificial intelligence. In the near future, in fact, all doctors will carry the world's medical knowledge in their pockets (with the question-answering capabilities of IBM's Watson) to augment their intelligence and intuition when treating you. While the quality of information available on popular medical websites can be inconsistent, there is little harm jumping in with your own research.

Suppose, for instance, that you have a new pain in your knee. By using digital diagnosis software (as on The Stone Clinic website), you can be guided through common questions about the pain. When did it start? Was there an injury? Did you hear a pop? Is there swelling? Does the knee give way? When there is an injury to the knee, for example, and you hear a pop and the knee swells, the data indicates there is a 90 percent chance you need surgery—because you have likely torn a key structure in the knee, such as the meniscus or cruciate ligaments. These don't usually heal on their own and if left untreated, lead to arthritis.

If, on the other hand, swelling occurs after kneeling—and there is no pop or specific trauma—then most likely, ice, soft-tissue massage, and NSAIDs will resolve the problem. These dramatically different reactions can all be determined by Googling your combination of symptoms, without seeking direct professional help.

Many people don't recall all of their symptoms when first asked in an examination room. Taking the time to be guided through various possibilities without time (or cost) pressure allows you to present a full narrative of your illness or injury. The more complete your information is, the more likely your diagnosis and treatment will be accurate. As internet tools for diagnostic specificity improve, our use of in-person medical services should become less frequent and more targeted.

In the past, doctors were wary of patients who came in with stacks of papers, newspaper articles, and *Reader's Digest* articles describing their diagnosis and home cures. Rolling their eyes, the doctors couldn't wait for the speech to be over so they could get to the real business of doctoring. What has changed is access to top-quality information. Patients can be stunningly well informed, and the more so, usually, the better.

Because patients realize that doctors can't know everything, that often their time is limited, and that at the end of the day, the patient who has thought deeply about their symptoms and possible causes is a better informant than the one who leaves the injury to the doctor to figure out. "The patient is almost always right" were the wisest words I learned from my physician father.

Yet it still takes a good doctor to listen and to think. The best doctors do both really well. Which brings me to: Google your doctor. Because just as you, the patient, bring your biases and information to the examining room, so does a doctor. Knowing his or her biases, skills, and experience will help you understand why one treatment is offered and not another. A doctor whose practice is mostly artificial joint replacements, for example, is highly likely to offer you drugs and relative rest advice until you are old enough for a joint replacement for your symptoms of knee arthritis. It is what he/she knows and does well. The doctor who does more biologic joint replacement procedures is more likely to offer injections of stem cells, growth factors, joint lubrication, exercises, or biologic replacement of your damaged meniscus or articular cartilage. The doctor who has had success with partial joint replacements will be more likely to offer that procedure than a full joint replacement. Their spheres of experience affect how they listen, what they hear, and what they recommend. Knowing your doctor's skills in advance will help you make the best choices in collaboration with the doctor. And this doesn't just apply to surgeons. Medical doctors who are attuned to environmental causes of disease will assess your mercury and magnesium levels, while "traditional" doctors may be more focused on your blood lipid and sugar levels.

Lastly—after you've performed due diligence with your symptoms and doctor—you'll want to Google your diagnosis and treatment. After you have received a treatment plan, whether drugs alone or surgery, the side effects are often scary and sometimes unpredicted. By Googling those symptoms, you effectively crowdsource your case to the vast group of people who have experienced the same symptoms after the same combination of treatments. The end result is that everyone becomes more knowledgeable by sharing information about what actually does occur, not just what was hoped for.

So use the internet to your best advantage. Google your symptoms and present as full a picture as possible to a doctor who will listen intently. Read widely and act wisely to achieve the best possible outcomes.

SHOULDERS

The shoulder is the most mobile joint in the body, and because of its extensive range of motion, it's susceptible to injury and pain. While the shoulder is not thought of as a weight-bearing joint, once you lift an object or roll over at night, the forces going through the shoulder joint exceed those of most joints; this is due to the long lever arm of the outstretched arm. The shoulder can hurt after it has been injured or for no apparent reason. Most shoulder problems are relatively short lived, but sometimes the pain is indicative of a more complex issue. Here's what might be wrong and whether or not it's a cause for concern.

- **No worries.** Slight pain with elevation and when playing overhead sports is common. The four tendons that make up the rotator cuff and the bicep tendon (the combined musculature that drives the shoulder motions) can be inflamed by activities such as throwing, shooting basketballs, and lifting bags overhead. The tendons are covered by a thin layer called a bursa, which swells when irritated. The bursa is then filled with inflammatory components that irritate the nerve fibers, sending pain signals to the brain. Mild use of anti-inflammatories and eliminating the overhead activities usually cures the mild bursitis, or tendonitis, and solves the problem. Exercises to strengthen posture are also commonly used by our physical therapists to fix mild shoulder irritations. Slumping at your desk, reaching for your mouse, and hunching over your keyboard, can all put extra strain on the shoulder, neck, or back and may be the cause of your shoulder pain. Stand with your shoulders at or behind your hips with your belly button tucked in and notice the difference.

- **Some concern.** Pain that does not go away or pain that occurs with every activity indicates the key tissues are irritated enough that they are sending pain signals even without motion. This degree of inflammation precedes more structural injuries, such as tears of the tissue or early arthritis. Treated fully, the tears and the arthritis can be prevented. The treatments are often injections of growth factors from platelets and lubricating fluid called hyaluronic acid. Physical therapy focuses on shoulder mechanics, muscle strengthening, and sports-specific training to help fix the activity that might be causing the injury. Often we see throwers with slight errors in their throwing mechanics or golfers with swing abnormalities that bring on the problems. Correction of the motion fixes the pain. We avoid cortisone as there is clear evidence that it weakens the tissues of the shoulder if used too frequently.

- **Real worry.** Pain at night and/or pain not improving with therapy after four weeks are red flags. Pain radiating down the arm, up to the neck, or to the back are also worrisome for injuries, not just in the shoulder but sometimes of the neck. These injuries need to be worked up with careful physical exams, X-rays, and MRIs. A full tear of the rotator cuff will often present with night pain because when you roll over, you push the arm up into the socket through the rotator cuff tear. Pain radiating down the arm or up to the neck can sometimes originate in the discs in the neck or the nerves at the front of the shoulder called the brachial plexus. Instability of the shoulder, with the shoulder popping in or out of the joint, is another area that is best treated with early repair of the torn ligaments.

Fortunately, most of the torn tissue in the shoulder can be repaired—under a local block with an arthroscope—as an outpatient procedure. Only severe arthritic cases require bionic replacement. The biologic treatments of anabolic stimulation of the tissues with injections, plus exercise, physical therapy, and activity coaching are becoming more effective, more targeted, and more widespread. The key is to treat shoulder injuries early before full tearing of tissues leads to disability.

Impingement

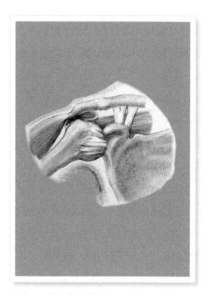

Upper arm pinching the shoulder bursa beneath the bony acromion

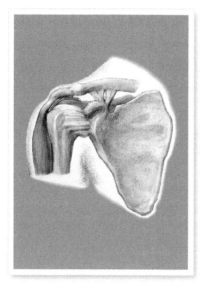

Normal, healthy subacromial bursa

Shoulder pain at night, pain when lifting a briefcase, pain with over-head activities, even pain while brushing your hair—all are most commonly caused by shoulder tissues pinching together, called impingement.

To understand shoulder pain, you first have to know a bit about how the shoulder is held together: in large part, by the rotator cuff tendons and covered by the acromion. The rotator cuff is made up of tendons from the four key muscles that lift and guide shoulder motion. The acromion is the bone on top of the shoulder. It acts as a roof to the shoulder joint. When the space between the tendons and that bony roof narrows—which can be caused by bone spurs or inflammation—impingement occurs. The pain of impingement comes from the tendons of the rotator cuff muscles impacting the underside of the acromion. Think of it as putting a thumbtack between your belt and your waist. Every time you stick your stomach out, pain occurs. (That might be a good training technique for your abdominal muscles but a little unwise!)

Figuring out the cause of the impingement drives the treatment. If the acromion has formed a spur beneath it, from arthritis or trauma, removing the spur fixes the impingement. If the lining of the tendons becomes inflamed from repetitive overhead activities, such as pitching or tennis, shrinking the lining solves it. If the mechanics of the shoulder are poor due to one muscle or another being weak (like a car whose tires are soft on one side), the shoulder moves abnormally, pinching the tissues. Strengthening those muscles solves that problem.

The key is to figure out what the cause is and to avoid damaging the structures when trying to repair them. A careful physical exam with a good history intake often results in a full, accurate diagnosis.

Each muscle can be tested individually, and the point of impingement is usually felt. A high-quality X-ray and MRI can differentiate between bony impingement and soft-tissue swelling or tearing. (Unfortunately, the X-rays and MRIs are often not of sufficient quality to make the best diagnosis. The imaging technique matters!) Sometimes, selective injections of the various tissues with short-acting anesthetics can be helpful, though they're usually not necessary.

Impingement is often caused by specific activities or imbalances of the shoulder, and a careful physical therapy and strengthening program repairs the damage in most cases. "Careful" is emphasized because we often see patients doing the wrong exercises due to the lack of an accurate diagnosis. Injections of joint lubrication plus growth factors and/or stem cells are replacing cortisone in our practice. They act as a natural anti-inflammatory, stimulate healing, and do not have cortisone's downside of weakening the tissues. Surgery to remove the spurs or chronically swollen bursa is almost always curative, but it's usually reserved for patients who fail our nonoperative approaches.

Life with shoulder pain is not fun. Fortunately, the most common causes are completely fixable.

Dislocation

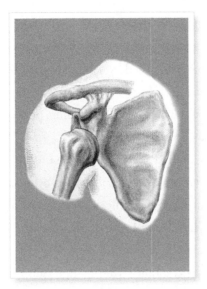

Anterior dislocation of the shoulder

The shoulder can dislocate or just subluxate—i.e., move partially in and out of the joint. The causes for these are most commonly a torn ligament or a lax capsule. The repair steps have improved dramatically and are worth doing early.

The shoulder joint, the upper arm (called the humerus), and the socket (called the glenoid) have a tremendous range of motion, much like a ball and socket joint. While the muscles and tendons crossing the joint are important, it is mainly the ligament and surrounding capsule (the bag of tissue that the joint sits in) that determine the stability of most shoulders. Once these are torn or stretched, the shoulder becomes unstable, unreliable, and susceptible to arthritis.

A fall on the outstretched arm drives the humerus backward. The high brace in kayaking, the high stick position when hit by another player in hockey, the fall while skiing with the arm out to the side, the football hit directly on the upper arm—all of these are mechanisms for tearing the ligament that holds the arm in place. With enough force, both the ligament and the surrounding capsular tissue may be injured. The instability caused by subluxation or dislocation is a risk factor for further injury. Surfers with unstable shoulders are at risk of drowning, mountaineers at risk of falling, police officers at risk of being overwhelmed in a confrontation.

It is not only trauma that leads to the unstable shoulder. Some people are born with more flexibility than others, and some with a tissue variant that causes hyperflexibility: tissues that stretch widely. These shoulders have capsules that are loose, like baggy shirts. The shoulder may move in and out of joints like these without tearing the ligament. Hypermobility from natural causes does not produce the sheer forces across the joints that create cartilage damage. New laxity from an injury in an otherwise tight joint, however, does.

Fortunately, the repairs for these conditions no longer require open surgery or even permanent implants. Current outpatient arthroscopic techniques permit sewing of the tissues back to the bone, reefing the loose capsules, and anchoring the repairs with suture knots buried into the bone. Healing of the tissues is now augmented with the addition of growth factors and progenitor cells. The rehabilitation programs have grown more sophisticated, with isolation of each muscle group and immediate strengthening under the guidance of rehabilitation specialists.

There remains an argument among some specialists as to whether a first-time dislocation should be surgically repaired or if it should be left alone to see if the shoulder dislocates again. In some people, it may not. My view is there are no key tissues in the body that are best left torn, and when the consequences of a new injury are as potentially great as an unexpected shoulder dislocation, and when the repair is so straightforward, the best idea is to fix it early and well, and rehab the heck out of it. Don't let a shoulder injury become a psychological crutch for giving up activities you love, and don't permit an avoidable disease like arthritis to surface in your future.

Frozen Shoulder

"Stuck on the side of you..." While those are not quite the lyrics of the Stealers Wheel song, that is what someone with frozen shoulder feels like. When they try to lift their arm, there is no free motion of the upper arm in the shoulder joint. Instead, the patient elevates the shoulder blade and twists the neck to get the motion they desire. It can be a painful affliction.

Since the shoulder is a ball-and-socket joint, it is the most mobile of all the joints in the body. It is surrounded by a capsule of tissue that contains synovial lubricating fluid. The muscles, tendons, cartilage, and soft-tissue attachments must all remain healthy, soft, and flexible. This way, the shoulder can move through its full range of motion, yet not fall out of the joint. Any injury or medical condition that causes inflammation can restrict the motion of the shoulder by tearing or stiffening the soft tissues, thickening the capsule, reducing the fluid, and tightening the joint. While there is an association between inflammatory arthritis, thyroid disease, and diabetes, even mild injuries such as a fall onto an outstretched hand can lead to the frozen shoulder presentation. It appears most commonly in middle-aged women and can be significantly disabling, with the worst pain occurring at night.

The diagnosis of frozen shoulder is usually made by a careful physical exam and augmented by X-rays and MRI. The MRI is useful because it can show the associated injuries, such as a torn rotator cuff. Our treatments have evolved to be personalized for each patient. There appears to be a cycle for a frozen shoulder beginning with a rapid loss of motion, a prolonged state of stable discomfort, and then resolution in many patients.

In the past, clear inflammatory presentations that we associated with rheumatoid or calcific arthritis were often treated with cortisone and anti-inflammatories and combined with physical therapy to help mobilize the joint. While the drugs improve the symptoms, it is not clear if they change the course of the disease. All anti-inflammatory drugs cause damage over time.

Injury-related causes of frozen shoulder, such as torn rotator cuffs, are sometimes best treated with prompt surgical release and repair followed by extensive physical therapy. What we don't know is where in the cycle of frozen shoulder intervention is most effective.

The newer therapies—cytokines and growth factor injections to recruit the body's own stem-cell-derived progenitor cells, combined with joint lubrication—present an interesting dilemma. The sons and daughters of stem cells, now most often called progenitor cells, are growth factor production factories. They stimulate the cells of the joint tissues. The hyaluronate lubricants are the natural oil of the joint. We now have easy access to high concentrations of these growth factors and hyaluronate, which can be administered in the office without taking the patient's own fat or bone marrow. But while this potent therapy is changing our treatment of many injured tissues, it is unclear in a frozen shoulder. Do we really want to stimulate more tissue "healing" if this might make more scar tissue? Or will the strong anti-inflammatory properties of the recruited progenitor cells, combined with the lubrication ability of hyaluronate injections, naturally move the frozen shoulder to a more rapid recovery?

One of the great wonders of medicine is that we can test these novel therapies with very little risk and potentially tremendous benefit. If our patients leave with a wave of their arm, we know we got the treatment right.

The Biceps Tendon

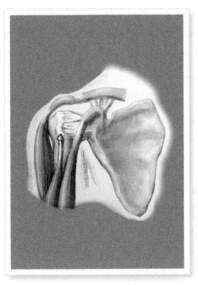

Long and short head of the biceps

The biceps tendon is not having a good era. It is frequently implicated in shoulder pain, injected with steroids, cut out at surgery, or severed and reattached, all in the belief that it is the primary generator of shoulder pain in active people. As with the meniscus tissue of olden days, top surgeons around the world believe that removing the tendon is the best way to affect a cure. How old-fashioned and unfortunate does that sound?

The bicep is the "Popeye" muscle of the arm. It not only flexes the arm but also stabilizes the shoulder by exerting downward pressure on the humeral head. The bicep is attached by a strong tendon inside the shoulder, just underneath the four tendons that make up the rotator cuff. It is this tendon that can become inflamed or partially torn when the arm is overused or when the rotator cuff is impinged from bony spurs or the swollen inflammation of bursitis. Athletes and others who use their arm in overhead activities often irritate the tendon and present to their doctor with shoulder pain.

Traditional treatments of shoulder pain from inflammation have been rest, ice, physical therapy, and cortisone injections. Unfortunately, cortisone weakens all the tissues of the shoulder while shutting down the inflammatory process. When these nonoperative methods fail, or if there is an associated tear of the rotator cuff, surgery is often deployed. The inflamed bicep tendon is removed from the shoulder by cutting it free or cutting and then re-anchoring it away from the rotator cuff.

The thinking behind this is that the inflamed tendon is a pain generator, and its role in shoulder function is not very important. This logic sounds uncomfortably similar to the reasoning once used to justify excising the meniscus cartilage when torn—a procedure we now know leads to arthritis in the knee joint. While tendon amputation may not lead to arthritis, the function of the shoulder cannot be normal without all of its key structures.

My insightful patients ask the following obvious question: "Why can't you doctors figure out a way to heal the inflamed or frayed tendon? It has been there for millions of years, and just because you don't understand its full role doesn't mean you should amputate it! Figure out how to repair it!"

The future, clearly, is not in the removal of major attachments of muscles. It will lie in novel ways of stimulating the healing of injured tendons, such as the bicep. These advances are on the way. They include the integration of new matrices (such as collagen sheets) preloaded with the patient's stem cells and growth factors and surgically wrapped around the injured tendons or injected into their sheaths. Another novel approach is to provide a self-assembling, injectable collagen material, which is then melded with ultraviolet light stimulation. A third approach will use a resorbable artificial material that will stimulate tendon regeneration.

Stay tuned for the new era of anabolic tissue healing—brought to you by biologists, chemists, and tissue engineers in the hopes of ending the primitive amputation of temporarily damaged joint structures.

Broken Collarbones

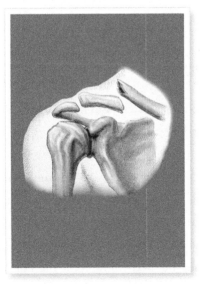

Midshaft fracture of the clavicle

Clavicle fractures hurt. The collarbone sticks up under the skin and moves around. It is scary. In the past, most fractures of this type were left alone to heal on their own. Today, many are being repaired. What changed?

First, some basic anatomy: The collarbone (clavicle) is a curved, twisted, partially flat bone that acts as a strut—or outrigger—stabilizing the shoulder. It is most commonly broken in the middle after falls off of bicycles, motorcycles, horses, or other moving objects. In children, the bone ends heal quickly and erase any deformity. In adults, it's different. The old belief was that most collarbones heal well without surgery. But newer data shows that if the bone is displaced more than 1.5 centimeters, or angled more than forty-five degrees, the healing is compromised. Either the clavicle doesn't heal at all, or it mends with a deformity that produces long-term weakness and intermittent pain. This data, combined with better repair techniques, has changed the approach to clavicle fractures.

Clavicle surgery, when it was previously performed, involved thick plates and screws. Since the bone is not flat along its length—in fact, it twists—such plates artificially affected the pattern of the clavicle as it healed. The surgery often involved cutting through a sensory nerve that crossed the clavicle, and most often, the plates had to be removed after healing since the skin overlying the collarbone is thin.

Even when the plates could remain, they were not always secure—so most athletes were prevented from returning to sports until healing occurred. This combination of negatives led many surgeons and patients to ignore most clavicle fractures.

Two technical advances have changed our strategy. First, today's plates—when they are used—now come pre-curved to match most clavicle shapes. Additionally, newly designed threads in the screw holes of the plate allow the screws to lock the plate in securely. This produces a much stronger construct than the older screws, which simply held the bone against the plate. Lastly, the materials used have changed to higher-quality steel or titanium, permitting thinner, lower-profile plates.

Most attractive for many patients is the improved technique called "intramedullary pinning." In this procedure, a screw is placed through the bore of the clavicle, eliminating the need for the plate altogether. While tricky to perform and not applicable to all fractures, pinning is performed as outpatient surgery through a miniature incision. Patients can quickly return to sports (one of our patients rode his bike in the Race Across America two weeks after surgery), though they're advised not to fall, if possible.

The outcomes of surgically repaired clavicle fractures are now proving to be better and less deforming than those of fractures left alone. The shoulder is better stabilized, the power increased, and the cosmetic appearance improved.

So, the next time you crash and break your collarbone, have confidence that your season may not be over. On the other hand, staying vertical has a much better outcome.

Diana Nyad Pushes the Limits

Legendary long-distance swimmer Diana Nyad gave the honorary presentation—a spectacularly inspirational speech —at an American Academy of Sports Medicine meeting in Seattle. Nyad came out of a thirty-year retirement to reattempt her nearly impossible goal of becoming the first person to swim 103 miles nonstop from Cuba to Florida, without the use of a shark cage. On her fifth attempt, at age sixty-four, she finally succeeded.

Part of her speech focused on her shoulders, often the weak link in overhead athletes (the windmilling of swimmers' shoulders makes them overhead athletes too). During the training leading up to her first attempt to swim the Cuba–Florida route at age sixty, she sought opinions from leading shoulder surgeons about whether or not her sore, aging shoulders would hold up—not just for the multi-day swim, but for the innumerable hours of training it would take just to start the swim.

As anyone with sore shoulders knows, sleeping at night and any simple overhead motion—raising your hands to lift a suitcase or wash your hair—can lead to pain as the muscles and tendons of the shoulder, primarily the rotator cuff and bicep tendons, engage and come into contact with the bones at the top of the shoulder. The pain is due to wear and inflammation. When that leads to tearing, the shoulder stops working correctly.

Diana was told multiple times to abandon any thought of the long-distance attempt. Her shoulders, she was warned, simply would not hold up. But a few doctors thought the shoulder wear wasn't all that bad, and the risk, given the athlete's desire, was worth it. In the end, it was. Recognizing that not every one of us has "Diana drive" though, how do you decide when to push it and when to hold back?

For shoulder injuries, there are definitely no black-and-white answers. Most soft-tissue injuries can be successfully treated with smart rehabilitation exercises, exercise technique modification, injections of growth factors (we rarely use cortisone anymore), and occasional anti-inflammatory medications. We surgically repair complete tears of the rotator cuff and shoulder dislocations, as they clearly get worse when untreated. However, for many of the in-between injuries, the jury is out. For instance, treatment of the inflamed bicep tendon has gone in multiple directions without clarity. Some surgeons cut the bicep tendon when inflamed; others reattach it in another place. I have most commonly left it alone and treated the surrounding injuries and the cause of the inflammation. There is still no clear consensus.

Ultimately, as Diana Nyad has clearly shown, the drive and desire of the patient may be the most important factor in deciding how to treat and when to push the limits.

ELBOWS

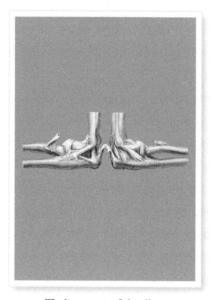

The ligaments of the elbow

The elbow joint between the upper arm (humerus) and forearm (radius and ulna) is crossed by the tendons that enable the arm to extend (tricep tendon) and bend (bicep tendon), and the wrist to bend (flexor tendons) and extend (extensor tendons). When excessive muscle loading occurs, the tendons can be stretched, partially torn, or completely ripped off the bone. Stretch injuries and partial tears most often heal without difficulty, yet sometimes the inflammation that occurs with any tissue injury persists, leading to pain, weakness, and swelling. Here are the most common examples at the elbow.

Inflammation of the extensor or flexor tendons of the elbow is lateral epicondylitis, often called tennis elbow. Pain is felt at the outside or inside of the elbow joint where the tendons insert on the bone. This common injury can arise from overuse, such as playing multiple sets of tennis in one day, or from a direct injury, such as hitting a ball hard and feeling sudden pain at the elbow. Activities causing epicondylitis are not tennis alone. It can stem from golf or repetitive activities, such as washing windows, which can cause inflammation on the inside or outside of the elbow. The condition is painful, it takes a long time to resolve, and it interferes with daily activities.

The syndrome is misnamed "epicondylitis"—misnamed because it is not an "-itis," which means inflammation, but an injury of the tendons in the forearm that insert at the outside (i.e., lateral) part of the elbow, which connect the muscles that enable the wrist and fingers to extend. One tendon, the extensor carpi radialis brevis, is most commonly the bad actor in the story of tennis elbow. While there are different theories about why this tendon, once injured, does not always heal properly, here is the basic story.

A tendon is made up of collagen fibers with specialized cells. These cells produce a range of charged molecules, growth factors, signaling factors, and other key components that keep the tissue healthy. The collagen fibers are crosslinked with chemical bridges. These permit the fibers to elongate and then return to their normal length. They provide just the right amount of tension to permit the muscles to act appropriately. Tension is the key to collagen function. Under tension, the collagen appropriately stretches and contracts. Without tension, the collagen degrades. A too-tight grip on the handle of a tennis racket, axe, bike bar, rowing machine—a seemingly infinite number of causes—can cause an overstretching of the tissue. This sudden lengthening may lead to micro- or macro-tears of the crosslinks that bind the fibers together, or even to the fibers themselves.

Then the interesting part begins. With normal activity, these small tears occur all the time. The body responds with increased blood flow.

Stem cells migrate to the site of the injury, where specialized repair cells take away the torn fibers and initiate the repair process, laying down new collagen. When done in an orderly fashion, the tissue is restored to normal and no scarring occurs. When these micro-tears occur in muscle fibers—from weight lifting, for example—the muscle heals with thicker fibers, leading to muscle building.

In the case of tennis elbow, however, something goes wrong; the reconstruction process loses its "general contractor," so to speak. It seems there are not enough stimuli to tell the body to recruit stem cells and initiate the normal healing response. The tearing away from the insertion on the bone at the elbow releases the tension in the fibers just enough to permit the degradation process to run amok; the torn tissue just lies there and slowly degrades. The chemical by-products of this degradation lead to the stimulation of pain neurons. If allowed to continue, cell death and permanent collagen fiber degeneration can occur.

Tennis elbow can be the kind of tearing that heals naturally, or the ugly kind that leaves weakened scar tissue and chronic pain. Treating the injury in a way that helps increase the probability of normal tissue healing is the goal. The classic treatment for tennis elbow—cortisone injections—actually makes the problem worse, though it relieves the pain in 50 percent of the cases. Cortisone inhibits cell metabolism, further shutting down the healing response. But it relieves pain by reducing the inflammatory agents at the site of the injury.

Soft-tissue massage to the damaged area breaks down scar tissue and stimulates the production of more collagen through a combination of cell stimulation and collagen fiber cycling. New collagen is laid down at the site of the injury. If careful stress is applied (in the form of gentle exercises), the collagen fibers line up along the lines of stress, leading to healthy healing of the tissue. Bracing the wrist, so as to decrease the distance the tendons are stretched, often helps—as does an elastic band wrapped around the forearm. If the joint is immobilized, however, scarring is more likely to form—with weakened tissue as a result.

Ice can reduce both pain and inflammation in tennis elbow. However, the relief is limited as the issue is not inflammation but tissue degeneration. It takes a new stimulus to remove this relatively dead tissue. The stimulus can take three forms: surgical, where the tissue is physically removed and sewn back to the proper length; manual, where massage therapy stimulates the repair; or chemical. Chemical stimulation today is best performed by the injection of stem cells and growth factors. These injections change the cellular environment surrounding the degraded tissues. In a recent study comparing the therapeutic results of cortisone injections to growth factors extracted from blood platelets, the growth factors appeared to be more effective. In another study, collagen fibers were restored to their normal mixture of small- and large-diameter fibrils under the stimulation of amniotic stem cells.

If not cured immediately after it appears, tennis elbow has a nasty habit of becoming chronic and painful. Attacking it early and often to prevent the death of the tendon tissue may be the best approach. It is always much easier to cure the injured than to resurrect the dead.

ANKLES

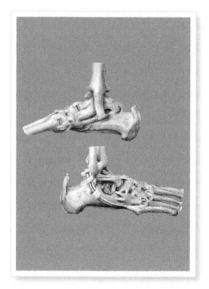

Ligaments and tendons of the ankle joint

If you have ever twisted your ankle, you'll know how agonizing that pain can be and how much the ankle can swell. Many people come to me after twisting their ankle inward, having landed badly from a jump, tripped over a curb, or just lost their footing on an uneven surface. It is a common injury, but thankfully it is usually minor and can heal without surgery. What you want to avoid is having it twist repeatedly afterward.

After a twist, you have most commonly damaged the anterior talo-fibular ligament of the ankle, which is the ligament at the front, on the outside. Put your hand on the bump on the outside of your ankle, the lateral malleolus. Now run your finger a little bit forward; that's where the anterior talofibular ligament is. This ligament is the key stabilizer of the ankle, and once it is twisted, the ankle may become unstable.

What I look for when I see a twisted ankle is the grade or degree of the sprain. Is it Grade 1 (a stretch), Grade 2 (a tear), or Grade 3 (a complete rupture)? Essentially, we need to know if the ankle is stable or unstable. If it is stable after a stretch or small tear, we can treat it with ice, soft-tissue massage, and ankle support. Ankles usually return to normal within a couple of weeks.

If the ankle is unstable after a more serious ligament tear, however, we will need to do a little more to help it heal. Otherwise, you are in danger of having the ankle twist again and again. This chronic instability is avoidable if specific treatments are started immediately after the injury. In these cases, often other ankle ligaments are torn, which means that the bones around the ankle might have shifted out of place. The nerve supply to the injured ligaments may also be compromised. These nerves provide proprioception, or position sense—in effect telling the brain where the foot is in space. In the healing process, it is critical to retrain the ligaments to regain the neural connections required for a stable ankle.

In the past, ankle injuries were often treated with cast immobilization for six weeks or longer. Unfortunately, this does not promote healing. The tissues that need to recover are weakened by the lack of normal motion and produce scar tissue instead of healthy tissue. Healing of the nerves is also compromised. Instead, we use an ankle brace or taping combined with a stabilization rehab program. Ankle training exercises help stimulate the ligament to heal along the lines of stress in a normal fashion rather than just a scar. We sometimes use electrical stimulation, and we have a host of balance and proprioception exercises.

Every now and then—one in five hundred or so ankle ligaments—we need to repair an unstable ankle surgically. This is because the ankle injury has caused more significant damage, sometimes the result of a single incident and sometimes caused over time by repeated twisted ankles. In these cases, I am able to sew the anterior ligament back into place using a technique I developed twenty years ago. It is an outpatient repair, which, when combined with a careful rehab program, has never failed to stabilize an unstable athletic ankle in our practice.

So remember, while ankle injuries are common and are usually minor, make sure you give your ankle the time and attention it needs to heal. This will help you avoid developing a chronically unstable ankle that gives out repeatedly.

Ankle Sprains

Ankle injuries are common. Sometimes they lead to chronically unstable ankles that give out repeatedly. Instability is avoidable if specific treatments are started immediately after the injury.

When an ankle is injured from twisting in toward the other foot —an inversion injury—most commonly, the anterior talofibular ligament is stretched or torn. If the two other primary ligaments on the outside of the ankle (the posterior talofibular ligament and the calcaneofibular ligament) are also injured, the primary bone of the ankle, the talus, can be displaced from beneath the tibia, and the ankle "shucks" out of joint.

A physician, physical therapist, or trainer examining the ankle soon after injury can compare the amount of "shuck" to the opposite ankle and develop a grade for the amount of injury suffered. Usually, if the injury is limited to one ligament, the instability is less. If all three ligaments are involved, the ankle is more unstable.

The nerve supply to injured ligaments can be compromised leading to loss of position sense, balance, and coordination. Specific exercises can counteract these effects.

Even soft-tissue injuries of the ankle were placed in casts in the past. We have found this to be detrimental to the healing tissues. When injured collagen tissues are immobilized, the collagen heals in a disorganized fashion, producing scar tissue. The tissues are weakened by the lack of normal motion and stress required for tissue nutrition and organization. The injured nerve fibers have difficulty reestablishing the proprioceptive sense for the ankle. The result is a higher incidence of chronic instability. The key is early diagnosis, swelling reduction, stabilization, and stimulation for healing.

Repeated Ankle Injuries

The Golden State Warriors' Steph Curry has suffered repeated ankle injuries, including post-surgery. The questions most often asked by athletes, coaches, trainers, and of course fans are the following: What can be done to speed healing? What can reduce the reinjury rate? Are there permanent solutions? The answers are evolving.

Most ankle sprains happen when the foot rolls inward and the leg keeps moving outward, tearing the ATFL ligament. Though the injury usually heals on its own, the best results occur when the ankle is braced and motion is directed to permit the fibers to heal in a tight fashion.

For those athletes who tear their ligament recurrently, it is best to repair it. Assuming it is the anterior ATFL that is torn, the most successful repair is a primary suturing of the ligament back onto the fibula. This is called a Brostrom repair. Over the years, we and other surgeons have modified the original technique in various ways to make the procedure more reliable.

Some more complicated ligament reconstructions involve weaving other tendons through the bones to both reconstruct and reinforce the torn ligaments. Other techniques use artificial materials to brace the bones—though these materials usually fail over time due to the repetitive motions of the ankle even under normal walking conditions, never mind sports.

In what I call the "anabolic era" of sports medicine, we now add growth factors and stem or progenitor cells to almost all injuries. There is a growing body of evidence that healing is both accelerated and improved by these supplements. While athletes used to travel to Germany, Mexico, or the Cayman Islands to get these treatments, there are now far better solutions available here in the US. Among these are improved versions of PRP (blood platelet concentrates), fat aspiration, and bone marrow concentrates.

Much of our recent work has focused upon amniotic fluid (since no one is growing faster than the fetus). The fluid surrounding the healthy newborn is loaded with the highest concentrations of both progenitor cells and growth factors, which make them excellent anti-inflammatories and anabolics. If carefully harvested, concentrated, and preserved, these growth factors and cells are so far the most potent stimulants for healing that we have tested and used clinically.

The old days of immobilization during recovery are long gone. We have discovered that lack of motion leads to disorganized scar formation rather than the well-aligned collagen fibers associated with normal ligament morphology. For injured and reinjured ankle ligaments, in-season treatments focus on the injection of growth factors into the torn tissues. This is followed by ice, compression, elevation, and massage to reduce swelling (swollen tissues are distorted and heal poorly). The faster the swelling resolves, the faster the healing. Bracing is combined with careful exercises to further stimulate the torn tissues to heal along the lines of stress. In addition, a total body fitness program is started on day one of the ankle injury. We want the injured to see themselves as athletes in training, not as patients in rehab. The ability to come back from an ankle injury better than you were before it occurred depends on all of these healing factors being applied to the injury site, along with the parts attached to it: namely, the entire body and mind.

Reducing repetitive injuries depends on a host of factors. Successful reconstruction of all the damaged tissues is important, but so is the brain/body training designed to improve the connection between the mind and the ankle position in space. Though this proprioception skill seems to be diminished in people who suffer frequent ankle sprains, it may be amenable to novel brain/body training programs.

The ultimate solution to recurrent ankle injuries, of course, would be the ability to avoid repeating the injury after the first successful repair. One can envision sensors placed in future athletes' shoes or socks, or even stuck to their skin, that could measure the force and direction of the ankle motion. Such sensors would signal the brain and stiffen the shoe, preventing the ankle from rolling into the injury position. Any tech venture capitalists own a basketball team?

Ankle Arthritis

Ever wonder why you don't hear about ankle arthritis or ankle replacements? The ankle doesn't get arthritis, except if injured. Why is this, when the entire body rests on these relatively small joints?

The bearing surface of joints is the articular cartilage. It is the white, shiny material you see when you crack open the chicken wing. When that surface wears down to the underlying bone, you have the most common type of arthritis: traumatic arthritis. The joint can wear down from an injury that kills the cells that keep it healthy, or from a loss of the normal alignment—leading to an irregular wear pattern. If the cartilage is repaired or the alignment fixed, arthritis can often be prevented.

In the ankle, cartilage looks just the same as it does in the hip or the knee. Yet something about it prevents it from wearing away without an initial injury. Despite being a quarter of the size of the larger joints, the degenerative disease called osteoarthritis rarely happens in the ankle. No one knows why. So if people never injure their ankles, they never end up with artificial ankle joints. But anyone who keeps twisting the joint is nonetheless asking for trouble.

When the ligaments surrounding the joint become stretched or torn, the bones move in and out of the joint. That abnormal motion means the force is not distributed evenly. The motion leads to high shear forces—the kind that scrape off the surface layers—and high local compression forces. These small changes lead to pressure points. The pressure points, in turn, kill the underlying cells. The cells stop making the matrix that absorbs the fluid in the joint to keep it spongy. Then the cartilage stiffens, there's a breakdown, and the bone is exposed.

This cycle is predictable, but it's also preventable. When the ankle ligaments are injured, they can be braced to permit healing, or repaired. The longer the ankle stays unstable, the more likely the damaging cycle begins. Our ability to repair ankle joints has been much improved by MRI-clarified understanding of anatomy, by the addition of growth factors and stem cells, and by the ability to regrow damaged articular cartilage with paste grafts. Another factor is our evolving understanding of rehabilitation. This combination makes the repairs of today substantially faster than the olden days, when a full year was often lost to such injuries and recoveries.

ARTHRITIS

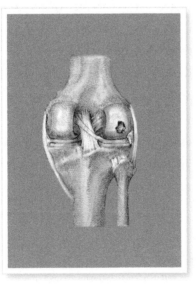

*Articular cartilage damage of the lateral
femoral condyle in the knee*

Arthritis is a silent, insidious, and painful joint disorder that ruins many lives. In the US, it's the most common cause of disability. Around fifty million American adults have some form of arthritis. That's one in four. By 2030, an estimated sixty-seven million American adults are projected to have doctor-diagnosed arthritis.[9]

Arthritis covers many conditions. What they have in common is joint pain that can be chronic, activity limiting, and ultimately disabling. There are two main categories, inflammatory and mechanical. Arthritis, as an inflammatory disease, is characterized by inflammation of joints that leads to destruction of the bone and cartilage. This includes gout, lupus, rheumatoid arthritis (RA), and fibromyalgia. (Lupus and RA are autoimmune diseases.) Arthritis as a degenerative condition is characterized by cartilage damaged as the result of an injury, or broken down over time by wear, exposing the underlying bone. Rubbing against the exposed bone produces symptomatic pain, inflammation, swelling, and stiffness. This is osteoarthritis (OA), the most common form of arthritis affecting twenty-seven million adults in the US.

The exact causes of osteoarthritis are not known, but many contributing factors are well understood. Traumatic arthritis comes from an injury that damages the articular cartilage. Arthritis also occurs when a patient's meniscus cartilage has been damaged or removed

---

[9] The CDC combined data from the National Health Interview Survey (NHIS) years 2013–2015 Sample Adult Core components to estimate average annual arthritis prevalence in the civilian, non-institutionalized US adult population aged eighteen years or older. Overall, an estimated 22.7 percent (54.4 million) of adults had doctor-diagnosed arthritis, with significantly higher age-adjusted prevalence in women (23.5 percent) than in men (18.1 percent). Arthritis prevalence increased with age. See: Kamil Barbour, Charles G. Helmick, Michael Boring, and Teresa J. Brady, "Vital Signs: Prevalence of Doctor-Diagnosed Arthritis and Arthritis-Attributable Activity Limitation—United States, 2013–2015," *Morbidity and Mortality Weekly Report* 66 no. 9 (2017): 246–253, https://www.cdc.gov/mmwr/volumes/66/wr/mm6609e1.htm; and Jennifer M. Hootman et al., "Updated projected prevalence of self-reported doctor-diagnosed arthritis and arthritis-attributable activity limitation among US adults, 2015–2040," *Arthritis & Rheumatology* 68 no. 7 (2016): 1582–1587, https://pubmed.ncbi.nlm.nih.gov/27015600/.

following a sports injury, leaving the knee exposed to increased forces that wear off the articular cartilage-bearing surface. We are approaching an annual patient load of 1.5 million Americans undergoing meniscus cartilage removal, leaving a large population without cartilage protection and prone to arthritis. A person's weight or bone malalignment are also contributing factors.

It may come as a surprise to learn that most arthritis may be preventable. Sports and activity-related injuries lead to arthritis later in life. While such injuries usually cannot be prevented, the subsequent arthritis would most likely not occur if the damage was repaired immediately using modern regeneration and replacement techniques.

But this doesn't often happen. Patients tend to ignore their injuries. Surgeons still remove the damaged tissue and tell their patients to come back when they need a knee replacement. Arthritis pain is treated with cortisone instead of growth factors and stem cells, and insurance companies don't pay for up-to-date tissue regeneration techniques. How do we change this?

First, don't ignore an injury. If you twist your knee, hear a pop, and then have swelling, there's a 90 percent chance you have torn a key tissue in the knee. If left alone, the injury will cause arthritis; if repaired properly, it may not. Getting an accurate, rapid diagnosis—often with MRI confirmation—is the critical first step. Not having the damaged tissue removed, if at all possible, is the next step.

Unfortunately, most surgeons still remove damaged knee tissues —usually the meniscus shock absorber and the articular cartilage surface—without applying the latest repair, regeneration, and replacement techniques. Why? Because those repair techniques are difficult, take extra operating time, are not reimbursed by insurance companies, and do not have enough large-scale studies to convince the entire medical establishment that they work. But here are the facts. We know that if joint cartilage is repaired or replaced when it is injured, the likelihood of arthritis is significantly less. In the US—where eight hundred thousand meniscus tears occur each year[10]—less than 10 percent are repaired,[11] and only about 0.25 percent of people receive a new meniscus.[12] That's because a future arthritis problem is not likely to cost the insurer money, as most people don't stay with the same insurance company for more than a few years. Surgeons tell the patients to expect arthritis to set in ten to twenty years in the future; sometimes it occurs much sooner.

After arthritis does occur, cartilage repair and replacement procedures can still be beneficial. They can reduce pain, improve functions, and prolong the time before an artificial joint is required. Our own data shows that on average, many severely arthritic joints can be biologically repaired (as long as it's not bone on bone). This can delay the need for an artificial joint by ten years, on average. (Since only the first artificial joint has the best outcome, and the joints last only a couple of decades, it is important to delay this procedure until patients are past sixty or older.) Again, biological repair is not in the interest of the insurance company. Most patients are told to live with their arthritic knee, and their pain, until they are older.

[10] David S. Logerstedt, et al., "Knee pain and mobility impairments: meniscal and articular cartilage lesions," *Journal of Orthopaedic and Sports Physical Therapy* 40 no. 6 (2010): A1–A35, DOI: 10.2519/jospt.2010.0304.

[11] Between 2005 and 2011, there were 23,640 meniscus repairs. Geoffrey D. Abrams, et al., "Trends in meniscus repair and meniscectomy in the United States, 2005–2011," *American Journal of Sports Medicine* 41 no. 10 (October 2013): 2333–9, DOI: 10.1177/0363546513495641.

[12] In 2011, there were 675 MAT procedures performed in the US. Gregory L. Cvetanovich et al., "Trends in meniscal allograft transplantation in the United States, 2007 to 2011," *Arthroscopy: The Journal of Arthroscopic & Related Surgery* 31 no. 6 (2015): 1123–1127, https://pubmed.ncbi.nlm.nih.gov/25682330/.

The nonoperative procedures for preventing arthritis are also exquisitely effective and underfunded. The joints are protected by the muscles that surround them. The forces absorbed by the joints are a multiple of body weight. Most people take two to three million steps per year at up to five times their body weight, depending on the height of the step.

Optimizing your body weight matters. Being ten pounds overweight leads to up to fifty pounds of extra force, two to three million times per year. The stronger the muscles around the joint, the better they absorb some of the force—rather than the joint surfaces. Preventing self-induced injury would significantly lower the arthritis rate.

Research funding would also help. Ninety-seven percent of arthritis diagnoses are the types that orthopaedic surgeons most commonly treat: osteoarthritis or traumatic arthritis. Only 3 percent are inflammatory; these are called rheumatoid arthritis (or related variants). Yet 97 percent of the funding of the Arthritis Foundation goes toward that 3 percent of diagnoses, for two reasons.[13] First, because that's where much of the money in pharmaceutical treatments of arthritis is to be made. Second, because rheumatologists control the Arthritis Foundation. A major effort to focus research dollars on improving techniques for injury repair would improve outcomes for millions of people.

Given the projected costs to society of $128 billion (or 1.2 percent of GDP) for arthritis treatment each year, one would think that a

---

[13] Arthritis Foundation,. "Arthritis Foundation Awards Nearly $5.5 Million in Scientific Discovery Funding," *PR Newswire*, February 4, 2016, https://www.prnewswire.com/news-releases/arthritis-foundation-awards-nearly-55-million-in-scientific-discovery-funding-300215019.html.

national program to prevent this disease would be a high priority.[14] Cancer may kill six hundred thousand people in the US this year, but arthritis ruins more lives.[15] And it doesn't have to.

Arthritis Riddles

You know that big, ugly bone spur that can grow on the side of a finger, toe, or knee, like a stalagmite in a cave? That growth is called an osteophyte—stimulated to form by osteoarthritis. As painful as they can become, these growths hold the secrets to the riddle of a cure for arthritis.

A bone spur, if you look under the often-tender, red area of skin that covers it, looks like a white, shiny, and perfect articular cartilage —the same material that covers the ends of the bones inside of our joints. Underneath the shiny surface is a column of new bone. It has the same architecture and cellular material of healthy bone and cartilage, but it is formed on the edges of the joint rather than in the middle.

Arthritis often follows this sequence: First, there is a wearing away of, or damage to, the cartilage surface. Next, the bone beneath becomes deformed as it loses its protective covering. The rough surfaces then spread particles around the joint, leading to inflammation of the surrounding tissues. Those tissues produce enzymes that accelerate the disease and cause more swelling.

---

[14] Louise B. Murphy, "Medical expenditures and earnings losses among US adults with arthritis in 2013," *Arthritis Care & Research* 70 (2017): 869–876, https://doi.org/10.1002/acr.23425.

[15] National Cancer Institute, "Cancer Stat Facts: Cancer of Any Site," https://seer.cancer.gov/statfacts/html/all.html; Barbour et al., "Vital Signs."

One of the body's reactions to this process is to spread the weight-bearing forces across the joint. This is done by increasing the surface area through the formation of these bone spurs.

In the past, treatments for arthritis have included drugs to decrease the inflammation, rest to diminish the painful grinding, surgery to clear away damaged tissue, and ultimately, artificial joint replacement—usually after years of suffering.

In today's anabolic era of orthopaedics, the preferred treatments are different. We use exercises to strengthen the muscles around the joints (and to increase the range of motion lost due to inflammation and tissue stiffness), injections of lubricants to decrease the friction, growth factors and stem cells to stimulate repair processes, and surgical replacement of the meniscus, articular cartilage, and ligaments to restore the knee joint's anatomy. But the future of treatment lies in harnessing the Vesuvian eruption of bone and cartilage that creates bone spurs.

Our bodies already know how to form healthy, nearly perfect tissue at the edges of joints. We must learn how to direct the body to form them where we want them: at the site of the worn or injured cartilage surfaces. We're discovering how to do this through a series of studies of the paste graft technique. This process involves first creating a local fracture in the arthritic lesion, then packing the area with marrow and progenitor, stem, and articular cartilage cells. It's almost as if we're nurturing a bone spur like a Bonsai tree and coaxing it to grow the way we want it to. Long-term data of arthritic patients followed for ten to twenty-three years after paste grafting demonstrated the success of this technique.

Other studies of the osteophyte itself will lead to additional novel techniques. It is clear that the body knows what to do, but it is directionally challenged. In this era of rapid technological advances, the call has gone out. Can our body learn to deliver cartilage where it's needed and supply its own cure for arthritis?

Researchers are making headway in discovering the biologic underpinnings of tissue injury. Recent research demonstrated that when a meniscus tissue is torn, pro-arthritis enzymes and factors are released, which stimulate the synovial lining cells of the joint to go into overdrive. The tissues talk to each other.[16] They are biologically, not just mechanically, active.

The enzymes and factors released into a joint after injury produce a degradative fluid. Degradative means that the compounds break down tissue, inhibit healing, cause swelling, and eventually cause arthritis. When people complain of joint swelling, the fluid is degradative and leads to more injury over time. Healing occurs when the swelling resolves and the body lays down new tissues.

This new biologic understanding of tissue injury is leading to novel approaches to repair. Most importantly, injured tissues need prompt repair. Left unrepaired, they continue to stimulate the surrounding tissues, leading to the cycle of breakdown and arthritis. Prompt repair can now sometimes mean not just surgical repair but injections of progenitor cells derived from stem cells. Data presented from the group in Tokyo, led by Dr. Ichiro Sekiya, convincingly demonstrated limited meniscus repair with injections of high numbers of synovial progenitor cells alone.[17] These cells migrate to the

---

[16] Betty Liu et al., "Matrix metalloproteinase activity and prostaglandin E2 are elevated in the synovial fluid of meniscus tear patients," *Connective Tissue Research* 58 no. 3–4 (2017): 305–316, DOI: 10.1080/03008207.2016.1256391.

[17] Masafumi Horie, "Implantation of allogenic synovial stem cells promotes meniscal regeneration in a rabbit meniscal defect model," *Journal of Bone and Joint Surgery* 94 no. 8 (April 2012): 701–12, https://pubmed.ncbi.nlm.nih.gov/22517386/.

site of injury and induce repair both directly and also indirectly by releasing growth factors and changing the degradative environment to an anabolic one.

The importance of the chemical environment of the joint, and its influence on healing, has wide-ranging implications. Drugs we take to reduce inflammation may sometimes inhibit healing (as non-steroid anti-inflammatories such as ibuprofen, have been shown to do). Arthritis may in fact be preventable if we are able to stop the production of the enzymes early after injury. A new compound (named IL1-Ra, or Anakinra) did just that in an unrepaired, displaced fracture that normally would have gone on to severe arthritis. Other compounds such as glucosamine and chondroitin also induce the production of normal joint lubrication and stimulate matrix repair. Supplements in the flavanol family may remove senescent cells, thereby decreasing the flood of degradative factors in the joint environment when aging cells die. Their mechanisms of action may now be accepted as valuable-therapeutic and, possibly, disease-modifying agents.

The biologic era of joint repair is evolving so rapidly that removing injured tissues may soon be a surgical procedure of the past. Repairing, regenerating, and replacing tissues with natural tissues as opposed to artificial materials is the path keeping biologics firmly ahead of bionics in orthopaedics.

Arthritis Prevention

In the past, without the benefit of high-resolution MRI, we relied on physical exams, history, and experience to determine whether or not surgical repair was necessary. We were often wrong. What has since come to light is that most joints perform poorly when important structures are injured, leading to arthritis. The consequences are huge, with arthritis now being the most common cause of disability in the US. Twenty-three percent of US adults (about fifty-four million people) have arthritis, and 60 percent of them are of working age (eighteen to sixty-four). Medical costs are $81 billion. Yet much of it is preventable.

Let's look at four joints together, each with a common injury, that were previously left to "heal on their own."

- **The ankle joint.** Ankle sprains are so common that people often do not seek medical attention at all. Many do "heal" on their own. Yet MRI imaging and careful examination reveal scarring at the torn anterior lateral ligaments. The scar does not stabilize the joint the way the injured normal ligament did. While ankle arthritis remains relatively rare, it is probably better to help the ligament heal normally. In this case, non-surgical methods are playing a major role. It appears that by bathing the injured ligament in growth factors, from PRP to amniotic fluids, then applying soft-tissue massage, careful rehabilitation exercises, and limited bracing, the ligaments may heal with a normal collagen fiber orientation rather than scar tissue. The key is treating the ligaments before they scar.
- **The hip joint labrum.** The hip was often the forgotten child of sports medicine. Imaging improvements led to a better understanding of the joint's components and to the realization that certain tears were correlated with bony spurs. If treated, patients could return to sports and possibly

diminish subsequent arthritis. This protocol is still a work in progress, but arthroscopic surgical techniques have advanced to a point where surgeons can repair hip tissue. A stable, non-painful hip is far more likely to remain healthy than its injured cousin.

- **The shoulder dislocation.** Shoulders dislocate when the ligament labrum complex, the tissue that holds the arm securely to the shoulder blade, is torn from the bony attachment. This often occurs during a fall, when the arm is unprotected. The dislocation sometimes relocates on its own, or it may need to be reset by a medical team. But the tissue does not heal normally. We know this thanks to high-quality MRI, which shows the damage to the bone and the scarring of ligaments when they are left to heal without repair. Our job is to rebuild the normal attachments, rehabilitate the joint, and try to restore normal motion. If we don't, the constant abnormal rotations of the shoulder will likely lead to arthritis.

- **The knee joint ACL.** Torn ACLs occur well over 300,000 times each year in the US. Approximately 250,000 of these are surgically repaired. If left untreated, there is an 80 percent chance of a subsequent meniscus tear, as the force distributors on the joint surface become more exposed when the ACL is torn. Even repaired, however, there is a 50 percent chance of developing arthritis in ten years after an ACL injury. This is due either to the initial injury, the subsequent damage to the meniscus, the harvest of the patient's patellar tendon or hamstrings to rebuild the ACL, or the misplacement of the ACL reconstruction tissue at surgery. Clearly, we need to advance the science of diagnosis and improve the repair strategy. Better surgical techniques with augmentation of donor tissue, along with growth factors and stem cells, may reduce the chance of arthritis. But left alone, the knee is often doomed.

So when you hear that pop and feel the "catch and give way," don't bury your head in the sand. Get thee to a surgeon! The key for all critical joint structures is to return them to their normal anatomy as rapidly as possible. Only then can we hope that arthritis may be prevented and that we can continue our active, athletic life with a smile rather than a crutch.

Don't Go Home and Rest

"Go home and rest. Wait for your joint replacement. Take ibuprofen. Then, after your procedure, rest some more. Walk, but don't exercise too much. Don't wear it out." These out-of-date responses to arthritic joint pain are flat-out wrong.

If you have arthritis, going home and resting produces muscle atrophy, bone loss, and loss of balance and coordination, and it increases obesity and leads to depression.

Exercise designed to protect the arthritic joint, while simultaneously building the muscles around it and the rest of the body, increases function and decreases the forces across the joint surface. It improves balance and coordination (limiting falls), helps control weight, and improves one's sense of well-being. So the logical treatment for arthritis is a program of smart, progressively increasing exercises.

Exercising alone, however, is not as effective as exercising under the guidance of a physical therapist or trainer. Objective measurements of your progress, instruction in new exercises, safe and efficient techniques, and a competitive motivation to improve are all factors that drive our progress. Meanwhile, the increased circulating testosterone, pheromones, and adrenaline generated by exercise drive well-being. Exercising outdoors has an improved wellness value over indoor exercise. Most outdoor exercises require balance, expose the skin to sunlight (needed for vitamin D production and bone formation), and are mentally expansive.

If you like using gym equipment, move your setup outside or find outdoor fitness stations.

After artificial, partial, or complete joint replacement, the advice is the same. We have never seen a well-placed artificial joint worn out from exercise. The most common cause of wear is loosening of the cement interface with the bone, most likely caused by a weakening of the bone with aging. The only known way to increase bone mass is by resistive exercise. So increase your walking, hiking, skiing, and weight lifting to save your artificial joints.

The most common question we hear about sports and joints concerns running. Be advised: our views on this subject are not shared by all doctors. First, a question. Which has more force on the knee joint, running a mile or walking a mile? The answer is that the quantity of force is about the same due to the fact that you take fewer steps when running. If you must run, use "Chi running" techniques. This involves short strides, midfoot landing, soft surfaces, and new running shoes. While running in general is not our favorite sport for artificial joints—and since most people with severely arthritic knees gave it up years ago—we prefer to encourage other activities such as skiing, hiking, biking, swimming, yoga, Pilates, and/or weight lifting, which load the bones and muscles without high-peak impacts. Some running is so pleasurable, however, and so unlikely to cause damage, the benefits outweigh the potential risks for our addicted runners.

As for anti-inflammatory drugs—ranging from over-the-counter drugs, such as Advil or Motrin to stronger prescription brands—these do work to reduce swelling and pain and are a godsend to many people suffering with arthritic symptoms. Yet the downsides must be managed as well. NSAIDs decrease collagen formation, leading to poor healing of soft-tissue injuries, and they inhibit bone formation, leading to stress fractures. Meanwhile, according to the American Gastroenterological Association, the serious side effects of NSAIDs, such as stomach bleeding, result in more than one hundred thousand hospitalizations and thousands of deaths each year in the US.

Additionally, when it comes to arthritis, NSAIDs can often exacerbate the problem by masking injuries that are sometimes fixable. A torn meniscus, for example, can lead to osteoarthritis, yet if it were treated, repaired, or replaced, it would diminish the arthritic damage that it produces in the joint. Where possible, it's best to address the cause of the arthritis by repairing the problem rather than taking painkillers to cover up the pain.

Some patients are able to improve their symptoms and cut down on their painkillers by taking supplements both orally, such as glucosamine, and by injection, such as hyaluronic acid. They help a subset, but not all, of patients with arthritis. Unfortunately, we cannot tell in advance who will benefit, yet trial and error with these treatments has no known downside. In our practice, before the addition of anabolic therapies including PRP and amniotic-fluid-derived growth factors and cytokines, approximately 30 percent of the patients were super responders to either glucosamine and/or hyaluronic acid injections or got up to a year of relief from a single injection. Thirty percent of our patients had a mixed response, and 30 percent seemed to gain no benefit. After we created a cocktail combining hyaluronic acid plus platelet-derived growth factors (PRP) from the patient, plus amniotic fluid, our efficacy in arthritic joints rose to 80 percent, with patients reporting significant symptom improvement at twelve months.

So go home and start exercising. Live long by being active.

Back Pain

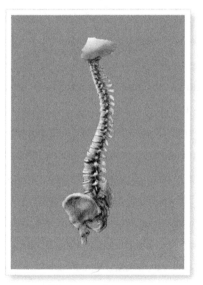

The bones of the spine

Low back pain connects with a special region in the brain and produces the fear that you will never be the same again. When we see a patient with back pain, the key questions we ask are, How and when did it happen? Is the pain localized to the low back, or does it radiate? Do you have numbness or weakness in the legs?

Assuming there wasn't a major accident or trauma to the back, the physician is trying to determine one of the following: Do you have a disc herniation that is pushing on the nerves that exit the back and go down the legs (sciatica)? Do you have bony narrowing in the spine from spurs or arthritis (stenosis)? Or is this more common, muscle-initiated back pain? (The most common things we find in a muscle physical exam are limitations of motion in the low back and tight hamstrings.) Other causes—like infections, tumors, and congenital problems—are rare.

If the exam and history of the back pain have a high probability of disc origin, an MRI is most helpful to shorten the process. A large, herniated disc pushing on the nerve root *may* respond to nonoperative measures but often does not. It is much faster to just remove the dislodged piece of disc through a minimally invasive outpatient surgery than to suffer with the pain for months.

Speaking of suffering, back pain that is not disc related falls into the realm of the Buddhist proverb that says, "pain is unavoidable, but suffering is optional." This is where the care plans get both interesting and controversial.

In the past, patients suffering from back pain were placed on bed rest with narcotic medication, often for weeks. There was nothing good about this treatment. Today, we focus on breaking the cycle of muscle injury, which leads to stiffness. The associated inflammation irritates the pain fibers, all of this creating fear and depression. This leads to even more limited activities, along with low testosterone or adrenaline stimulation. On top of all that, the common pain medications taken by many patients actually increase their depression.

Our preference is immediate, hands-on physical therapy, focusing on a range of treatments undertaken all at once. First, we work on mobilizing the stiff muscles and joints, contracting counterbalancing muscles. Selectively exercising them breaks the muscle spasm of the pain-generating muscles. Second, we use hands-on soft-tissue and muscle massage—focused on trigger points and fascial release—combined with manual traction. This directly relaxes both the treated muscle and the mind. Third, we supervise specific exercises that do not irritate the back but help the patient achieve a sweat workout—thereby increasing testosterone, adrenaline, pheromones, and a sense of well-being. Fourth, we have started a new program of injecting biologically active growth factors into the injured areas of the spine to naturally shut down the inflammation and hopefully induce healing.

Physical therapy should also focus on exercises to increase the function of lower back stabilization and to support muscles with vague names like the transverse abdominus and multifidi. It should also ensure you have adequate hip and upper back mobility. Stiffness and tightness above or below the lower back will add to the excessive pressure on the discs or nerve roots during movement. Performing daily tasks with proper body mechanics will also help reduce unnecessary pressure on the low back. Ideally, daily physical therapy should be taken advantage of until the episode is relieved. Pool, hot tub, and hot shower exercises help keep the therapeutic exercises going after the patient leaves the clinic.

For pain relief, alternating ice and heat, combined with acetaminophen and ibuprofen, are effective. With acute pain, having the physician add a shot of ketorolac (Toradol) can often immediately break the spasms.

People with back pain often suffer for a long time, and this changes

their lives. The key is immediate treatment. The faster that back pain
is relieved, the less likely it becomes a chronic problem. It is because
of both fear and the fact that the pain cycle is often left to "heal itself"
for weeks before treatment that the patterns become embedded, and
the pain raises to a level where it cannot be ignored. If you want back
pain behind you, deal with it up front.

Stress Fractures

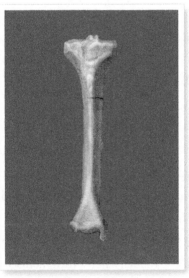

Stress fracture of the proximal tibia

Stress fractures happen to athletes at the worst of times. Usually, it is
just when they're increasing training, starting a new sport, or landing awkwardly from a jump. The bones of the feet and the shins are
most at risk, but occasionally the hip or spine is injured. The knee is
also exposed to such fractures, mostly during ligament ruptures and
after meniscus removals. Here is the current thinking on what to do.

When force exceeds the strength of the bone, a fracture occurs. Certain bones seem more susceptible—such as the small bones of the feet, which must accept a load of up to five times the body weight when a runner lands on one foot. These bones and the anterior cortex of the tibia (shin bone) see forces that exceed the mechanical ability to absorb them. When this happens, they may break rather than bend.

Knee injuries—especially those involving cruciate ligament ruptures—almost always bruise the bone. It is hard to have enough force to elongate the knee ligaments to the point that they rupture without smashing the tibia onto the femur (thigh bone). The hairline cracks and swelling that occur within the bone are best seen on MRIs. (Bone scans were commonly used in the past, until the radiation doses were realized to be toxic.)

Unfortunately, these kinds of bone injuries often cause long-term problems. First, they can take a long time to heal—even after the ligament surgery is completed. The bruises, which are essentially stress fractures, cause pain. The articular cartilage that overlies the bone is often damaged when the bone is impacted, and this damage can lead to post-traumatic arthritis.

It doesn't take the major force of a ligament rupture to produce a bone injury. In some patients, when a torn meniscus cartilage is surgically removed, the load on the tibia is now concentrated in a smaller zone. This can lead to a sudden breakdown of bone and cartilage called spontaneous osteonecrosis—often abbreviated as SPONK or SONK. We call these "knees that have gone to hell," since a patient who showed up six months earlier with a simple meniscus tear now returns with a severely painful arthritic knee.

The problem of a stress injury to the bone may be a much more important cause of later-stage arthritis than we previously realized.

For this reason, dramatic efforts to repair the bony lesions when they occur have grown in importance.

Bone injuries heal by recruiting bone-forming cells (osteoblasts), by suppression of bone-resorbing cells (osteoclasts), and by the orchestrated laying down of new bone. This coordination can be accelerated by subtle forces, including bone-specific magnetic waves, ultrasound, electrical current, and weight-bearing exercises. All of these stimulate cells to release bone-friendly growth hormones, peptides, and stem cell recruitment factors. These "chemical" agents can now be augmented by injecting the anabolic factors found in PRP, as well as from fat- and bone-derived progenitor cells, amniotic-fluid-derived growth factors, and other stimulants directly into the bone.

Abnormal forces bearing down on the joint surfaces can be modified in a number of ways. These include using heel wedge inserts that change the angle of the joint, osteotomies, or bone angle adjustment surgery, and braces that unload the joint, as well as gait and muscle training under the guidance of an expert physical therapist. If the meniscus cartilage in the knee is partially missing, it can be regrown with a collagen scaffold (CMI or collagen meniscus implant). If it is completely gone, a new meniscus from a donor can be inserted to rebalance the joint and distribute the loads more equitably. Recent long-term data from our research group has shown a seventeen-year benefit from meniscus replacement in cartilage-damaged knees, specifically when the articular cartilage is simultaneously repaired using a paste graft technique.

No single way has proved optimal for rapid healing of bone bruises and stress fractures. That's why we employ all of the techniques at once, when possible. The consequences of unhealed stress fractures are so severe that we now consider this problem a "bony emergency."

Stress fractures should produce stress in the medical system. Early repair will lead to later serenity.

Achilles Tendon

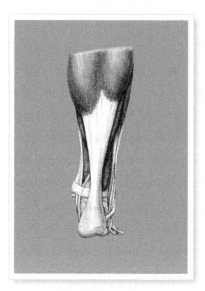

The Achilles tendon

Achilles tendons must have been rupturing since the time of Achilles. How else would every forty- to sixty-year-old male weekend warrior (and a number of pro basketball players) have learned to recognize and dread that classic gunshot sound of the tendon snapping?

The Achilles tendon is a broad, strong, fibrous band connecting the calf muscles to the heel. It is designed to stretch and contract, which permits a forceful push off from the foot while walking. It ruptures most commonly in males over fifty when landing from a basketball jump or lunging for an errant tennis ball. But it can also occur in elite athletes—like DeMarcus Cousins and Kevin Durant of the Golden State Warriors. In younger athletes and women, the tear is more commonly associated with the use of fluoroquinolone antibiotics such as Cipro (why this happens is unknown).

Why does it vex men in the fourth and fifth decades? The answer, like most in medicine, is multifactorial—an awful word that means "many contributing causes." Men traditionally play ballistic sports, at levels beyond what their fitness might warrant, well into their later years. A testosterone-driven, competitive edge pushes them to leap higher, land harder, and lunge further going for that shot that is just out of reach. Their risk factors seem clear.

What about women athletes? It's not fully understood. Though women are often also super fit, they are less likely than men to rupture their Achilles tendon. According to one study, the Achilles tendons of women may be more elastic than those of men, which may contribute to their reduced incidence of tearing.

While the Achilles tendon can potentially heal without surgery, the healing occurs with scar tissue filling in the rupture gap. This makes the tendon weaker. Few athletes want that outcome or the risk of the tendon not healing at all. Regarding surgery, medical debate focuses on whether or not to repair the tendon and whether to perform the repair using open or percutaneous, closed surgical techniques. We do not open the Achilles to repair it. When it ruptures, the sheath containing the tendon remains intact. The bleeding that occurs—with all of the progenitor cells and growth factors that blood brings—bathes the ruptured fiber ends. Many surgeons prefer the open technique so they can see the ends of the tendon, but open surgery dissipates those healing factors and causes scarring of the sheath. The percutaneous technique uses strong, absorbable sutures that we weave into the tissues through several small skin punctures.

The ends of the ruptured tendon are pulled together, permitting healing at the tendon's normal length. The sutures dissolve, and the tendon, sheath, and muscle-to-tendon length all return to normal. We see no reason to use permanent sutures, devices, or other implants that increase the risk of infection or scarring.

The frustrating part, however, is that the healing takes so long. We try to accelerate the process by adding growth factors and progenitor cells. Yet while it makes sense to do this, we still don't have the data to confirm that these interventions make a significant difference.

A second depressing factor is the degree of muscle atrophy we see in the calf during the healing time. The injury, the surgery itself, and the non-weight-bearing interval all conspire to weaken the calf muscles. While we try to exercise the quad and hamstrings—using stretch cords and other devices that isolate these muscles while not loading the calf muscles themselves—the leg weakness is still significant. Pharmaceutical interventions could prevent some of this, but these are still in the testing phase.

The Achilles tendon rupture remains a major injury with a slow recovery process. No wonder it is a feared event and a huge motivation for us to find better solutions. Achilles's mother didn't understand anatomy. If you are going to be dipped into the river Styx, ask your mom to hold you by the big toe, not the heel.

Calf Strains

Calf strains are in the air. No, not different kinds of baby cows, but the strained muscle kind that sidelines great basketball players like Kevin Durant. Here is what is known and new about them.

The calf muscles are primarily the two heads of the gastrocnemius and the deeper soleus muscle. They connect to the foot through the Achilles tendon. Strains of the muscle are code words for tearing. When it is just the muscle that tears, treatments do not involve surgery. When the tendon tears, most commonly we repair it with a percutaneous (through the skin) tendon repair. Open surgery is rarely required.

Calf muscle strains (i.e., tears of varying degrees) are defined by muscle fiber separation. They usually occur after landing awkwardly from a jump or a sudden push off in a sprint—actions where the muscle contraction is more forceful than the individual fibers can withstand. Small amounts of fiber disruption are called mild sprains. The more fibers disrupted, the more severe the label—moderate, severe, or complete rupture. In top athletes trying to hide the severity of their injury, the "strain" label is often used when, in fact, there is a complete tear of the muscle—or even worse, of the tendon attached to it.

Muscle injuries, unlike tendon or ligament ruptures, are typically followed by profuse bleeding, inflammation, remodeling, and regeneration. Muscles have an abundant blood supply, so that when the fibers tear, there is an immediate rush of blood to the site of injury, and with the blood comes stem and reparative cells. While one might think this would lead to rapid healing, the repair cells directing such healing are in fact inhibited by unique cells that lay down scar tissue rather than normal muscle fibers. The healing of the muscle is initially somewhat disordered, and only over time—with exercise and hormonal stimulation—can it be remodeled. Exercise induces hypertrophy (enlargement) of the muscle fibers while the hormones, with their specialized growth factors, direct individual fiber regeneration.

Until recently, it was believed that most injured muscles could not be fully restored to normal. This misconception has been overturned by encouraging studies of heart muscles. After the heart's blood supply is temporarily interrupted (which is called myocardial infarction), injured heart muscles have been restored with a direct injection of stem cells.

So the calf strain is really a "mini model" of every injury and of most repair processes. And the treatment is evolving. We are moving beyond rest, ice, and anti-inflammatories to a more active protocol that includes controlled exercise to induce remodeling. The goal is to induce more rapid tissue regeneration by treatments such as alternating ice and heat to improve blood flow and injections of tissue-specific growth factors to recruit muscle-specific stem cell derived cells to the site of injury.

As long as a calf strain is *really* a strain—rather than a complete tear of the muscle and tendon requiring surgical repair—nonoperative interventions can cure the injury. Only the athlete, agent, surgeon, and MRI know for sure. In Kevin Durant's case, the proof is in the jumping.

Leg Curvature

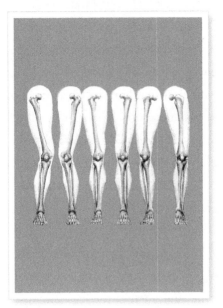

Knock knees, straight legs, and bowlegs

The fastest runners in the world often have bowed legs and toes that point in. Football running backs are all bowlegged. Many football linemen, who must squat and be forceful, are neutral to knock-kneed.

If so many great athletes have these leg angles, why do doctors so often recommend to the rest of us a "corrective" osteotomy: a cutting of the tibia, and occasionally the femur, to change the alignment of their legs?

Because of arthritis and dogma. People have curvature in the legs for a number of reasons. Some are born with curved legs, become great athletes, and never have a problem. Other people with bowed legs or knock-knees develop significant pain, particularly when they lose their cartilage shock absorbers. For many, the curvature worsens over time as a result of gradual cartilage loss and development of arthritis in one side of the knee, usually after an injury. The legs either become bowed or knock-kneed, consistent with either an inside or outside meniscus and articular cartilage loss. Like an engine that is out of tune, the wear patterns dramatically accelerate.

Loss of the meniscus and articular cartilage often happens to the young when playing sports. Traditionally, the torn meniscus is partially removed or the damaged articular cartilage shaved smooth. While we have always known that this cartilage loss leads to the arthritis pain of later life and to the subsequent curvature of the bones, there weren't alternatives.

Orthopaedic surgery students are taught that bad biomechanics will destroy good biology any day of the week. So if a patient complains of knee pain with bowed legs, the recommendation has often been to change the alignment of the legs and distribute more force to the center or the outside of the knee. Or if a patient has injured their weight-bearing surface articular cartilage or lost a portion of their meniscus cartilage, traditional orthopaedic advice is to rearrange the tibia, a procedure called an osteotomy—a polite term for cutting the bone in half and wedging it open. The foot is pushed over to the centerline, a plate and screws are applied, and six months of healing begins. This technique is designed to straighten the leg and make the person attached to it put more weight on the opposite side of the knee, hopefully reducing the wear, tear, and pain in the affected side.

While many patients and doctors have been happy with this, my view is that the real problem is the loss of the cartilage shock absorbers that led to the curvature. Therefore, it makes much more sense, and involves much less risk, to replace the missing tissues. Tissue replacement partially corrects the curvature, relieves the pain, and most importantly, can restore the person to sports activities without the risk of the osteotomy or angle-changing procedures.

In fact, data published by our research group demonstrated no effect of "mal-alignment" on the improvement in pain and function in arthritic patients who underwent meniscus cartilage replacement with articular cartilage repair.[18] At the end of the study, 79 percent of the 120 patients were still enjoying all the benefits of their meniscus replacement up to twelve years from surgery, independent of the amount of curvature in their legs. Based on the results seen up to the end of the study, we estimated that patients can expect an average of nearly ten years of pain and function improvements if they have the cartilage replaced before having to consider joint replacement. (Our current data now shows that this is seventeen years of improvement.) Next we went back and looked at our most active high-level athletic patients and found that they too were able to enjoy the same (in fact better) long-lasting benefits from meniscus transplantation. Again, the amount of curvature in the legs did not affect the outcome.

So, in my view, while I understand that curved legs lead to bad biomechanical alignment, and that this abnormal pressure can ruin good biology, it is better to repair the bad biology first and see if the repair is good enough. Why? Because realigning the legs of people who have lived with their curvatures all their lives is asking for trouble with not just their knees, but with all the rest of the body that has grown up with their unique shapes. And trouble does happen. In one major study, the complications of leg realignment (loss of motion,

---

[18] Kevin R. Stone et al., "Long-term survival of concurrent meniscus allograft transplantation and repair of the articular cartilage: a prospective two- to 12-year follow-up report," *The Journal of Bone and Joint Surgery* 92 no. 7 (2010): 941–948, https://pubmed.ncbi.nlm.nih.gov /20595111/.

infection, pain, stiffness) occurred in up to 40 percent of corrections.[19] While infection can occur in any surgery, if it occurs in cartilage replacement procedures, the knee can be washed out and the process started over. It is not so easy for bony procedures.

The knee joint does poorly after cartilage injury and loss. Fortunately, we have now become experienced in replacement and regeneration of these crucial tissues. It is now possible to solve these problems as soon as they arise rather than waiting for the inevitable increased curvatures and arthritis with pain and loss of function. Ultimately, the solution is to repair, regenerate, or replace the missing or injured tissues when they first present with injury. If this becomes the standard of care, we will not be "correcting" the curved legs after the cartilage horse has left the barn.

---

[19] Bruce Miller et al., "Patient satisfaction after medial opening high tibial osteotomy and microfracture," *The Journal of Knee Surgery* 20 no. 2 (April 2007), DOI: 10.1055/s-0030-1248031.

CHAPTER 5

FOCUS ON YOUR JOINTS: KNEES

The magical knee joint combines the femur of the thigh, the tibia of the shin, and the patella of the knee cap. These bones are tied together with the primary ligaments: the anterior and posterior cruciates, and the medial and lateral collaterals. The bones are covered by shiny, white articular cartilage and protected by soft, fibrous meniscus tissues. The joint is surrounded by a capsule with a wonderful lining called the synovium, which produces lubricants that keep the joint moving. The entire complex bears your weight over two to three million steps per year for a lifetime, and up to five times the body weight when you land from a jump. If it is not injured or affected by a disease, the joint can tolerate a lifetime of running. Unfortunately, once any one of these key structures are injured, the entire joint is placed at risk of degeneration. Here are a few of the common injuries and novel thinking about them.

BIOLOGIC TREATMENTS

Anterior Cruciate Ligament (ACL)

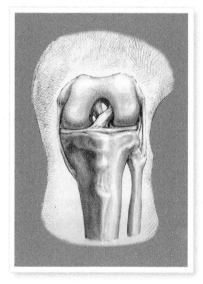

The knee joint

The ACL is a broad, thick cord the size of your index finger, with long collagen strands woven together in a way that allows it to withstand up to five hundred pounds of force in young, healthy people. It connects the thigh bone to the shin bone and is a key stabilizer of your knee, guiding your tibia (shin bone) through a normal, stable range of motion. When the ACL tears, it unravels like a braided rope and does not heal on its own.

The ACL is the most commonly injured ligament in the knee—three hundred thousand tears each year in the US alone. Females, for many different reasons, are more likely to injure their ACL than males. People often tear the ACL by twisting the knee while changing direction rapidly, slowing down from running, or landing from a jump. The thigh bone moves past where the ligament can stretch, producing the famous "pop." Once broken, it may partially heal to the surrounding tissues, but the ligament rarely regains its normal connections. While some patients have "ACL independent" knees and don't develop significant instability after rupture, most athletic people need their ACL to provide stability and to protect the meniscus tissues that rest upon the tibial plateau. Left unstable, approximately 80 percent of injured people will eventually go on to develop meniscus tears and 50 percent will develop knee joint arthritis.

Once torn, the optimal time to restore stability is immediately. While there has been considerable debate about the timing of surgery, all collagen-based tissues start scarring and shrinking within minutes of tearing. The ACL fibers are similar to a climbing rope, which once stretched past their limit, suffer from internal disruptions of most of the fibers—even when the outside sheath looks intact.

Efforts to perform suture repair of the torn ACL tissue have had only selective success, despite efforts to add scaffolds, stem cells, and growth factors to the injured tissue. And those limited successes were obtained only when most of the ligament was still intact, acting as a scaffold to which the injured tissues could adhere.

In my hands, primary repair works well when the tear is partial, located near the ligament origin on the femur, and the patients are older. Young, healthy, aggressive males rarely protect their primary repairs long enough to provide a successful outcome. Future devices most likely will be designed to work as temporary ligaments while inducing normal tissue remodeling.

In the initial assessment of ACL injuries, a common diagnostic error is missing associated knee injuries when confronted with the more obvious ACL rupture. When the ACL ruptures, more than just the ACL is stretched. The most common secondary injuries involve the meniscus, the articular cartilage, and the secondary ligamentous tissues, such as the outside back corner of the knee. If these tissues are ignored or resected, and not surgically repaired, the knees fail quickly.

ACL reconstructions with patients' own tissues—usually hamstring or patella tendon grafts—have not evolved very much. In the twenty-first century, we should not be taking one part of a person to rebuild another part. The harvesting of patients' tissues permanently damages and weakens their knees, sacrificing normal anatomy. Surgical techniques have improved, and most surgeons have the tools to replace the original ligament anatomically—with tissue at its origin on the femur and insertion point on the tibia—to avoid the errors of placement that led to failure in the past.

Surgeons' traditional reconstruction techniques involve taking away a part of the patellar tendon at the front of the knee or the hamstring tendons at the back and side of the knee. Harvesting those critical tissues induces a second injury to the patient, resulting in permanent weakness and abnormal knee mechanics. The body of evidence shows that using one part of a patient's knee to fix another part is a bad idea. This is driving both the increasing use of donor tissue and the search for better alternatives.

Many surgeons and patients choose to use the patient's own tissue because they believe that donor tissues have a higher failure rate than autogenous tissues. I disagree with this logic. Donor tissues may have a higher rupture rate if the tissues are not of ideal quality and anatomically placed. Thirty percent of people under twenty re-rupture their ACL-reconstructed knee within a few years, irrespective of whether donor tissue or their own tissue was used. Given this high repeat injury rate of young people with ACL injuries, I would prefer that my patient reinjure the donated tissue instead of their own. Harvesting their own tissue produces a guaranteed second injury to knees that never fully recover, and may be associated with a higher arthritis rate from tissue harvest and resulting leg weakness.

The pressing questions are: Why are we still robbing Peter to pay Paul by harvesting one part of the knee to fix another? Why are ligaments taking a full year to remodel? Why is there still a high reinjury rate? And why so much arthritis? Can't we put in tissues that are stronger and able to resist this devastating injury?

Allograft (donor) tissue is increasing in ACL reconstruction surgery. The tissue, when harvested from young donors (usually people who die from motorcycle accidents or gunshot wounds), is very rarely rejected. However, the industry is not well regulated, and a variety of tissues and tissue sterilization treatments exist—producing a mixed bag of quality. For example, if irradiation is used to sterilize tissue, it is permanently weakened. Certain tissue—such as a graft from the patella tendon (called bone-patellar tendon-bone)—is much stronger than tissue from hamstrings or Achilles tendons, which are designed to stretch during normal walking. These tissues have poorer outcomes when used to reconstruct an ACL (which is not designed to stretch).

In our experience, the use of bone-patellar tendon-bone donor tissue is the best choice for now. Bone-patellar tendon-bone taken from animal tissue, called Z-Lig, was tested successfully in Europe and South Africa in a rigorous prospective double-blind trial. The tissue had been treated to remove the key antigens that cause rejection. The US trial for approval has not yet begun. The addition of growth factors and stem cells to donor tissue is also under investigation in our facility and others.

The hope is that stem-cell-derived progenitor cells and growth factors will accelerate the healing of ACL donor grafts, and that improved collagen structures created in the lab will be better than the native ACL. Animal tissues that are stronger than human tissues (and treated to reduce rejection) will play a role. Faster healing and stronger grafts should lead to better joint protection.

We also now understand how to diminish arthritis by repairing and replacing the missing meniscus and regrowing the damaged articular cartilage within the knee. Altogether, these efforts to biologically replace the knee joint have already made a difference. We are aggressively working on improving these approaches, as the current state of the ACL surgery art is still a work in progress.

When Your Knee Goes
Snap, Crackle, Pop

A question I am asked a lot is, "When I hear clicking and popping in my knee, is this something I should be concerned about?"

Joint noise in the form of crackling, clicking, or popping is very common. It may be from simple soft-tissue catching, or more serious damage to the bearing surface of the joint, the articular cartilage. It occurs not just in knees but also in ankles, hips, and shoulders. Here are the messages the percussionists in your joints communicate to me.

Snaps. Snaps are most often the clicking of a scar tissue band over the edge of the upper thigh bone (the femur). These are usually not serious, though they can sometimes be painful. Scar bands can respond to physical therapy; soft-tissue manipulation stimulates collagen cells to produce collagenase, which breaks down scar tissue and can also promote collagen formation in the healing process. Manual therapy is highly effective for many snaps.

Crackles. Muscles attach to bones through tendons. The tendons are covered in thin sheaths, which normally provide smooth gliding surfaces. When these sheaths get irritated, they swell, and the thickened tissue increases the resistance for the tendon. The pulling and sliding of tendons against the swollen tissue of these inflamed sheaths produce crackles, which can be both felt and heard. When severe, this is called crepitus. The patellar tendon and the pes anserine tendons—the insertions of the hamstrings on the inner side of the knee—are most susceptible. Treatment is by ice, massage, injection of growth factors called PRP, and anti-inflammatory medications. We no longer inject cortisone into these tendons as the cortisone weakens them and can lead to rupture.

Pops. Popping when you pull your knuckle is a release of gas from the joint. This is different from the knee pop. When a pop is loud enough, it's usually caused by a piece of tissue getting caught between bones—often a torn piece of meniscus, or a loose body being pushed out from between the femur and the tibia.

"Doc, I hurt my knee and heard a pop, and then my knee swelled." When I hear this from a patient, I know the injury is potentially serious. Overwhelming data reveals that with a popping sound at the time of injury and subsequent swelling, the patient has almost certainly injured either ligaments—anterior cruciate ligament, posterior cruciate ligament, or medial collateral liga-ment—or the meniscus or articular cartilage. Ninety percent of the time, surgical repair of the injured tissues will be required for the optimal outcome—especially when pops are associated with pain or are reproducible during an exam. So pay attention to the pops!

Grinds. A common cause of grinding is loss of smooth articular cartilage in the kneecap (the patella) due to a previous injury or arthritis. The rough bone underneath, or the fragmented cartilage bits themselves, grind against the top of the femur (the trochlea).

Put your hand on your kneecap and do a squat. You can feel (and often hear) the grind. It can also happen between the femur and the tibia, usually after the meniscus cartilage has been torn or removed. Such grinding eventually leads to pain and often swelling.

This is due to the small bits of cartilage being sprayed around the joint during the grind, which land in the joint capsule. Fluid is produced in response to this irritation. The knee swells, limiting the range of motion. Grinds are not good in coffee *or* in knee joints.

So what are your knees saying to you? Often, nothing at all. Most of the time, these noises are natural and do not mean you will develop arthritis or be prone to injury. When popping sounds are accompanied by swelling and pain, or they produce a catching sensation, or the joint gives way, these are times when we worry about a possible injury. A physician should examine you to make a clear diagnosis.

If there is pain, swelling, or giving way of the knee, we will do a careful exam, history, and an X-ray and/or an MRI to study the cartilage and the soft tissue within the knee and determine if the tissues need to be repaired. If the important tissues of the knee are torn, we will plan to repair that tissue. When key tissues are not torn, careful physical therapy, sometimes combined with growth factor injections, can often fix the problem and help you avoid surgery.

So remember, if you hear clicks and pops in your knee but feel no pain or swelling, don't worry. It is normal. If you have pain, instability, or swelling, make sure you check it out to avoid further damage to the joint. The philosophy on this has changed from "rest your knee and wait until you are older for a joint replacement" to fixing the problem by repairing or replacing the missing cartilage immediately—so that you may never develop arthritis or need a knee replacement.

Why ACL Repairs Fail

For decades, efforts to repair the ACL after rupture have been unsuccessful. This is because the forces required to tear the complex weave of the ACL's collagen fibers involve both tearing and pulling apart. Think of a climbing rope. When overstretched, the rope fails within its sheath, not just at a single clean edge. Here is why the ruptured anterior cruciate ligament is most often replaced (reconstructed) rather than repaired.

The ACL stretches from the femur to the tibia, guiding the knee through its range of motion. The fibers are interspersed with blood vessels, nerves, and cells that provide life and sensation to the ligament. To rupture it, the tibia must shift forward, often with abnormal excessive rotation.

Imagine if you were inside this ligament during a ski fall. You would first see and feel the majority of the fibers around you tightening rapidly and stretching to their limit. Then—at different areas along the length of the taut ligament—breaks would occur: first at the shortest fibers, then twisting up through the rope-like structure with each sequential fiber giving way. Depending on the position of the tibia at the moment of impact, and the relative strength of the bone versus the ligament, the majority of the torn fibers might be close to the femur, close to the tibia, or in between. In any case, most of the fibers would have experienced forces that come close to or exceed their stretching limits.

With milder injuries, the sheath surrounding the ACL may stay intact, holding the unfortunate ends of the once beautiful, interwoven fiber linkages. But if the sheath ruptures, you may see (from your viewpoint inside this ligament) the joint fill with blood. The ruptured blood vessels then leak their fluid into the injury, causing swelling and pushing apart the native structure. Almost as fast as the rupture occurs, the body's defenses respond to the alarm. The brain sends protective signals to splint the joint with the surrounding structures. Stem cells—those that live within the joint, and those called into action by the chemicals and proteins released by the cells of the ACL—rush to the site. Other cells, designed to remove damaged fibers and lay down scar tissue, also race to the injury. But just as the ends of a frayed rope shrink when a lit match is held to them, the fibers of the ACL retract. And without the natural tension of being strung from one end to the other, the body's ineffective repair process leads to shortened, scarred tissue. This is often attached to the nearby posterior cruciate ligament like gum stuck to a wall.

Enter the young surgeon into this bloody field of disarray. He or she arrives with the knowledge that ACL reconstruction is often performed by using part of the patient's own knee, the patellar tendon, or the hamstrings. Though these procedures are often relatively successful, harm is done to the donor—and follow-up visits show a disappointing level of reinjury and arthritis down the line. This leads to the unfortunate decision to simply repair the frayed "rope." Sutures are put in place, while clots of blood or combinations of resorbable collagen are stuffed between the ruptured ends of the ligament and femur from which the ACL originates—all in the hope that this complex structure will magically reform itself.

Yet, over the past one hundred years, study after study has shown that while certain very small tears of the ACL (generally in women over the age of forty) can be healed effectively with sutures and scaffolds, all the others stretch out the repair over time—leaving the knee vulnerable to reinjury when the patient returns to sports. My own experience with suturing ligaments, in the enthusiasm of my early career, led to exactly the same results. A few do very well. Most do not.

The reason is obvious. The forces involved in rupturing the ACL —a key linkage between very large bones—do damage to the entire ligament. The human body's repair process cannot effectively recreate this ligament, except under perfect tension and biologic conditions. Suturing a cruciate ligament, even with an additional scaffold, does not solve the majority of the joint's problems. The solution lies in better replacement tissues, better surgery, and better rehabilitation techniques.

ACL Disasters in Football

ACL injuries in professional football are on the rise. The injury is at least as serious as the "concussion" disaster story we've been hearing about, but players haven't changed behaviors that often lead to knee damage. The outcomes may be even worse than from head injuries.

Each year, there are about thirty ACL injuries in the NFL—that's in the preseason alone. The upward trend continues possibly due to bigger, faster players. Conventional wisdom maintains that strengthening leg muscles will protect the knee, but this clearly doesn't hold true with mass and power increases. No one in athletics is stronger than American football players, yet they rupture their ligaments regularly.

Braces to protect the knee have never worked, despite brace manufacturers' best efforts to market them as "protective gear." The braces strap onto the large muscles of the thigh and calf in an attempt to limit ligament rupturing during extremes of motion. The knee joint must bend and rotate to function normally. However, there simply is no external brace that can control the motion of the femur on the tibia without being screwed into the bone itself. Other than using braces for resistance to bruises and providing warmth, athletes in most sports—including skiing—have given them up. Surgeons use them only temporarily in the immediate postoperative period.

A pro football player's average career length is only three years, and an ACL injury is not benign. Fifty percent of people with

ACL injuries develop osteoarthritis within ten years, whether or not they have surgery. At the end of the day, losing a key structure that guides the knee causes devastation to normal knee mechanics. Twenty-seven million Americans have knee arthritis after soft-tissue injuries. While it's true that concussions may lead to brain degeneration in some athletes, ACL injuries occur three hundred thousand times a year in the US alone and lead to arthritis that now affects millions of people. Concussions can be debilitating, but arthritis always is. Both need better care.

ACL Recovery: Why Does It Take So Long?

When San Francisco 49ers quarterback Jimmy Garoppolo tore his ACL in the second game of the 2018 season, the immediate verdict was, "He's out for the season. He'll be back next year." When Klay Thompson fell in the Toronto Raptors championship series in 2019, rupturing his ACL, fans felt the same resignation, wondering: Will he ever return? If so, at what level?

Why does it take so long to recover from a simple ligament rupture? Answer: it's not just the injury; it's the surgery, the muscle atrophy, the lost neurologic connections that lead to coordination, and the mindset, part of which is fear of reinjury.

The injury, the tearing of the ACL from the bone or the rupture of it in the middle of the ligament, sets off a cascade of biologic consequences. Immediately the brain is informed of the rupture by the complex signaling of pain fibers. Often athletes note that there wasn't much pain with the injury, just a pop or a sickening feeling when the tibia shifted unnaturally on the femur. Within the ACL, there are mechanoreceptors attached to nerves that convey not just pain but also proprioception, or the knowledge of where the joint is in space. The sickening feeling so often reported by patients may be the brain recognizing the disruption of the normal signals from the knee joint structures. Chemical signals travel from the ruptured tissue through the blood vessels that penetrate the ligament as well as from the hypersensitive joint lining called the synovium. The ruptured ligament cells are recognized by the synovium, which then releases its own macrophages to rush to the site of injury and initiate the repair process. The patient often perceives this release of stored cells as joint swelling.

Combining all of these biochemical and neurologic events leads to two other debilitating consequences. First, the brain and other tissues release stress hormones, predominantly cortisol. Among other reactions, this hormone binds to muscle cells in the leg, and within eight hours, muscle atrophy begins. Why this occurs is not known, but this is one of the more discouraging aspects of an ACL injury. It takes a year to rebuild lost muscle. Two major stress events lead to muscle loss: the initial injury and the surgery itself. If the patient's own tissues are used to repair the ACL, a second round of pain, stress hormone release, and muscle atrophy ensues.

Lastly but importantly, fear enters the brain. Fear of the loss of sports activity, fear of reinjury, fear of surgery, worries that the body will never be the same again…and other rational fears. Overcoming these reactions often determines the timeline for return to sports and is a major reason why so many athletes never return to the same level of performance after an ACL injury.

A number of athletes have chosen to ignore their ACL injuries and have returned to play in a few weeks. Unfortunately, they often go on to tear their meniscus cartilage and stretch other ligaments around the knee joint.

ACL recovery takes many months because the new tissue used to replace the native ACL is tendon, not ligament. The tendon tissue undergoes "remodeling," meaning that blood vessels grow into it, cells are released, old collagen is broken down, and new collagen fibers replace it. Gradually the tendon graft turns into a ligament. This process, called ligamentization, takes up to a year, and the tissue is weakened when the vessels penetrate it. Speeding up ligamentization is a major goal of the new anabolic therapies using growth factors and cells.

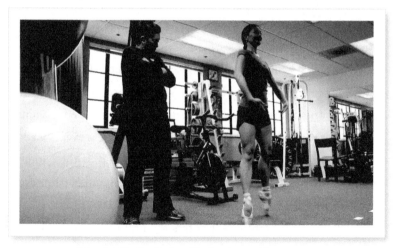

Natalya V. • Professional ballet dancer & instructor
after ACL repair by Dr. Stone

Doctors are developing novel approaches to combating proprioception loss, muscle atrophy, and fear responses. We focus on reducing swelling, accelerating tissue healing by introducing stem cells and growth factors, and introducing neurofeedback through balance training, sometimes using virtual reality headsets. Muscle atrophy may be partially preventable by blocking muscle receptors. This is a work in progress.

Artificial ligaments remain popular in some areas of Europe, Australia, and Asia for top-level professional athletes. While most artificial ligaments will fail over time, they often permit the athlete to return to sports activity in the same season. They have not yet caught on in the US, although research is ongoing. Given the amount of money and prestige on the line for NFL quarterbacks, for example, it is easy to see how pro players might favor this choice.

Xenograft ligaments using pig tissue were approved in Europe (after extensive testing here at our clinic and a wide clinical trial outside the US) and are awaiting commercialization. Pig tissue can be stronger than human tissue, and thus it may help prevent second-site surgeries sometimes needed when a patients' own tissue is used as graft material. Remodeling would still need to occur over the course of a year.

Related injuries also slow the recovery process. Often the corner of the knee is stretched with an ACL injury. If this is not identified and repaired, it can lead to a high ACL failure rate. If the meniscus tissue is torn, it too must be repaired, and if a significant piece is removed, the knee is doomed to develop arthritis.

The state of the art is not very artful, unfortunately. The best treatment would involve immediate repair of all injured tissues with augmented rapid healing. We are developing combinations of better tissues loaded with stem cells, better scaffolds for regrowing tissues that are partially torn, and novel artificial materials that may support regeneration while functioning immediately as successful replacements.

For now, the quarterback's choice is to either go short for a sure gain with an artificial ligament—providing immediate stability but an uncertain future—or to go long with natural tissues from their own bodies or donor tissues, augmented by growth factors and progenitor cells, and hope for the best. Which would you choose?

Opt In

I f all of us were organ donors, there would not be a shortage of the life-saving tissues that go to waste every day. I'm talking about more than kidneys, hearts, and lungs. Orthopaedic tissues, such as meniscus and articular cartilage, are also in short supply. Here is a little insight into a solvable problem.

Opting in takes an act of mild courage and intention. You must choose to donate your tissues upon death. Because so few take this step, other people languish on waiting lists, often dying before the tissue they need becomes available. The numbers are staggering. Some 120,000 people are on waiting lists for organ donation in the US each year.

The choice to opt out makes one feel a little guilty about wasting one's organs and allowing them to rot in a cemetery or be burned up in a crematorium. But in places such as Austria, the United Kingdom, and Chile—where everyone is automatically opted in—90 percent of people are organ donors.

Donated organs, as well as non-life-saving tissues, are badly needed here in America. This need not be the case. In the US, approximately 10,000–25,000 healthy young people, all potential organ donors, die each year. If each had a pair of healthy knee joints, as many as 20,000–50,000 medial and lateral meniscus cartilages could be made available for donation each year. But they are not, and so there is a shortage.

In the US currently, only about two thousand meniscus transplants are performed annually. Clearly, there is a large and unmet need. There are several reasons for this sorry state of affairs. First, though, it's important to know that the actual cost of harvesting a meniscus from a cadaver is no higher today than it was ten years ago. The cadavers are donated for free, so the costs are mainly for harvesting (and dozens of other tissues, such as hearts, lungs, eyes, and bone, are harvested at the same time), testing for infectious disease, packaging, and storing. FedEx distributes the tissue, often with an extra charge given directly to the recipient.

So why the shortage? Because the worldwide demand for meniscus tissues and other orthopaedic reconstructions is soaring, and US tissue banks can sell their donated tissues to overseas surgeons and hospitals at a hefty premium, especially since most other countries do not have regulated tissue banks of our quality.

All of this has vastly inflated the cost of a donor meniscus replacement. Tissue banks have increased the price from around $1,500 in 2010 to approximately $5,000 today. Even so, it sometimes takes months to supply the tissue.

That brings us to another sad part of this story: it is unclear if those Americans who *do* opt in would want to see their donated tissues distributed randomly around the world (and sold for a high markup). While we are a generous nation, when there is a real shortage here at home, I think most people would want to see their fellow Americans' needs met first.

Tissue donation, and the use of these tissues to replace injured parts, is an important field that needs wide utilization and improvement. We, along with other research sites, are actively engaged in teaching surgeons the techniques of meniscus transplantation, educating doctors and patients about the importance of replacing the tissue as soon as it is removed, and adding stem cells, progenitor cells, growth factors, and other additives to these tissues to help incorporate them into their recipients in a faster and stronger manner. These programs will not advance, however, if the costs of tissue acquisition are pushed so high that few surgeons use them, insurance companies balk at the high cost, and tissue banks focus only on the highest bidders.

One solution: make opting in as an organ donor universal, so that you must opt *out* to not be a donor. Overwhelm the system with supply, train surgeons to replace tissues, and convince patients to reject a "wait until my body falls apart" attitude. Today, in the twenty-first century, we should not be taking tissue from one part of an injured person's body to replace another part when off-the-shelf tissues could be ubiquitous and effective.

The Posterior Cruciate Ligament (PCL)

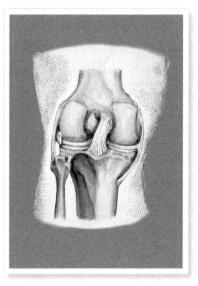

The knee joint from behind showing the posterior cruciate ligament,
meniscus cartilages and collateral ligaments

The knee is tied together by more than just the anterior cruciate ligament (ACL), though you might not know that from hearing regular reports of ACL injuries from football, soccer, basketball, and skiing. The "other" ligaments matter just as much, and though injured less frequently, their care and feeding determine the function of the knee.

The posterior cruciate ligament (PCL) extends from the back of the tibia to the front of the femur, inside the knee. It stops the tibia from going backwards when hit from the front, and it guides the rotation of the knee in synchrony with the ligaments that surround it. The PCL is often ruptured in car accidents when the knee hits the dashboard and in ski accidents when knees are impacted in wild falls. For years, surgeons advised patients to live with their injured ligament as repair or reconstruction were difficult and the disability was not too bad. Yet over time, those untreated knees degraded, arthritis set in, and knee replacements ensued.

Today we understand that the PCL can sometimes be repaired. This is done with sutures anchored to the bone (when partially torn) or reconstructed with donor tissues (when completely ruptured). The best repairs and reconstructions are those done immediately after the injury when the tissues are fresh and the joint is not further stretched out. Insertions of the PCL extend over such a wide area that it has become mandatory to use large tissue replacements to get an optimum result. The more collagen and the thicker the tissue used in these insertions, the better. And the sooner the better because over time, the PCL tissues scar down, and the supporting structures become stretched out.

Our donor tissues are now preloaded with anabolic growth factors from both concentrated blood (PRP) and from amniotic tissues containing growth factors at the time of implantation. It is believed that by boosting the early healing response, the thick replacement tissues may heal faster, though the definitive data is not yet in.

It has become clear that a PCL injury is rarely an isolated injury. If there is enough force on the knee joint to rupture this key structure, then it is likely that other supporting ligaments and tissues have also given way. We rarely see a torn PCL without an injury to the corners of the knee. These typically occur in the posterolateral corner which, if ignored, leaves the patient with only a partially functioning knee. Meniscus tissues are also frequently torn along with the PCL and are best treated with an immediate suture repair. Left alone, they become more degenerated and less repairable.

In sum, the knee joint works because a wide range of tissues collaborate to guide the joint through a complex series of rotations and flexion that encompass normal knee motion. As we deepen our understanding of the relationships between the tissues, we appreciate how important it is to restore *all* of the supporting actors when the lead actor is obviously disabled. And once repaired—unless the tissues are then rehabilitated with exercises that stimulate normal maturation—scar tissue forms, degrading the final outcome.

There are no simple knee injuries that are big enough to tear a key guiding ligament. As MRI imaging techniques improve and mechanical testing becomes more refined, our surgical tasks will increase in complexity. Beware of insurance companies and healthcare guidelines that limit repairs and restrict rehabilitation, that insist on generalist surgeons and not specialists, and that delay the time of injury repair. They may seem simple and cost-effective for the payer, but they doom the patient to an unnecessary lifetime of disabilities. Cost-effective can often become health-defective.

Steph Curry's Knees

W hen the Golden State Warriors take the court, their speed and precision is second to none. You watch the ball; I watch the knees. Both are doing remarkable things, especially under the guidance of point guard Steph Curry. Here is what's happening from an orthopaedic surgeon's perspective.

Curry plays an average of thirty-four minutes each game. Players take about 175 steps per minute during a game. So, in Curry's case, that's 5,950 steps per game. (While calculated measurements of professional basketball players' steps per minute or per game vary, I am using reported averages.) While he is running (which is most of those steps), he lands on a single leg, with a force up to three times his body weight. If Curry's playing weight is 185 pounds, that's up to 550 pounds of force with each step distributed through his feet, knees, and lower body. Now you know another reason why the coach limits the minutes Curry is on the floor.

When Curry jumps—and he makes at least twenty jump-shot attempts per game—he lands with even greater force. (Fortunately, he usually lands on both legs.)

To the surprise of many, the cartilage of the knee joints (and other joints of our bodies) can take these forces without developing arthritis. Unless the joint is injured, there is no evidence that the forces of running or jumping damage carti-lage. This remarkable substance is made up of collagen fibers and a sugar matrix that absorb and release water with every compression. The natural lubricants of the joint, hyaluronic acid and lubricin, are ultra-slippery. As long as those surfaces stay intact, the stresses of sports are handled well.

Weight matters. A ten-pound increase can add up to fifty pounds on each knee joint during the two to three million steps people typically take each year. Curry compensates for his increased weight by increasing his musculature. The muscles, when well developed, can shield the joints to a degree by absorbing the energy of the jumps and landings. Coordination matters too. Watch Curry hit the court after a shot: he lands softly. Years of training to be smooth in the jump shot and coordinated in all the running motions diminishes off-balance or awkward landings and disperses the forces on the joints evenly.

It is when an injury occurs—such as a torn meniscus, a nick in the surface of the cartilage, or a torn ACL—that the mechanics of the joint become abnormal. Unless the compromised element is repaired or replaced immediately, degradation, called traumatic arthritis, sets in. Much of the new era of orthopaedics involves the biologic replacement of such damaged cartilage. This includes the meniscus and the ligaments, in addition to the lubricants, growth factors, and cells that restore health to the joints.

For Curry, the key is to not get injured in the first place, and if he does, to repair the damage and replace the injured tissues promptly. For the rest of us, building muscle to protect the joints, thereby improving our fitness to diminish the chances of injury, are our best tools. We have remarkable bodies with capabilities that exceed our wildest imaginations. But their vulnerabilities must inspire us to train, prepare, and enjoy every day. We may not be the athletic equals of Steph Curry, but there's a lot of warrior in every one of us.

The Medial Collateral Ligament (MCL)

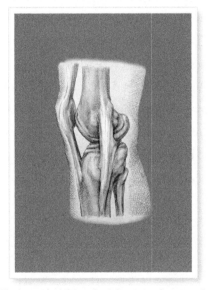

The knee joint from the side view, showing the medial collateral ligament

The medial collateral ligament (MCL) is the third major ligament of the knee. It is a broad, flat, membranous band, situated slightly posterior (back) on the medial (inner) side of the knee joint and extending from the thigh bone to the shin bone. It stops the joint from opening like a book, yet permits enough freedom for the joint to both bend and extend fully.

The ligament has two major components: a set of deep fibers and a shallower band. These tissues are made up of cross-linked collagen with the ability to stretch slightly without breaking, fold without ripping off the bone, and rotate as the knee itself bends and rotates through its full range of motion. This fibrous collagen structure, however, is not inert. The fibers are interspersed with cells that have mechanoreceptors: pressure gauges and chemical sensors. When the cells are stimulated by the compression or stretching associated with various movements, they send signals to the brain and release growth factors. Thus, the dynamic cellular and fibrous structure of the MCL updates itself with every slight motion of the knee.

When the MCL is stretched by a misplaced foot—or by another player crashing into it—a physiologic general alarm is issued, unleashing a cascade of responses. If the stretch is slight, no tearing of fibers occurs. Still, pain is sensed by the overstimulation of the cells and by the nerve endings in the tissue. A call for a small amount of growth factors goes out. Cells release recruiting factors, blood vessels leak a little fluid, and a tiny amount of swelling occurs. The swollen area is filled with enzymes that remodel any injured fibers and with anabolic factors that—if necessary—stimulate repair of the stretched fibers.

If the stretch is moderate but not complete, a greater call to action is released. There is more pain and responsive swelling, and more robust collagen formation and healing responses are initiated. If the stretch is so extreme that the ligament ruptures, a blood clot forms at the broken ends of the vessels and tissues. The joint remains unstable until natural healing forms new fibers across the gap or a surgeon sews the ends together.

Fortunately, the medial collateral ligament has a great blood supply. Unlike the ACL, the MCL can usually heal on its own. Today, given the availability of stem cells from various sources, we can accelerate the healing by injecting these cells and their potent growth factors into the injured tissues. These work by recruiting more cells, by stimulating cells to lay down new collagen, and by reducing scarring and inflammation. Amniotic tissues have two to sixty times the growth factors found in normal circulating blood. They are currently the most powerful tool we have to return torn tissues to their healed status. Unfortunately, in June of 2021, the FDA placed a pause on the use of birth-tissue-derived cells and growth factors.

However, data suggests that the addition of amniotic tissue to torn ligaments may drive them to heal with the normal concentration of small- and large-diameter fibers. This is a big improvement over the usual stiff scar tissue, which has only large-diameter fibers. Healing MCL bands can then be exposed to careful motion that stimulates but does not further stretch the tissue. This, along with soft-tissue manipulation by qualified physical therapists, stimulates the mechanoreceptors on the cells to lay down additional collagen—and may promote faster, stronger healing.

Other Knee Ligaments

There are a lot of structures guiding the knee, all of which must be evaluated in any complex knee injury. We've covered injuries to the ACL, the PCL, and the MCL. Here are the other knee ligaments, how they come to be injured, and current treatment methods:

- **The posterolateral corner of the knee (PLC)** is not truly a ligament but a merger of soft tissues at the back (posterior), outside (lateral) corner of the knee. The area is significantly injured in up to 30 percent of ACL injuries, yet the injury is often missed, even when an MRI has been obtained. It is diagnosed by a careful examination of the knee that demonstrates a rotating of the tibia off the femur when the leg is bent. Missing the diagnosis and failing to repair this corner when the ACL is reconstructed is a common cause of recurrent knee instability and ACL failure. We rebuild this corner with a donor ligament, which almost always makes the knee feel more stable and protects the central ligaments.

- **The lateral collateral ligament (LCL)** is injured much less frequently in sports, though an injury can occur if somebody were to cartwheel down a ski slope or get taken out with a side hit in football or soccer. The LCL can heal on its own if the injury is isolated to the LCL, but when found in combination with ACL or PCL tears, the injury often needs to be repaired. The repair is usually done with sutures and augmented by a donor tendon.

- **The anterolateral ligament (ALL)** is a thickening of the synovium (a layer of tissue which lines the joints and tendon sheaths) at the front outside of the knee. It may be injured when the ACL is torn and can be diagnosed with an MRI. Reinforcing this area with sutures, or on occasion with a graft, can provide additional stability to the ACL reconstruction, though we suspect it most often heals on its own.

The Patella

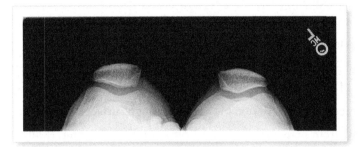

The patellofemoral joint

The patella, more familiarly known as the kneecap, is a sesamoid bone, meaning it is embedded in a tendon. In this case, it's the tendon that connects the thigh muscle to the tibia. Unlike other bones, the patella is mostly dense, compact cortical bone. Its best function is to act as a lever arm, permitting the thigh quadriceps muscle contractions to elevate the lower leg. When it is injured and painful, the thigh muscle weakens, the patella moves abnormally, and the cycle worsens.

The patella holds relatively little marrow, the spongy tissue that helps other bones absorb impact. The underside of the kneecap, which rubs against the femur, has a thick layer of articular cartilage, the bearing surface of joints. If an injury to the patella damages or roughens that surface, small bits of cartilage break off into the knee. This irritates the joint lining, called the synovium, and produces joint fluid that swells the knee. The rough cartilage causes the familiar grinding sensation, and the swollen knee forms scar tissue. Patients often complain of "catching" from the rough damaged cartilage surface and experience pain when bending or going up stairs.

Injuries to the kneecap heal poorly, if at all. While treatments for other parts of the knee have evolved, the patella remains in the old school of frustratingly vague treatment options. When the cartilage is damaged enough to warrant repair, it can be smoothed down with shavers or heating devices, but neither of these actually repairs the tissue. If the wear increases, the bone of the patella is exposed and pain can become chronic.

Temporizing steps, such as injecting lubricants, appear to help by reducing the friction between the rough surfaces. Growth factors and stem cells may promote some cartilage healing, though not enough to cure really significant injuries. Physical therapy helps by strengthening the muscles that guide the kneecap in the groove on the femur and by helping to align the leg and soft tissues. But nothing really cures the damage. Over time, kneecap cartilage injuries lead to painful arthritis.

Cartilage repair techniques developed over the last twenty-five years are excellent for the groove in which the kneecap tracks, successfully treating the damage and arthritis that develops there. But these techniques are less successful for the kneecap articular cartilage. There are simply not enough stem cells or marrow for the marrow-stimulating procedures to grow thick enough repair tissue over the kneecap surface.

Treating significant areas of cartilage loss on the patella surface with paste grafting has worked successfully for many patients. Still, we always warn the patient that there is a possibility that any surgery designed to stimulate the patella cartilage to heal will fail and make the problem worse instead of better.

For the most severe cases, where the arthritis has progressed to bone-on-bone contact at the kneecap, the most remarkable recent advance has been the introduction of the Mako robot for isolated patellofemoral bionic (or artificial) replacement. This robot brings an extremely high level of accuracy to the process of creating and installing a prosthetic knee joint.

As biologically biased as our clinic may be, this robotic method truly superseded what we could do with biology alone at the kneecap. In the past, there were several limitations to artificial patellofemoral joint replacements. The shape of the joint was so complicated and so individualized to each person that our handheld guides and surgical methods did not permit us to place the replacement parts accurately enough. Computer-generated modeling, followed by robotic guidance of the surgeon's hand, helped us overcome those obstacles.

Once the joint is replaced, patients can return to full activity and sports without pain. The downside is that these new parts (like all artificial materials) will eventually fail, but hopefully not for decades.

Where to from here? The future lies in better cartilage replacement. Our team and others are dedicated to advancing this science. Stopping the arthritis before it progresses is the first step, with biologic surface replacement being the ultimate solution.

In the meantime, protect your kneecaps, treat minor injuries immediately, smooth down the more serious ones before they grind away the surfaces, and employ the best lessons of physical therapy and muscle development on a daily basis. If you kneel to pray, pray to be able to kneel forever.

Tonya Harding and Mob gangsters had it right. Take out the kneecaps, and you eliminate your opponent. Today, with customized and accurate placement, people suffering from damage leading to arthritis of the kneecap can overcome the lifelong curse of the gangsters' wrath.

The Meniscus

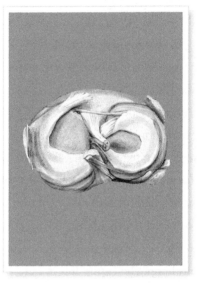

The meniscus cartilages seen from the top down

The meniscus is the key fibrous shock absorber in the knee joint. Its crescent shape rests on top of the tibia (the shin bone) and cups the femur (the thigh bone). The meniscus can be compared to a gasket in a hose. If it is cut, water leaks out, and it fails to diffuse the force that presses through the knee joint when you walk or run. A torn meniscus is often painful, requiring arthroscopic surgery. Most commonly, the surgeon removes the torn tissue, which relieves the immediate pain.

The meniscus gets torn by being pinched between the femur and the tibia. This can happen during sports or through any bending or twisting motion—sometimes just getting out of a car is enough. Often a pop or sudden pain occurs, sometimes with swelling. The torn tissue acts like a windshield wiper in the knee joint, mechanically causing pain and wearing away the opposing articular cartilage surface. The cells of the torn, unstable meniscus also release factors that speed up the onset of arthritis. Thus we often remove the torn part, and sometimes suture it.

Meniscus removal is a procedure called a partial or total meniscectomy. Regrettably, this procedure is performed five hundred thousand times each year in the US alone.[20] Why regrettably? Because it often leads to arthritis. Actual *repair* of the torn meniscus has become easier with new surgical tools and better training of surgeons, yet repairs are performed in less than 10 percent of all meniscus tears. The reasons given are varied. Often the surgeon does not believe that the torn meniscus tissue is healthy enough to heal after repair or that the defect left behind is great enough to produce disability. We now know, however, that when a surgeon removes a significant amount of the torn meniscus, the knee is left unprotected from weight-bearing forces. Removing as little as 20 percent of the meniscus tissue leads to a 160 percent increase in force transferred to the tibia.

The force on the knee concentrated on a narrow part of the joint causes arthritis to ensue.

When symptoms of arthritis first appear, the area exposed is usually small. The symptoms can be moderate with little impact on one's lifestyle. But if it remains untreated, the wear continues. As the damaged area increases, the symptoms and pain increase as well, interfering with work and leisure activities.

It's a serious problem, and the data is stunning. A recent study reported that the lifetime risk of developing symptomatic knee osteoarthritis is 44.7 percent. The current standard of care is artificial knee

---

[20] Sunny Kim et al., "Increase in outpatient knee arthroscopy in the United States: a comparison of National Surveys of Ambulatory Surgery, 1996 and 2006," *Journal of Bone and Joint Surgery* 93 no. 11 (2011): 944–1000, https://pubmed.ncbi.nlm.nih.gov/21531866/.

replacement.[21] While the average age of the first diagnosis of knee arthritis is fifty-four, knee replacement is not usually performed until an average age of sixty-six, leaving 9.3 million people suffering for an average of twelve years.[22]

Studies cited by journalists in recent stories look at this population and conclude that meniscectomy alone does not change their outcome. On this point, they are correct. Removing more of the key shock absorber in the knee does not help cure or prevent the pain of arthritis and probably accelerates it. What is not mentioned is that during the last twenty years, other methods of repair have evolved. Reconstruction and replacement of the meniscus cartilage and the articular cartilage have advanced to the point where a number of long-term studies document excellent pain relief and a return not only to daily activities but to sports as well.

In the past, these now-common techniques were difficult and time consuming. Many were not reimbursed by insurance. So only 3 percent of all meniscus tears were properly repaired, despite the knowledge that meniscectomy can indeed lead to arthritis. Today's repair techniques use new surgical tools that allow surgeons to repair the meniscus even in tight knees and to place sutures in almost all types of tears. At this time, more meniscus tears are being repaired.

---

[21] Louise Murphy et al., "Lifetime risk of symptomatic knee osteoarthritis," *Arthritis and Rheumatism* 59 no. 9 (2001): 1207–1213, https://pubmed.ncbi.nlm.nih.gov/18759314/.

[22] Elena Losina et al., "Lifetime risk and age at diagnosis of symptomatic knee osteoarthritis in the US," *Arthritis Care & Research* 65 no. 5 (2013): 703–711, https://pubmed.ncbi.nlm. nih.gov/23203864/.

ANNUAL MENISCUS SURGERIES IN US

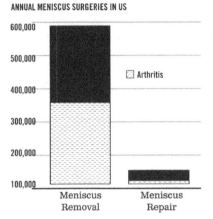

The Problem:

• 605,000 meniscus removal,
  60% progress to arthritis

• 37,000 meniscus repair,
  20% progress to arthritis

Repair, or replace...not remove.

Meniscus reconstruction—using a combination of a collagen scaffold with stem cells or growth factors to regrow portions of the meniscus for patients who have pain after meniscectomy—is currently possible as well. The collagen meniscus implant (CMI) is a regeneration scaffold that has been used in more than six thousand cases in Europe and is available in the US as well.

Meniscus replacement using allograft, or donor meniscus, has been practiced selectively since the late 1980s. Several centers have extensive experience and have produced long-term studies showing improvement in pain and function as well as a return to sports. One study documents the remarkable reduction in artificial joint replacements for arthritic patients who underwent meniscus replacement with articular cartilage repair.

In addition to significantly improving a patient's quality of life, reducing osteoarthritis has direct and indirect cost benefits. The average outpatient treatment and drug cost for chronic osteoarthritis is $5,133 per year. The average indirect cost (disability, lost wages, etc.)

is $6,340 annually. This means a five-year remission of symptoms can save $58,000 per patient. If you extend this over the average life expectancy from sixty-six—about ten years for men and fifteen for women—the savings is an impressive $160,000 per patient.[23]

So when meniscus surgery is reported as useless, remember: not all meniscus surgery is the same. Evolution over millions of years refined the meniscus cartilage to protect the wonderful knee joint we all depend on. Surgeons now have the skills and tools to restore the injured meniscus. Patients, surgeons, and insurance companies should all be motivated to expand the utilization of these tools. By doing so, they can reduce arthritis, delay or prevent the need for artificial joint replacement, and return people to active lifestyles.

---

[23] See Sara Burbine et al., "Projecting the Future Public Health Impact of the Trend Toward Earlier Onset of Knee Osteoarthritis in the Past 20 Years" (presentation, American College of Rheumatology Annual Scientific Meeting, Chicago, IL, November 8, 2011); Losina, "Lifetime risk and age at diagnosis"; and Le Kim et al., "Healthcare costs in US patients with and without a diagnosis of osteoarthritis," *Journal of Pain Research* 5 (2012): 23–30.

No Meniscus Procedure Is Ever Standard

A surgeon should never treat a meniscus repair as an assembly-line process. When I hear a patient say, "The doctor told me it's a standard procedure," I often think that means there isn't much thought being put into it. In my mind, there is no such thing as a standard procedure. Patients commonly say to me, "I was told I have a torn meniscus cartilage in my knee. The doctor said it's simple to just remove the torn part. He does it all the time."

Ugh, I think. Actually, each person is different. Each knee is different. Each torn meniscus cartilage is different. And most importantly, the outcome of each procedure is different. Let me explain.

The meniscus is the key shock absorber in the knee. When even small amounts of it are removed, the force concentration on the tibia goes up, wearing away the bearing surface and leading to early arthritis. When torn, the goal is to save as much of the meniscus as possible, preferably by repairing it or, if it's truly irreparable, by removing as little as necessary to recreate a smooth surface from the frayed edges. Even the most common tears often have extra side tears or hidden degenerative areas that can affect the results.

The artistry of the surgeon determines how smooth and shaped the remaining tissue is. The surgeon's scientific understanding of how important the tissue is, how to stimulate a new blood supply, how to use stem cells and growth factors to augment healing, how to suture the torn edges, or if necessary, how to replace the meniscus with a new donor meniscus all pre-determine how the surgeon is going to act when faced with the unique tear inside your knee.

Your own preferences also contribute to making your case unique. Are you willing to have a longer rehab period in order to permit tissue healing? Are you okay if an effort to save your meniscus fails and you need a follow-up procedure? Do you just want to get back to work quickly and aren't concerned with the long-term outcomes? Do you want to run marathons and need every bit of shock absorption possible? Have you and your surgeon agreed on the goals of the surgery?

I believe there is tremendous art to surgery and science to the artistry. I believe every patient and every problem—not just meniscus injury—is unique, and that it's important to try to match the surgeon's skills with the patient's needs. Part of a surgeon's job is to educate patients not just about what we can do today but what the future is bringing in terms of new techniques and understanding. If you're told that your procedure is standard, remember to ask, "Whose standard?"

Meniscus Implant

Patients often ask me, "Isn't there a shock absorber you can put back in my knee?" The answer is yes. A meniscus transplant uses donor tissue to replace a missing meniscus. But this approach relies on a supply of healthy, young donor tissue (not always easy to acquire) and a highly specialized surgical procedure.

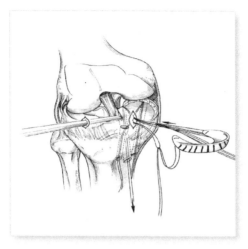

Replacing the meniscus

Now, however, there is a new approach to fixing torn and missing meniscus tissue, called the collagen meniscus implant (CMI). The CMI is a biological device made of highly purified collagen, which acts in two ways. First, it is a physical scaffold upon which new meniscus tissue can grow. Second, it contains growth factors and stem cell holders able to actually stimulate regrowth in areas previously not repairable. In fact, the CMI is not so new; I invented and patented it in 1986.[24] This was the world's first orthopaedic tissue regeneration template. It was tested extensively in animals and people and was found to be safe and effective.

A private company ultimately developed the device and conducted further trials, gaining Europe's CE mark of approval in 2000. It has been available in Europe ever since, with over four thousand procedures performed. It was briefly available in the US (2008–2010),

---

[24] "Prosthetic Meniscus" US Patent # 4,880,429. Issued November 14, 1989.

but a dispute with the FDA meant the implant was off the market for almost five years. This dispute was resolved, and the CMI is once again available to patients in the US. I don't benefit financially from the recent FDA decision, but it brings a smile to my face and warmth to my heart that good science can eventually prevail over politics, and devices that benefit patients eventually can be used by surgeons.

The CMI's availability is important to the more than 1.4 million Americans who tear their meniscus tissue each year and to millions more around the world. In multiple studies of patients who had a meniscectomy alone versus a meniscus reconstruction with the implant, the latter group did better.[25] People who had previously had a resection of their meniscus and had continued pain also benefited. Whether or not the progression to arthritis is prevented has not yet been demonstrated, but intuitively, we understand that more tissue is better than less. In our practice, the CMI was also used as a stem cell and growth factor carrier to augment difficult-to-repair meniscus tears.

The availability of the CMI is good news for people who badly tear their meniscus cartilage. Ideally, meniscus cartilage tears must be repaired and reconstructed when they are freshly diagnosed. In all replacement and repair scenarios, there is a race between healing and

---

[25] See Kevin R. Stone et al., "Development of a Prosthetic Meniscal Replacement," in *Knee Meniscus: Basic and Clinical Foundations*, edited by V.C. Mow (New York: Raven Press, 1992), 165–173; Kevin R. Stone et al., "Meniscal Regeneration with a Co-polymeric Collagen Scaffold," *The American Journal of Sports Medicine* 20 no. 2 (1992): 104–111; Juan Carlos Monllau et al., "Outcome After Partial Medial Meniscus Substitution With the Collagen Meniscal Implant at a Minimum of 10 Years' Follow-Up" *Arthroscopy* 27 no. 7 (July 2011):933–43, DOI: 10.1016/j.arthro.2011.02.018; and Stefano Zaffagnini et al., "Prospective Long-Term Outcomes of the Medial Collagen Meniscus Implant Versus Partial Medial Meniscectomy: A Minimum 10-Year Follow-Up Study," *American Journal of Sports Medicine* 39 no. 5 (February 2011):977–85, https://doi.org/10.1177/0363546510391179.

a return to normal life. While the body is remodeling the implant into normal meniscus tissue, the patient risks tearing the implant by pivoting or twisting. The challenge now is to get surgeons to deploy and insurance companies to approve such tools—not just for the patients with refractory pain but also to help patients avoid arthritis, a problem that may not appear for a decade or more.

Meniscus Replacement in Children

When children tear the meniscus, it often can be repaired. But when it is torn badly, it is often resected (cut out), leaving the child without this key structure. The lateral (outside) part of the knee is the most sensitive to any meniscus cartilage loss in children—but loss of any significant portion of the meniscus cartilage leads to pain, swelling, and early arthritis. The incidence of such tears is about sixty-one per one hundred thousand people each year. Yet the repair/replacement ratio is low—between 10–20 percent for repair and 0.25 percent for replacement.[26] Why?

Meniscus regeneration and replacement in children is a growing field, though unfortunately still small. In children who still have open growth plates (i.e., their bones are still growing), surgeons sometimes tell parents to wait until growth is finished before risking surgery. Their concern is that the growth plate might be injured, leading to growth arrest and deformity. This fear, however, must be balanced against the following facts.

First, there is nearly a 100 percent chance of early arthritis if a child loses the entire meniscus, and probably a greater than 90 percent chance if they lose the posterior horn of the tissue. The earlier the

---

[26] Logerstedt et al, "Knee pain and mobility impairments"; Cvetanovich et al, "Trends in meniscal allograft transplantation."

tissue is repaired, regenerated, or replaced, the less damage occurs. Modern techniques of meniscus transplantation do not require permanent stitches to be used. The growth plates can be protected by creating very small drill holes above the plate. So waiting for further growth is unwise.

Another concern is whether or not a donor meniscus will grow with the child or how long it will last. There are no long-term studies of meniscus replacement in children published in the medical literature, but what we have seen in our meniscus replacement practice over the last twenty-five years has been promising.

The story is similar for meniscus regeneration. As discussed earlier, a collagen meniscus implant (CMI) that can induce regrowth of the meniscus tissue upon a trellis-like structure is now available. Logically, children should be able to regrow their tissue even better than adults. Yet unfortunately, there are no reported cases of the CMI being used in children.

Surgical techniques and instruments for meniscus repair, regeneration, and replacement have improved dramatically. The reasons for not utilizing these techniques to protect injured knees should override excuses from the past, especially given the consequences of tissue removal alone.

Sometimes, in medicine and surgery, all that parents and doctors have to go on is common sense, experience, and probabilities of success. We know that meniscus injuries are devastating to the knee. We know how to regenerate and replace them even if we cannot yet guarantee they will last or protect the joint the way the original meniscus did. But without a large multicenter research trial with long-term data, many insurance plans won't agree to reimburse the procedure. Common sense says they should. Children's knees say they must.

Fractures

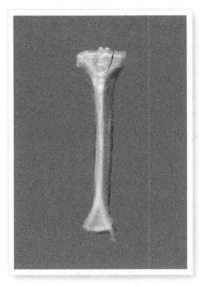

Tibial fracture

Bone fractures around the knee fall into two groups: those that lead to arthritis and those that heal just fine. Here is a brief guide to which is which.

When a fracture of a supporting bone such as the tibia in the knee occurs from trauma or excessive load, a key variable is whether or not the crack is wide or narrow and whether the surface of the joint is intact or depressed. Since the coefficient of friction of the smooth articular cartilage that covers the ends of the bones in joints is slicker than ice sliding on ice, any disruption increases the friction, wears away the surface, and leads to arthritis. Separations or depressions of more than two millimeters are significant enough that they warrant immediate surgical repair as an attempt to restore the congruency of the joint surface.

Fractures from trauma to the knee joint can be described as clean breaks—where a single crack occurs without damage to surrounding soft tissues, such as the meniscus or ligaments, and without depression of the surfaces—or as complex fractures with multiple fracture lines and a variety of associated injuries. Defining which is which often depends on the quality of the imaging techniques available. X-rays show the obvious bony fractures, CT scans define the bony injury patterns and degrees of depression (and permit 3D models to be computer generated), while high-quality MRIs best define the soft tissues. It is common for us to obtain all three to refine our repair techniques. Each one—X-ray, CT, and MRI—has advantages and limitations. Given that we cannot accept more than a couple of millimeters of offset and that soft-tissue repair is as important as the healing of the bone, incomplete information may lead to an unfortunate outcome.

Fractures from mild impact, or stress fractures, raise the question of underlying bone disease, weakness, or osteoporosis. Here we must understand the biology of the patient to find the cause of the bone softness and treat it in conjunction with the injury. Only resistance exercise has been consistently shown to build bone, and relative disuse always leads to bone weakness. Unfortunately, the drugs for treating osteoporosis have not been overwhelmingly successful. Other causes of bone weakness, such as dietary restrictions and hormonal imbalances, must be discovered and corrected. The challenge with a stress or insufficiency fracture is how to apply just enough force to stimulate the bone cells to heal without further deforming the bone. We often do this with pool exercises, where water provides resistance to deformation of the bone during healing. Outside stimulation—by electrical current, ultrasound, magnetic fields, and vibrating plates—play a supportive role to exercise and are helpful in many cases.

Fractures from major trauma and those where the ligaments, meniscus, and articular cartilage are damaged heal the best when reassembled as anatomically as possible. Immediate surgery is often the best approach with a careful reconstruction of all the injured tissues. It may come as a surprise to some, but the skillset and biases of the surgeon are the first components of optimizing the outcome. If the surgeon is an athlete or understands the needs of athletes, he or she is more likely to repair and reconstruct the tissues necessary for high-level sports. If the surgeon is a trauma surgeon alone and not particularly attuned to the demands of an athlete, the bones may heal but the joints may not work as well as needed.

The second most important factor is the attitude of the patient. Upbeat patients with can-do attitudes, who get themselves immediately to physical therapy and use their injury as motivation to return to sports better than they were before they were injured, are those who heal the best. Patients who feel victimized by their injuries are often immobilized psychologically and physically, leading to poorer outcomes.

Ultimately it is not just the injury, and not just the surgeon, and not just the patient. It is the interplay of all three that makes the healing happen. Breaking bad does not have to mean healing worse.

Cartilage Paste Grafts

From the earliest descriptions of cartilage injuries in the Hippocratic era, holes in the cartilage-bearing surface of joints were thought to be irreparable. In the words of physician William Hunter, in 1743, "Cartilage is a troublesome thing, once injured never repaired."

This was the dogma that all orthopaedic surgeons were taught. The holes, or divots, often enlarged over time, and arthritis of the joints—so it was believed—was the inevitable outcome.

Yet isolated cartilage injuries did not always fall down this rabbit hole. Several investigators noted that these injuries sometimes healed on their own, and at other times never caused a problem. But the path the injury took was unpredictable.

For most of the twentieth century, methods for repairing cartilage injuries focused on bone marrow stimulation. Drill bits or awls were used to create passageways for the marrow cells to exit onto the fractured surface and create a "super clot." This freed the pluripotential progenitor and marrow cells within the marrow to form healing tissue on the divot in the bone.

These liberated marrow cells were believed to have all the healing powers necessary to form new cartilage. When continuous motion was applied (using machines, pool exercises, or stationary bikes), the newly formed tissue received mechanical signals, inducing the production of new cartilage rather than bone or scar tissue. Unfortunately, this release of potent healing cells often fell short of forming true cartilage. The repair tissue usually looked like scar tissue and, in the joints of athletes, failed to provide the durability necessary for impact sports.

In the early 1990s, two major approaches were initiated to solve the problem of cartilage healing. The most popular—and most expensive —was an effort to grow cartilage cells called chondrocytes in the lab, squirt them onto the cartilage defect, and cover them with a layer of fibrous tissue from the bone. This sequence required two surgical procedures and expensive laboratory work. It relied on the wishful thinking that the cells would actually stay in place and somehow make enough surrounding tissue to form cartilage before the patient's activity squished it out of the knee. Tens of millions of dollars were spent on this effort. It was eventually abandoned in favor of pre-loading cells onto matrices of resorbable material. A version of this technique, called MACI, was recently approved by the FDA—though the results from studies in Europe have been decidedly mixed.

A second approach involved extracting plugs of intact cartilage and bone—from other parts of the knee or from donors—and placing them like hair transplants into the defects. These plugs sometimes worked but rarely fused with the surrounding cartilage. The donor surfaces never quite matched the patient's own geometry and when they failed, they left large holes in the knee.

A third approach was pioneered, by me, in 1991. It is called articular cartilage paste grafting. This technique relied on turning the dead divot or arthritic area of the joint into a full, fresh fracture, then pasting on a mixture of the patient's own articular cartilage, bone, and underlying cells. A core of cartilage and bone was taken from the intercondylar notch of the knee (where it is not needed and grows back on its own, in any case). This core was mashed into a paste in the operating room and immediately packed into the defect. Mashing was shown to activate the cartilage cells to release growth factors, while the matrix of cartilage was shown to stimulate more normal healing when motion was applied.

This "paste graft" technique has been validated independently in multiple animal models and has shown to be superior to marrow stimulation alone. It requires nothing more than routine operating room tools. The absence of commercial support has caused it to be ignored by much of the orthopaedic industry. Yet now, three decades later, the results of articular cartilage paste grafting in humans and animals match or exceed that of any other technique.

(A side note on the science of paste grafting: Doctors traditionally believed that when cartilage was hit with a hammer, the impacted cells would die. Now, however, studies done on impacted cartilage in collaboration with Dan Grande, PhD, have demonstrated that the cells in the articular cartilage of the paste graft were first upregulated, meaning they were stimulated to increase their production of extracellular matrix and initiate a repair process over the first forty-eight hours. This explains the proliferative repair response we see in the chondral lesions treated with the paste graft technique.)

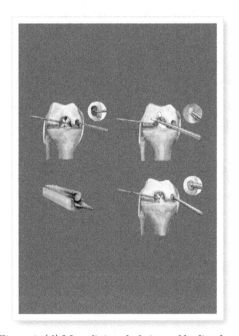

Figure 1. (A) Morselizing the lesion to bleeding bone
(B) Harvesting of articular cartilage and cancellous
bone from the intercondylar notch
(C) Manually crushing the graft into paste
(D) Impacting the paste graft into the morselized lesion

An excellent example of the impact of articular cartilage paste grafting can be seen in conditions like osteochondritis dissecans (OCD). This condition usually occurs in kids and more commonly in adolescents. When kids get persistent knee pain, an X-ray may show a lesion of the articular cartilage, which is the bearing surface of the joint. That lesion is usually called osteochondritis dissecans. It's a terrible and misleading name that implies inflammation (itis) and drying out (dissecans), though neither is present in the condition. Instead, a portion of the weight-bearing surface of the joint—the articular cartilage, with a small layer of underlying bone—becomes unstable or completely dislodged. This leads to pain and swelling.

Spontaneous healing of OCD can occur when the patient is very young. But if it shows up in the teen years, the symptoms often become worse. An X-ray or MRI reveals the damage, and a decision must be made about whether to wait for healing or repair the lesion. When surgery is chosen, usually based on continued pain and a desire to return to sports, various methods are traditionally employed. These include pinning the loose bone back in place, microfracturing the base of the lesion to stimulate healing, cartilage replacement, or complete cartilage and bone replacement.

Unfortunately, none of these has a consistently high rate of uniform healing. The reason is that the bone and cartilage may be partially "dead"—a condition that led to the lesion in the first place. Re-fixing abnormal tissue has an uncertain outcome.

We've found that articular cartilage paste grafting can be applied successfully, even in large lesions that have failed other methods. Long-term data, now over twenty-five years, confirms the success of the paste graft treatment in these lesions. There is no commercial product involved and no harm done by this attempt at repair. In fact, the procedure can be repeated if the healing is incomplete. OCD occurs not just in the knee but in the ankle and elbow as well, and while the cause is still unknown, the same treatment is possible.

We are working to expand and improve the efficacy of the cartilage repair technique, with the goal of achieving full biologic joint replacements for people with severe sports injuries and arthritis. The addition of stem cells and growth factors will also be tested to determine if these factors alone are enough to improve the outcomes for cartilage repair.

More compelling data will push the adoption of paste grafting. Meanwhile, we strongly believe, based on current research, that isolated divots in the cartilage and wider areas of cartilage damage can be repaired with simple, inexpensive, outpatient techniques—when doctors use them.

Why Microfracture Fails

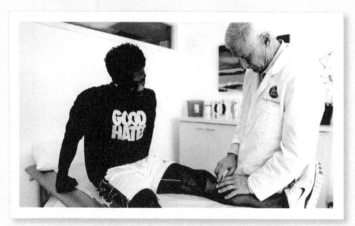

Tracy Porter • Super Bowl–winning cornerback.
Dr. Stone performed a meniscus transplant and an articular
cartilage paste graft to repair Tracy's knee after a
failed microfracture and meniscectomy.

Microfracture—the puncturing of holes to release marrow blood in joint surfaces with cartilage injuries—is reported to be failing in most cases after a few years. Multiple studies provide the reason and offer solutions.

Here's how microfracture works. Holes created in the joint bone release marrow cells and blood that form a clot on the surface of the fractured bone. This clot contains healing factors that lead to the formation of collagen repair tissue. Similar to a clot on the skin, the collagen that forms is scar tissue: disorganized fibers of protein that, over time, remodel into fairly good-looking tissue.

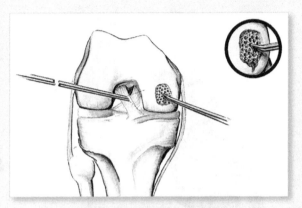

*Making holes in articular cartilage with a pick
in the microfracture technique*

But microfracturing the bone alone, especially in the setting
of arthritis, fails to heal normally at multiple levels. First, the bone
cavities created by the fracture process sometimes fail to heal,
leading to cysts in the bone. These cysts eventually lead to pain
and deformity of the bone. Second, the structure of the bone
above the cysts fails to form a rigid base. This base is comparable
to the subflooring in your house—it's required so that the protective layer of tissue that forms above it can absorb force and wear
properly. Third, the collagen formed is usually in a scar pattern
that sometimes—but not always—forms into the normal cartilage
structure required for lasting durability.

For athletes, the temporary repair provided by the microfracture process often breaks down after a few years of playing on the
joints. No amount of subsequent stem cell or other injections will
bring back a complete, healthy structure of bone and cartilage.

What's Hot and What's Not in Knee Surgery

In ending this section on biologic treatments, let's summarize the current state of knee care art.

Stem cells are both in and out. It was once thought that if these cells were injected into joints, they would turn into cartilage. Two problems arose. First, when stem cells are stimulated, they divide into asymmetric daughters, one of which is a clone of the parent cell and one of which is called a progenitor cell. The progenitor migrates to the site of injury and induces tissue repair but does not actually form new cartilage directly. Secondly, when grown outside the body and then injected, the cells may die rather rapidly after injection. What we have learned is that an increasing number of concentrated growth factors, cytokines, immune stimulants, and even some drugs can induce the migration of the body's own progenitor cells—cells that direct healing—to the injured area. These cells then optimize the environment around the injury and may be instructional to the local cells to effect healing. Since the body has billions of these cells, it makes the most sense to us to inject the recruitment factors (cytokines and growth factors) rather than the cells directly.

PRP and growth factors are still in. PRP is a concentrate formed from platelets in the blood. The platelets have vesicles that contain vast amounts of varied growth (and other) factors that modulate the healing area. Formulations with and without white cells may have different effects on the tissues. Growth factors from fat cells, bone marrow concentrates, and amniotic fluid are all potent. While there's no clear superiority of one over the other at this time, the concentrations of growth factors in birth tissues, amniotic fluid, and Wharton's jelly far exceed those of fat, PRP, and bone.

Meniscus treatments are evolving. Despite evidence that removing even a small portion of the meniscus leads to arthritis, more than 90 percent of meniscus treatments are partial removals called meniscectomies. Insurance companies, by paying only for tissue removal, essentially kick the can down the road in the hope that some other insurance company will have to pay for a joint replacement. But more advanced techniques of meniscus repair, regeneration, and replacement are now making the procedures easier and faster, and surgeons are finally using them. Still, there remains only one scaffold to regrow the meniscus—the collagen meniscus implant (CMI)—but it is not being marketed or used widely enough yet. Meniscus replacement, or transplantation, has been shown in long-term studies to reduce pain and improve function in both pristine young knees and in older arthritic knees. But very few centers are deploying them regularly as the surgical technique is difficult and time-consuming.

Articular cartilage repair with microfracture has fallen out of favor. The results don't hold up in athletes for more than a few years. One scaffold, called MACI, has been approved in the US to hold cells and growth factors at the site of chondral lesions. The articular cartilage paste grafting technique that we pioneered thirty years ago has shown long-term effective results and is gaining traction with podium presentations at many major orthopaedic meetings. It still lacks commercial support, since it is free (i.e., without implants to charge for). Thus, it will likely lag behind in surgeon uptake until a wide clinical trial is performed and more surgeons are trained.

ACL treatments should be changing faster. ACL tears are still occurring at a rate of about three hundred thousand per year, and most are reconstructed with the patients' own tissues, though high-quality allografts are more widely available now. These have the same outcomes in some surgeons' hands and avoid the second-site surgery pain and weakness that the harvest of the patellar tendon or hamstrings produces. It remains shocking to me that, in the twenty-first century, we are still robbing one part of the body to rebuild another. No new artificial ligaments have come on the market, though there are several supporting scaffolds or bands being used (despite a lack of outcome data). Pig tissue we developed is approved in Europe but not yet commercialized. The arthritis rate after ACL surgery is reported at 50 percent after ten years, with the failure rate in young people at 30 percent. So there is a lot of room for improvement. Adding growth factors and progenitor cells should help, but data is pending.

Robots are more accurate than surgeons; they just lack judgment. Robotic assistance has permitted highly accurate outpatient partial and total knee replacements, and younger people are choosing these options. There is now a dramatic shift to cementless knee replacement devices thanks to robot-assisted surgeries. When these were tried in the past, the pain and failure rates were too high as gaps were present between the implant and the bone. The high accuracy of the robotic saws now permits near-perfect interfaces, thereby eliminating the need for cement. No cement may mean less chance of loosening, allowing patients to return to sports. This has major implications for patients, surgeons, and quality of life.

Real-time outcome data is rapidly entering the field. Thanks to the advent of personal fitness devices, ubiquitous electronic medical records, and artificial-intelligence-driven data-mining programs, we now have the ability to evaluate treatments much more effectively. Since nearly all patients now have smartphones, apps that can collect outcome data can soon be installed on those phones. They will monitor, in real time, the progress or problems with any medical or surgical intervention, collecting much valuable information over long spans of time.

What's hottest in medicine is technology and progress. What is not is a head-in-the-sand approach, repeating the same procedures with average or unknown outcomes. In my personal view, it is no longer acceptable for a doctor to perform a procedure on a patient, or put something in a patient, without knowing its outcome—either through others' research or the doctor's own results tracking. The question, "Doc, how do you know this works?" should be answered with, "Here is my data."

BIONIC KNEE REPLACEMENT

Partial and Total Joint Replacements

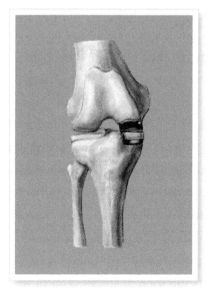

Partial knee replacement

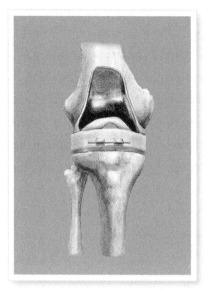

Total knee replacement

A total knee replacement means swapping the worn-out, painful knee joint surfaces with metal and plastic components. It involves placing a metal end on the thigh bone (the femur) and a metal and plastic tray on the shinbone (the tibia). However, knees do not necessarily wear out evenly. (In fact, they don't wear out at all unless there is an underlying injury. This could be a meniscus or ligament tear or a disease process, such as osteoarthritis. The cartilage in the knee is extremely durable, and if not damaged, lasts a lifetime.) Often, one part of the knee can be perfectly fine while another part is completely destroyed. If only part of the knee joint is worn out, why replace all of it?

Many patients with arthritic knees are told they need a full knee replacement when, in fact, there is another option: a biologic solution that involves replacing the meniscus and regrowing the articular cartilage, a procedure called BioKnee™. It's also possible that resurfacing only the worn part with a metal and plastic implant would do just fine. Partial knee replacement—also called unicondylar replacement—wasn't commonly performed in the past because of the difficulty in accurately matching the resurfaced parts to the uninjured knee. Computerized models and robotic arms have changed all that. Today, with robotic assistance, we can resurface the worn-out portion of the joint, either the inside, outside, or kneecap, and leave the rest of the joint alone. To work properly, the components must be put in extremely accurately. Even a millimeter or two of tilt or rotation dramatically affects the wear patterns and longevity of the components. (Think of how cars out of alignment cause rapid tire wear.)

With my robotic assistant, I can plan the surgery on a computer screen with a virtual model of the patient's own knee (built in 3D from their CT scans). I can put the components in place virtually and adjust them before making only a small incision. During surgery, the robotic arm and computer navigation provide me with pinpoint precision to enable optimal implant positioning and alignment that results in a more natural knee motion.

With a partial knee replacement, there is no need for freehand saws, drills, or guides. In fact, the procedure is so minimal that you can walk out of the surgery center one and a half hours after surgery and begin physical therapy the next day. Later, patients tell me that their knees feel normal, which almost never occurs after a full knee replacement.

I've dedicated much of my career to developing new ways to preserve the natural biology of the knee, to offer an alternative to artificial joint replacement. My bias is toward biologic knee solutions, which can rebuild and regenerate joints using donor tissue and stem cells. Sometimes the damage is too much for a BioKnee™, but it still does not warrant a total knee replacement. Just as for a cavity in your tooth, you would want a filling, not a set of dentures. For a partially worn-out knee, you would want a partial knee replacement, not a total replacement.

How to avoid a total knee replacement? First of all: don't get hurt. Once you injure your knee—if the meniscus cartilage, articular cartilage, or ligaments do not heal normally, or are not repaired, reconstructed, or replaced quickly—arthritis may develop. That's because loss of function of any of these key tissues means an increase in concentrated force on the joint surface and early wear.

If you do get hurt, insist on an accurate diagnosis with the latest diagnostic tools: high-quality MRI, X-ray, and physical therapy with gait analysis. If surgical reconstruction is necessary, your specific goal will be to restore full function. Don't accept less.

When patients come in with knee injuries, we typically hear four stories. The most common is, "I injured my meniscus cartilage, and they took out part of it. Now I have arthritis. Isn't there just a shock absorber you can put in my knee?" The answer is yes. It is available as a collagen scaffold (to regrow part of the meniscus) or as a full allograft (human tissue) to actually replace the meniscus.

The second most common story is, "I tore my ACL, and it was reconstructed. Now I have arthritis." The data shows that 50 percent of people with an ACL injury will get arthritis. This is partly due to the force of the original injury, but also due to the inaccuracies of ACL reconstruction techniques. The surgery either fails to restore normal biomechanics, or the harvesting of the patient's hamstrings or patella tendon (to rebuild the ACL) weakens the knee—leading to abnormal motion and early wear. The answer here is anatomic ACL reconstruction, which restores the original knee anatomy as closely as possible. This includes the use of off-the-shelf ACL replacement devices. In the US, this will be an allograft; in Europe, either an allograft or the newly available Z-Lig animal-derived tissue. Long-term data will be needed to determine if these alternatives diminish the arthritis. In any case, by using an off-the-shelf device, you are not injuring one part of the knee to restore another part.

The third story is, "I damaged my articular cartilage, and the doctor shaved it away." Cartilage restoration procedures have advanced to the point where damaged cartilage can now be repaired rather than removed. At The Stone Clinic, we often use a cartilage paste graft technique. We have more than twenty-five years of data demonstrating that paste grafting the lesion leads to effective cartilage repair. Other orthopaedic centers have other techniques that also have promising long-term data.

The days of hearing, "Remove the meniscus," "Cartilage cannot be repaired," and "Live with your arthritic knee until you have a knee replacement" are in the past.

The fourth most-heard story is, "I have arthritis and have been told I need surgery." This scenario has four possible outcomes. One, the joint spaces are still open. In this case, the patient can be treated with lubrication, growth factors, and physical therapy to diminish many of the symptoms but not cure the problem. Two, the joint spaces are open, and the cartilage can be restored with a biologic knee replacement. Three, the X-ray shows only one part of the knee is bone-on-bone. Here, a partial knee replacement using a MAKO robot can be performed, saving the rest of the knee. Four, the arthritis has progressed to severe deformity in multiple parts of the knee, in which case a total knee replacement really is the best option.

The reason this is the last option is because 50 percent of people with a total knee replacement have pain at ten years, and there is a high revision rate in the first two years. The replacement knees are not normal, and there is no going back to a biologic solution once the knee is completely replaced.

So while a total knee replacement is a great solution when and if the knee is completely worn out, we advocate exhausting the other options first. The best advice is if you get hurt, fix the damage immediately and avoid arthritis.

What Is a Partial Knee Replacement?

The knee is generally divided into three compartments: the medial, the lateral, and the patellofemoral. The medial is located on the inside of the knee, the lateral by the fibula, and the patellofemoral by the kneecap. Most arthritis cases involve one or two of these compartments. We now have access to a variety of implants to mediate the effects of knee osteoarthritis. Metal implants made of cobalt chrome are available to cover the individual ends of the femur. Titanium plates are used to cover the top of one side of the tibia. High-molecular-weight polyethylene buttons are used to cover the patella, and polyethylene trays to sit on top of the tibial plates. By resurfacing just the worn-out part of the knee, the remainder, including the ligaments, is left untouched. Knees with partial replacements feel more normal than those that require full replacements because the geometry of the knee remains intact and the ligaments guide the knee in the natural fashion.

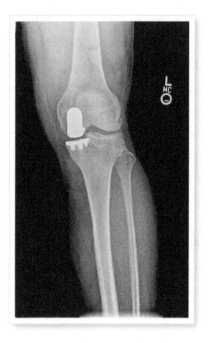

X-ray of partial knee replacement

To perform a partial replacement using twenty-first century surgical techniques, we obtain X-ray, MRI, and CT scan images. The X-ray shows the bony alignment and joint space. The MRI shows the articular and meniscus cartilage and the health of the ligaments. We usually know that the worn part of the knee, with bone-on-bone appearance on X-rays, has no functional cartilage left—but we are curious about the health of the remaining compartments of the knee. If they are healthy, there is no need to replace them. If not, we determine whether to provide a soft-tissue repair at the time of the partial replacement, a ligament replacement, or a multi-compartment resurfacing.

The CT scan is used to build a 3D model of the knee. On that virtual model, the metal and plastic components of the partial knee replacement are positioned. The ability to move the components to the optimal position in all planes, especially in rotation, is what makes computerized partial replacement superior to the old hand-held guides.

At the outpatient surgery center, the surgeon controls a robotic arm programmed to match the patient's 3D knee image. The tip of the robotic arm has a high-speed burr that removes only the area of damage shown on the imaging. Implants are then placed into the prepared area, effectively resurfacing the joint. To adjust for side-to-side joint balance, the surgeon chooses high-molecular-weight polyethylene implants of various sizes, testing each thickness until the ligaments on each side of the knee have the optimal tension. This, along with fine adjustments of the implants and careful handling of the soft tissues at the time of surgery, differentiates top-quality partial replacements from more average procedures. If the patella is worn down, the judgment as to whether or not to do a bicompartmental replacement (both the medial or lateral, plus the patellofemoral joint) is a challenging one. Many patients do fine without resurfacing the patella as most of the pain often comes from the medial or lateral sides. In fact, when we do a full knee replacement, we rarely resurface the patella. However, when only the patella is worn down and there is bone-on-bone appearance on the X-ray, then an isolated patellofemoral replacement solves the problem.

At this time, all partial replacements are cemented in place. The technology for making the undersurface of the implants in partial replacements porous to accept bony ingrowth has not yet been approved by the FDA. Hopefully, this will change shortly.

Surgeon judgment, experience, and bias influence these decisions. Knowing the bias of your surgeon is important. Is he or she an athlete? Do their patients return to sports? Are they more interested in total knee replacements rather than partials? Are they comfortable with robotic assistance? All of these factors affect the outcome. We encourage our patients to return to full sports because weight-bearing activity builds bone and strengthens muscles, thereby protecting the joint over time. The old advice, to rest your knee, leads to osteoporosis, muscle atrophy, and eventual failure of either the joint or the patient.

So if it ain't broke, don't fix it. If it is partially broken, fix only what needs fixing.

Know the Bias of Your Surgeon

S urgeons are like any other skilled professional. They like to do what they are best at, what works in their hands, and what they have observed over a lifetime of practice. They chafe at the bit when told, by insurance companies and/or hospital administrators, what they can and cannot offer to patients or which implants they are allowed to use. They want the best outcomes for their patients and for themselves. Their desires are often well-aligned with their patients' interests—and sometimes at odds with the system.

That being said, it is important to know what a doctor's biases are so that you, the patient, can decide if these fit with your own desires. This can dramatically affect the care you receive. Here are a few examples of how a surgeon's bias might affect you.

Total Knee Replacement versus Partial Knee Replacement

As discussed previously, if you show up with an arthritic knee that shows bone-on-bone contact in all or part of the joint, the surgeon may suggest a total joint replacement to replace all of the exposed surfaces with metal and plastic. This surgeon's experience with partial knee replacements may be minimal, or they may have heard about poor outcomes.

The truth is that the results of full knee replacement are not as good as advertised, with 50 percent of people having pain after ten years. What has also changed is that today, with robotic surgery, partial knee replacements are much more accurate, and most are performed as outpatient procedures. So knowing the surgeon's bias in advance will determine which procedure you are offered.

Biologic versus Artificial Joint Replacement

Arthritis develops over time. Knees begin to wear out due to loss first of the meniscus, then ligaments, and then articular cartilage. A surgeon who has experience replacing tissue will offer the suffering knee patient these soft-tissue replacement options. The surgeon without this experience may offer an osteotomy, a surgical procedure where the angle of the leg is changed by cutting the bone and wedging it open or closed in order to buy time before a knee replacement is required. They might also offer a distraction procedure where an external frame is placed to stretch out the compartment and combine the distraction with a biologic tissue replacement. (Or they may offer an artificial knee replacement up front.) The surgeon's skillset determines, in part, what you are offered.

Injections versus Cortisone or Surgery

Recent interest in biologic stimulation of joint healing has led to a plethora of new joint injections. These include growth factors called PRP; progenitor cells from fat, bone, birth tissues, and amniotic fluids; and lubricating injections (usually using hyaluronic acid). The data and outcomes of these injections are variable. However, in our most recent study, 80 percent of patients receiving a combination cocktail of HA, PRP, and amniotic fluid received relief lasting twelve months. If you are a responder, the benefits of pain relief and improved function are dramatic. Surgeons without this bias may offer cortisone—which shuts down inflammation and provides pain relief but also damages the tissues and does not stimulate healing—or just progress to a surgical solution.

Rehab versus Surgery

Rehabilitation techniques have improved significantly over the years. All of the patients in our clinic work with our rehab team, in addition to the medical and surgical team, to either optimize their recovery or avoid surgery completely. The team works with them not just to the recovery stage but beyond, to achieve a "fitter, faster, stronger" goal. If a surgeon does not have a rehab team or experience working closely with physical therapists, the option of avoiding surgery may not be offered as frequently, and physical therapy might not even be prescribed at any point in the care.

In sum, bias is a good thing. Surgeons generally stick to what works best in their hands. But knowing this bias is important for understanding why you are offered some solutions and not others.

Partial Knee Replacement for Athletes

The results of partial knee replacement have become so good that my patients often ask if they can run, play sports, and return to a full range of activities. My answer is often, "Yes, but…" Here is why.

Unfortunately, by the time many patients come in for resurfacing of the knee, they have limped for years. Their muscles are weak, their hip and back mechanics have compensated for the arthritic knee, and their range of motion is limited. To return to sports without damaging their knee joint, each of these limitations must be addressed with extensive physical therapy and fitness training.

Their ability to return to running specifically depends on their style and technique. Soft surfaces, smooth, short stride, and midfoot landing all contribute to safe running.

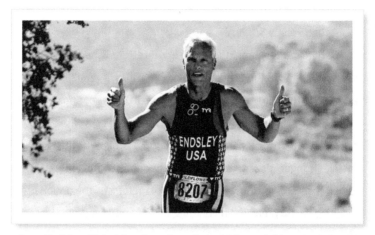

Scott Endsley • Triathlon champion after robotic partial knee replacement

Patients also ask if they will wear out or loosen their implants by playing sports. The answer is, "Not likely." While loosening has a number of causes, we believe that one of the most frequent is the weakening of the bone with aging and disuse. People have traditionally been told to limit their activities as they get older. In fact, by increasing weight training and loading of the joint, the bone mass increases; thus, the risk of loosening decreases. But even if things go south, the plastic-based inserts between the metal resurfacings are now replaceable if they wear out—though they rarely do.

So with modern outpatient techniques, partial knee replacements and sports can be complementary. But as with other activities, the quality of the motion affects the outcome.

CHAPTER 6

ANABOLIC THERAPIES

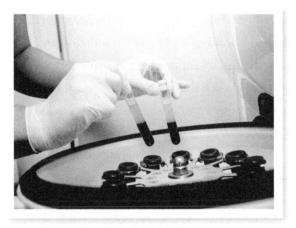

PRP preparation

The era of anabolic medicine is here. Now, when we are injured, we no longer have to wait for Mother Nature to do her job. We have the technology to augment and accelerate healing. Tissues once thought to be irreparable can now be repaired, regenerated, and replaced with active sutures, regeneration templates as scaffolds, and donor tissues often younger than the injured ones. These restorative devices are amplified by the addition of growth factors, cytokines, and progenitor cells. The days of just injecting cortisone and taking out damaged tissues are over.

Let's take a look at this novel landscape of healing, understand its many players, and examine its different applications.

HOW OUR BODIES HEAL

To truly understand why anabolic therapies are so exciting and how they work, you need to know how our bodies naturally heal themselves. Biologic healing works like a football team. When all the players play their roles, supporting the team at the right times and in the right ways, when the indefinable chemistry is just right, when coaches provide proper encouragement, when preparation and fitness are ideal, winning—or healing—occurs. Without all of these facets in place, random events may still lead the team to victory, but more likely, the result will be disorganized failure.

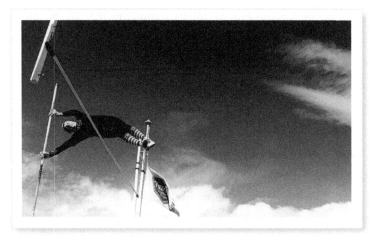

Kenneth S.C. • Pole vaulter and growth factor injection study patient

Injuries are like spontaneous game times. The injury occurs, and the call goes out to the team: jump into action. Multiple events occur simultaneously at the moment of injury. The cells of the injured tissues leak their contents into surrounding tissues. These materials are chemotactic. This means that they call other cells (progenitor cells derived from the body's stem cells) and blood factors to the site of healing. First they clean up and carry away the damaged tissues, and then they lay down new collagen, the backbone of all tissues in the body. Next, nerve endings in the tissues send signals to the brain, recording both the pain and the site of the injury. This provides directional information, prompting the body to protect the injury with limping, muscle contraction, or natural splinting of the area.

A sequence of healing usually characterized by inflammation, tissue remodeling, and (eventually) scar formation follows. The quality of the healing depends on the guidance and coaching of rehabilitation and exercise, along with physical, chemical, and hormonal influences.

All of these sequences occur successfully only if all the components are working. The creation of life on Earth required an all-star team of all the right chemical, biological, and physical players, along with energy from the sun to create and stimulate living organisms. The re-creation of healthy tissues is the same.

Plenty of things can go wrong. If the body is low on red cells (a condition called anemia), the healing is sometimes poor due to the low delivery of oxygen to the injury site. If the injured person is depressed, endorphins may not be released in the right combination to stimulate a healthy tissue response. The point is, healing occurs due to the collection of all the players on the team. Only when all the members are present and ready does the natural healing response work ideally.

HOW ANABOLIC HEALING WORKS

This brings us to stem cells. Much is written in the press on their medical uses, and millions of dollars are being spent on stem cell injections for nearly every injury. Yet only a very few truly effective outcomes from stem cell injections alone have been documented—and most are in the eye. Those that have been documented in joints have occurred only when the tissues are already in the repair process or can be stimulated to start healing, and the stem cells—which are now more correctly identified as progenitor cells—are used to assist and possibly accelerate healing.

The current understanding, based on a sequence of well-controlled studies, reveals that stem cells, when activated by the cytokines the body normally releases at the time of injury, divide into daughter cells, one of which is the same as the parent cell, and one of which is a progenitor cell that migrates to the site of injury. These cells exert their influence in adults by releasing packets of information called exosomes and vesicles. The exosomes are made by the machinery inside the cell, and vesicles are part of the cell fluid and cell wall. So it is these delivery vehicles of the cells rather than the cells themselves that stimulate the repair and regeneration of new tissue. These packets contain a large variety of growth factors and messenger RNA, the coding units of genetic information, that then merge with local cells at the site of an injury. The information packets stimulate those cells to induce healing, reduce scarring, delay apoptosis or early death, and restore health.

The reason for the failure of "stem cell" injections alone is the lack of the team. A progenitor cell is a growth factor engine, called to the site of injury to release growth factors that stimulate or augment the repair process and modify the behavior of other cells. When an injury site has all the other factors necessary for repair to occur, the progenitor cell can encourage the process. But when injected alone—especially into sites that do not have the healing stimulus, such as an arthritic joint—they have little chance of being effective. To address this deficit, we add combinations of additional factors to these injections, including using birth tissues with a native regenerative ability to induce a healing response.

The progenitor cell is like a star quarterback. Without a line in front of him and a talented receiver, without momentum and coaching, his team often fails to win. The biology of healing is no different. The successful biologic therapies of today combine recruitment of progenitor cells with other techniques and implants to create a complete healing environment.

Thus, the anabolic injection tsunami overwhelming all of medicine is evolving. Where once it was thought that these cells could morph into anything and cure everything, our new understanding of their behavior will change how they are used. Here is where we are on the learning curve.

Stem cells from embryonic tissue are the primordial cells from which all tissues in all animals grow. These pluripotent cells contain the genetic information and cellular machinery that develops into the healthy tissues that make up our organs—and the unhealthy ones that create tumors. Guiding their evolution is the primordial soup that they live in and the genetic programming it contains. The use of these embryonic stem cells in medicine is severely restricted due to religious beliefs as well as political issues—overlaid with ethical questions and the fear that new humans, built by mad designers, will overrun the world.

Once the embryo has grown into a fetus, the cells found surrounding the fetus, which are unique to the amniotic fluid, Wharton's jelly, and other birth tissues, have another level of potency. These amniotic fetal cells and growth factors guide this stage of development with potent anabolic, anti-inflammatory, anti-scarring, and antibiotic behaviors. They are the reason the mother's body does not reject the fetus, even though the fetus is genetically only half the mother (except, of course, in the case of immaculate conception).

One step further along in the development pathway are other types of stem or progenitor cells. These are programmed to develop into tissues such as bone, cartilage, and soft tissues, the mesenchyme of the body. These mesenchymal cells, or MSCs, are found on the walls of blood vessels, waiting to spring into action when injuries occur. Vascular tissues, such as fat and bone marrow, have the largest number of these cells.

The tsunami of stem cell optimism and application occurred

because scientists and physicians hoped that by injecting these cells into various injured organs, such as the heart, the spinal cord, or the knee joint, the injured tissues would regrow under the influence of the magical cells. So far, this hope has turned out to be only partially true.

Many studies have noted that without millions of progenitor cells, the tissue healing effects are not as effective. Thus, there have been furious efforts to grow more cells in culture prior to implanting them. However, with our emerging understanding that the tip of the spear in healing is not the cell itself but the weapons contained inside it, a whole new effort to isolate and manufacture those elements is underway.

Just as it takes a village to grow a healthy child, it will most likely take all of the cellular and growth factor players involved in injury and tissue regeneration to rebuild an entire organ or to cure arthritis. For now, our clinical strategy is to inject the most potent mixture of growth factors and cytokines from the platelets of the patient's own blood and hyaluronic acid (the lubricant of the joint). Access to birth tissues is currently limited by the FDA to controlled drug development studies. This mixed cell, growth factor, and lubricant therapeutic approach most closely represents that primordial chicken soup from which all sprang. Such injections may or may not be more targeted in the future.

The most fascinating part of this story is that almost no one has been hurt by the partial successes in treating tissue injury and arthritis achieved so far. There have been no downsides (except cost) to the wonderful, aggressive efforts to heal people with nature's tools. With the enthusiasm for this research felt by our team and many others, progress will be steady. You may look forward to sliding into the home plate of life a little worse for wear, but with a healthy smile.

INGREDIENTS FOR HEALING

As we saw in the last section, the science of joint repair is in full swing. There is a frenzy of activity around stem cells, growth factors, exosomes, and all forms of stimulation therapies. The bottom line is that no one factor does it all; joint repair takes a village. The environment for healing must include the right materials, the stimulation of the correct cells at the optimum moments, and the physiology and psychology of the patient to accept and promote a healing process. When any one of these factors is not present, the process of healing is incomplete. As our grandmothers figured out, when you treat a cold with chicken soup, you warm the body, calm the mind, and promote healing. The primordial soup surrounding injury repair needs a modern version of our grandmothers' wisdom.

Let's pause here and examine (or reexamine) each of these individual factors in tissue healing. A brief summary will help you keep track of the many players and recognize their role in the repair process.

Stem Cells

Stem cells are pluripotent self-renewing cells believed to be the precursor cell of all cell types, meaning that they can transform into the specific cell type of the tissue they are trying to repair. They have unique markers on their surfaces that identify them.

As discussed above, stem-cell-based therapies, in which the body's own cells are stimulated to contribute to the repair process, continue to evolve. In orthopaedics, many doctors have thought (and some advertise) that stem cells alone are able to make new cartilage and cure arthritis. However, senior scientist Arnold Caplan, PhD, (who popularized the theory that bone marrow stem cells are the precursors to all tissues) points to a new understanding of how stem cells—or "medicinal signaling cells," as Caplan calls them—go about making healing happen.

Stem cells predominantly live on the walls of blood vessels in addition to specialized stem cells that live within tissues, such as articular cartilage. The more vessels, the more cells. Fat contains the most stem cells, and bone marrow is also an excellent source. At the time of an injury to a joint, or an insult to the body such as an infection, the cells are called into action. Local cells respond to local trauma, but they also send signals, which recruit the army of stem cells lying in wait on the walls of vessels everywhere in the body. The stem cells, when activated, divide and send a daughter called a progenitor cell to the site of injury and release growth factors, antibiotics, and other proteins and factors necessary for repair. The cells are so powerful that together with the normal immune system cells, the drugs they release kill most invading bacteria long before the host feels a reaction. (An example of these antibiotic-like proteins are the "defensins" living in your mouth, which protect you from nasty food contaminants and scary remnants of your dog's unexpected mouth-to-mouth kiss.)

When bones break or ligaments tear, the stem-cell-derived progenitors release the anabolic factors that kick off the healing response. They stay around or recruit their friends to release other factors sequentially in the healing process. One factor is specific to taking away broken fragments and another to rebuilding tissue. The progenitor cells are the general contractors, calling in subs like plumbers and painters at just the right time.

Progenitor cells are potent growth factor producers and also participate in tissue healing and remodeling. With aging, there is some debate about stem cell potency. Does it really decline each year? The younger you are, the more stem cells you have, but their ability to affect repair may or may not change depending on the type of tissue injured. At surgery, we often release the marrow stem cells to assist in the repair of torn tissues. In the near future, pending FDA approval, we will add a frozen source of very young amniotic-fluid-derived growth factors. If processed properly, one cc of amniotic fluid contains two to sixty times the concentration of growth factors found in the patient's own blood platelet preparations. We plan to take advantage of both types of preparations by combining them with hyaluronic acid and then injecting them into the arthritic joint or injured tissues.

Progenitor Cells

Progenitor cells are one step down from true stem cells in that they can transform into many cell lines but are not self-renewing. Most of the adult so-called stem cell therapies are taking advantage of these progenitor cells. Progenitor cells release growth factors and guide the healing process after injury.

Monocytes and Macrophages

Monocytes are specialized white blood cells that consume invading bacteria, viruses, and fungi. They are the first responders of the body's immune system. They can also convert themselves into a larger cell form called a macrophage. At least two forms of these cells, it appears, are critical to driving the healing response down a healthy pathway rather than a tissue-rejection pathway. Certain stimuli can induce the formation of M2 macrophages, the repair type. We currently believe that progenitor cells, by releasing instructional growth factors, may direct this healing response. It may also be that certain cytokines induce the M2 transformation, which may be why having a lot of cells injected into an injured area may not be necessary as it is these factors and local cells that regulate the process. And there is a new focus on the abundant macrophages that live in the lining of joints called the synovium. This rich source of reparative cells may prove to be the most potent of the human responses to joint injury.

Osteoblasts, Osteoclasts, and Osteocytes

These cells make, break down, and maintain bone. The balance between osteoblasts (which generate bone) and osteoclasts (which remove it) is what maintains bone strength. With aging, all men and women lose bone density, women faster than men. Drugs developed to stop bone loss have had significant associated complications. Only resistance exercise has been shown to be effective; osteoblasts respond to stress such as weight lifting by producing more bone. Certain hormones, such as the parathyroid hormone, can be used to stimulate bone formation. The future of anabolic therapy will be to optimize these stimulants.

Chondrocytes

Chondrocytes are the cells that maintain the remarkable elastic characteristics of cartilage tissue: extreme lubricity and the ability to resist compression and shear forces, enabling us to walk or even run for a lifetime. Once thought incapable of instigating effective repair of damaged cartilage, we now know that chondrocytes, with the right conditions, can be induced to grow and repair articular cartilage. A unique articular cartilage stem cell has also been identified and may be the local director of the cartilage repair process.

Fibrochondrocytes

The unique cells of tissues, such as meniscus cartilage, both maintain the health of the tissue and migrate to the site of injury to attempt to effect repair once the meniscus is torn. All tissues that insert into bones have a zone where fibrochondrocytes manage the transition from soft tissue to hard tissue. There are several types, and these cells are the key to better tissue repair in the future.

Growth Factors

Growth factors are mostly proteins with names like transforming growth factor beta, insulin-like growth factor, and fibroblast growth factor. These proteins are the vitamins for tissue healing. Without them, injury can occur, but healing cannot.

Growth factors act to both directly stimulate healing and to recruit stem cells from the walls of vessels to migrate to the site of injury. Today, growth factors from platelets drawn from the patient in the office constitute an important part of our injection therapies. These are known as platelet-rich plasma, or PRP. Your blood contains hundreds of thousands of platelets per microliter. Inside these platelets reside packets of growth factors called alpha granules. A physician can spin your blood in a centrifuge, concentrate the platelets, and then inject them into the injured tissues or joints.

Platelet-derived growth factors are usually the least expensive and most available of anabolic therapies, yet other sources of growth factors have much higher concentrations and a wider variety of proteins and cytokines involved in the healing process. Because no complex organ grows faster than a fetus in a mother's womb, amniotic fluid,

Wharton's jelly, and other birth tissues are a particularly potent source of growth factors (and a few types of unique stem cells).

Cytokines

Cytokines are growth factors that induce changes in the chemistry of a tissue or the behavior of a cell. They travel or induce other cells to travel to the site of injury. In general, they promote growth, though some specific cytokines direct the processes of senescence (when cells cease replicating) and apoptosis (the death and removal of cells). An active area of research at this time involves rapid removal of dying cells before they actually die. The thinking is that during the process of death, the cells release degradative enzymes that are a major cause of tissue aging. If removed, the aging process may be delayed.

Lubricating Factors

Patients describe their arthritic joints as feeling dry, stiff, and crackly. This is due to a change in the chemical composition of the tissues and a decrease in hyaluronic acid (HA), the major natural lubricant of the joints. This acid is actually a charged sugar molecule, which means that it can attract and hold on to water, thereby plumping up tissues, such as skin, ligaments, and the meniscus. The amount of hyaluronic acid increases with age, but its thickness or density decreases. HA responds to stress, such as sunburn and other tissue injuries. While originally concentrated from rooster combs, it is now synthesized in the lab using genetic engineering techniques.

A syringe full of HA injected into the knee brings many patients relief from pain and inflammation, but the response is variable. We choose to augment the lubrication injections with growth factors from platelets to potentiate the biologic response. Our current belief is that growth factors stimulate the synovial lining cells to produce more HA. Data from a recent prospective double-blind trial of HA alone versus HA plus amniotic fluid supported this concept that the growth factors of the amniotic fluid stimulated an increased production of natural HA in the joint, leading to pain relief lasting up to one year.

Over the past ten years, numerous companies and doctors have developed their own stem cell and growth factor injection preparations. Claims by various doctors have induced athletes to travel to various countries to obtain what they hoped were the most advanced injections.

So which are the best? Here's what we know at this point. Current data shows that most stem cell injections have very few true colony-forming units, the measure of effectiveness of such cells. Worse, preparations of stem cells that were previously frozen are composed almost entirely of dead cells. Finally, the injected cells from many donor preparations—including most of the controversial fetal cell preparations—do not stay alive after injection into the joints long enough to produce a benefit.

That said, some stem cell preparations that are probably progenitor cell preparations are quite effective at augmenting repair of tissues after injection and have produced remarkable results. Which ones to use, which applications, and when it is best to combine cells with growth factors—these combinations are still under evaluation. Our current bias is to use a combination of PRP-derived growth factors with hyaluronic acid and marrow cells released at the time of surgery.

Huge amounts of research dollars and effort are being applied to optimize this new anabolic era of orthopaedic medicine. With more research, we expect that stimulating injections will accelerate the healing of a wide range of injuries, and that the outcomes of surgical procedures will be similarly improved.

SOURCES OF STEM CELLS AND GROWTH FACTORS

Here is a short list of the pros and cons of the stem cell sources that we can use to revitalize transplanted tissues today.

Fat	PROS: highly vascular, with many cells CONS: requires a separate surgical procedure; cell numbers and possible activity decline with age
Bone	PROS: marrow cells are more similar to cartilage and bone CONS: painful bone-marrow biopsy procedure; cell numbers decline with age
PRP	PROS: easy access with a needle puncture; less expensive; growth factors two to five times higher than normal CONS: variable growth factor concentrations based on the time of day the PRP is drawn and the platelet concentrations of the patient
Birth tissues, including amniotic fluid, Wharton's jelly, and membranes	PROS: growth factor two to sixty times higher concentration of key growth factors and cytokines; presence of amniotic cells depends on preparation; no second surgery CONS: cost; lack of cells (when filtered for sterility); quality control essential; FDA regulatory status unresolved (the FDA has placed a pause on further use of birth tissues until investigational drug trials are completed)

Let's expand on each of these sources. As a source of cells, fat is attractive—almost everyone has a little extra. It is highly vascular and therefore has many pericytes or cells living on the walls of the vessels. Those cells can be released from the vessels by mechanical shaking or by chemical release in the operating room (the FDA, at this time, only permits mechanical release for orthopaedic applications). The fact that the fat is from the same patient who is to receive the injection makes the risks of infection or rejection minimal. Numerous studies have shown that fat-derived cells can effectively release growth factors after injection into sites of injury and can help healing. A disadvantage is that the extra surgical procedure to harvest the fat creates a second site of potential surgical harm, sometimes deformity, and occasionally pain. It is not easy to do in an office setting. There is some concern that the cells derived from fat do not produce the same effect on musculoskeletal tissue as do the progenitor cells derived from bone. Lastly, the solution of fat cells is primarily cells and not growth factors, and thus leaves us relying on the cells to produce enough growth factors after injection.

Bone marrow is a rich source of musculoskeletal-derived stem cells in young people. The cells target injured tissues, release potent growth factors, and direct healing. Unfortunately, the number of stem cells declines rapidly with aging. Harvesting the cells requires a bone marrow needle stick, which is painful; therefore, only a limited number of cells are available.

PRP is platelet-rich plasma. Platelets are plentiful in most people's bloodstream. They play a major role in blood clotting (to stop bleeding from wounds), and they carry specialized vesicles called alpha granules loaded with growth factors. Drawing blood from a patient, spinning the blood in a centrifuge, and then concentrating and activating the platelets to cause release of the growth factors is the predominant method of utilizing this source of healing agents. There is tremendous variability in the preparation techniques. For example, other blood products, such as white blood cells, may be included. The process is relatively inexpensive, the science clear but highly variable, and the efficacy is most likely specific to each tissue injected.

Birth tissue products, such as membranes, cells, and fluids donated by the mothers when they give birth, are the new fountain of youth used in many fields of medicine. Tissues, cells, and fluids that provide protection for the fetus are rich in growth factors, unique fetal and maternal progenitor cells, lubricants, and a variety of other bioactive factors. The FDA currently does not know how to regulate these therapies. Are they drugs? Local devices? Do they have systemic effects in the recipients? What are the risks?

One major differentiator between birth tissue choices is the presence or absence of maternal cells, fetal cells, or growth (and other) factors. Maternal cells may be more likely to induce a rejection response or carry other unwanted characteristics. Fetal cells, Wharton's jelly, and amniotic fluid, on the other hand, have remarkable immuno-modulatory characteristics. These cells are antimicrobial (kill bacteria), antifibrotic (stop scarring), anti-inflammatory, and immune modulating to inhibit rejection of the fetus. Used as therapy, these growth factors—whether injected or released by cells—treat injured tissues and recruit the recipient's own healing cells to the site of the injection.

Pending FDA approval, some of the most potent birth tissue injections are the following:

- **Wharton's jelly.** This thick, gelatinous fluid, which surrounds the umbilical cord, is rich in growth factors and cells from both the mother and the fetus. For the cells to remain alive, the jelly must be stored in liquid nitrogen and defrosted immediately before injection.

- **Amniotic membranes.** The two layers of the amniotic membrane have different cell types and functions. The chorion (the maternal side of the membrane) is loaded with maternal cells, while the amnion (which faces the fetus) has fewer cells—but they are unique ones, believed to function as fetal stem cells. Companies that procure these membranes provide different products: chorion alone, chorion plus amnion, and amnion alone. The processing of the tissues determines whether or not the cells themselves stay alive, or only the growth factors. Cryopreserving the tissues (keeping them in extremely cold conditions in liquid nitrogen) keeps the cells active, while freeze-drying only keeps the growth factors active.

- **Amniotic fluid.** This is a potent, cost-effective anabolic injection. Depending on how it is processed, amniotic fluid may have two to sixty times the major growth factors found within a patient's own blood platelets. It contains a few unique fetal stem cells. If the fluid is obtained during a C-section and filtered through a 0.25-micron filter, it is sterile, acellular, growth-factor rich, and immediately available for use. With little processing required, amniotic fluid should be the least expensive product.

- **Exosomes.** These extracellular packets of growth factors and cytokines, released by progenitor cells, are also being packaged for therapeutic use. Their great potential is that specific packets of stimulating compounds may be selectively harvested for targeted therapies.

- **Cord blood and other placental tissues.** They most likely retain too many characteristics of the mother rather than those of the rapidly growing fetus and thus risk rejection.

If you are not yet confused by this plethora of choices, you are well ahead of the game. But don't think that these treatments are new. General surgeons have known since 1900 that amniotic membranes could be used to reduce adhesions in abdominal surgery. When the HIV/AIDS epidemic in the 1980s reduced the use of allograft (donor) tissues, tissue banks developed tests to screen out potentially infected donors. The tissues are now a remarkably safe alternative to cortisone, which damages tissues and shuts down healing. In contrast, the birth tissue derivatives stimulate healing, act as anti-inflammatories and antibiotics, help prevent scarring, and provide lubrication. Maybe not an actual fountain of youth, but certainly a potent therapy as we wait for more studies to define their optimal applications.

In the "do no harm" mindset of medicine, the use of birth tissues, once they become approved and cost-effective, would appear to be well within both safety and efficacy boundaries.

Given the wide range of helpful effects of stimulatory injections, it seems likely that the use of these active supplements to effect healing will expand rapidly in clinical care. In fact, we are seeing a reduction in surgical volume as we guide patients in regenerative medicine. Is a therapeutic version of the *Star Trek* medical tricorder far off? Or an MRI that not just captures images of injured body parts but also treats them? Or will we induce our own DNA to replicate our body parts the way salamanders do? Living in this anabolic era of sports medicine and arthritis care, we clearly have the capacity to heal and regenerate parts so you may live long and prosper.

Reincarnation:
Not Just for the Soul?

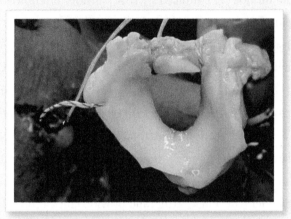

Donor lateral meniscus being transplanted by Dr. Stone
to replace the damaged or missing meniscus

Orthopaedic tissues transplanted into humans are dead tissues. That's right. Other than hearts, livers, and kidneys, which must be kept alive for immediate transplantation, any tissue that is removed from a donor or a cadaver is frozen, washed, sterilized, and delivered to a surgeon. From there, it may be used in new ACL grafts, meniscus replacements, rotator cuff patches, tendons for the hands and feet, and the list goes on.

The surgeon relies on the patient's healing ability to recognize and revive the dead donor graft. The body does this by sending scavenger cells that open up pores for the new blood vessels to bore into, lacing new blood vessels into the tissue, and finally sending specialized cells that lay down new collagen and restore the graft to life. In ligaments, this wonderful tissue regeneration process is called "ligamentization"; in other tissues, it's called "remodeling."

But the process of remodeling takes time, and during that period of restoration, the tissue is at its weakest stage. A new injury doesn't need to be very forceful to tear the healing tissue. Any illness might slow down the process. An early return to sports might put too much stress on the graft, leading to stretching or, in the worst case, a complete failure to remodel.

But why, in the twenty-first century, do we rely on nature's timeline alone to heal our repaired and replaced tissues? Fortunately, the entire field of tissue regeneration is changing rapidly.

Over the last few years, we concentrated and combined patients' own stem-derived cells and growth factors with donor tissues before using them to rebuild ACLs and meniscus tissue.

Today, tissues transplanted at surgery in our clinic are often preloaded with growth factors and patients' own marrow cells. They are then released into the joint at the time of surgery by making small holes in the bone. We must now do the basic science to determine the optimal concentrations of these factors when infused into tissues, and the clinical science to demonstrate if, and how much faster, the body heals with the use of these tissues.

INJECTION CHOICES FOR PAIN

Pain sucks. Pain is debilitating. It is hard to think straight, make good decisions, be a happy person, or contribute to society when you are in pain. There is no advantage to having pain after surgery. In fact, pain is a major cause of muscle inhibition, which leads to muscle atrophy and loss of joint motion, which leads to stiffness. Yet pain is still one of the most poorly understood sensations.

Why do we feel some kinds of discomfort and not others? For instance, you might wake instantly when rolling over onto a sharp edge of a bed frame, but not awaken when a surgical knife slices open your skin. Why do some people not feel pain at all? A full understanding of the how, why, when, and where of pain generation remains elusive. We do know that if pain is treated with opioid narcotics, the pain is still there but the patient doesn't care about it and may become addicted to the drugs. With this reality, we do all we can to block the brain from feeling pain by reducing it as much as possible with every safe therapy we can find.

Here are a few of the more novel ways to reduce pain using injections.

PRP or growth factor injections. One component of the blood stream is platelets, the cell-like particles, smaller than red or white blood cells, that release a soup of growth factors at the site of injury, sometimes in packets called exosomes. As explained earlier, platelets help in the clotting process by sticking to the walls of the damaged blood vessels and plugging the rupture. One of the most important compounds of the platelet is called platelet-derived growth factor (PDGF). This compound activates stem cells to produce progenitor cells, release from vessel walls, and migrate to the site of injury. The

progenitor cells and the growth factors released from the platelets have potent anti-inflammatory factors that reduce swelling and
thereby reduce pain.

White cells, the immune cells of the bloodstream, can be selectively
added or removed from PRP preparations. It is currently believed
that white cells can be used to increase the inflammatory response
when tissues are in more degenerative states and need a boost. Or,
they can be deployed in a two-step process, an initial increase and
then decrease in inflammation, thereby reducing pain.

An interesting side note: PRP is not new. It has been used for
more than thirty years in dentistry to speed the healing of reconstruc-
tive oral surgeries and by veterinarians to heal animals. While there
was some early fear in the sports world that the injections could be
a performance-enhancing substance, the fear seems to have been put
to rest. Major League Baseball, the NFL and the NBA, as well as the
World Anti-Doping Agency, have all declared that PRP is a safe and
legal treatment. So for now, blood doping with your own platelets
is legal, though blood doping with whole blood is not. Go figure.

Stem cell injections for pain relief. In arthritic joints, patients
report pain relief from injections of growth factors combined with
hyaluronic acid, often experiencing relief equal to that offered by
anti-inflammatory drugs. How does this work? The injected growth
factors activate the body's stem cells. The cells divide, producing
progenitor cells, which migrate to the joint and act by releasing
factors that modulate joint chemistry and influence local cells such
as macrophages. The stem-derived progenitor cells direct the anti-
inflammatory process by releasing specific proteins that: 1) reduce
degradative enzymes (factors that break down tissues); 2) shut down
the release of pro-inflammatory agents into the joint; and 3) stimulate

production of new collagen repair tissues. These factors also increase the production of lubrication in the joint by directly modulating the synovial cells lining the joint.

Anti-inflammatory injections. Compounds in the blood repair soup that most influence inflammation can be isolated in a unique incubation method that permits a potentially higher concentration of the factor called IL1Ra to be delivered to a site of injury. Additional anti-inflammation factors can be packaged into exosomes. The inducement of site- and action-specific growth-factor cocktails that target nerve endings are the hottest area of research in this space.

Lubrication injections for pain. The body's natural joint lubricant is called hyaluronic acid. This oil has been used to diminish the symptoms of arthritis by a series of injections. The lubricant decreases the release of small particles called wear particles, which irritate the lining of the joint, producing inflammation. More lubrication equals fewer particles, which means less inflammation, which equals less pain. Unfortunately, the lubricant only lasts in the joint for a few hours. Fortunately, when it works, the effect seems to last for months. The joint can be stimulated to produce more native lubrication by the addition of specific growth factors.

A Little Prick

Injections to the knee joint used to be scary and almost always involved pain. No more.

Knee injections can be nearly painless if several techniques are used. First, the patient must be relaxed. This way the muscles don't contract, forcing the kneecap against the femur and tightening the joint. Multiple deep, slow breaths usually do the trick, but sometimes a distracting nurse holding the patient's hand and telling a story does the job.

After the skin is thoroughly cleaned, we administer a local anesthetic (either as a topical ointment or injected with a dental microneedle). This step is critical to having a painless injection. Waiting a few minutes and letting the anesthetic drug work is the key. Stretching the skin overwhelms nerve stretch receptors. Placing strong pressure on the opposite side of the knee with a finger desensitizes the remaining nerve fibers. Additionally, having a patient count backwards from one hundred, out loud, especially in a second language if they speak one, has a dramatic effect on shifting the brain focus to a part of the brain that then selectively ignores the pain stimulus from the injection. The effect is quite remarkable. Last, a fast and accurate placement of the needle diminishes any residual pain.

WHY HA JOINT LUBRICATION WORKS

As part of a large, electrically charged sugar molecule, hyaluronic acid—the natural lubricant of the human joint—permits water to be absorbed and released from the cartilage surface of the joints. This provides durability and compressibility. Without HA we would all grind to a halt.

Recent work has clarified the many reasons why an injection of HA into a painful or arthritic joint helps relieve symptoms. These reasons include both mechanical lubrication and biochemical effects. Here are some of the highlights of this research.

- **Friction.** HA reduces friction, thereby decreasing the release of wear particles—bits of cartilage and bone that are rubbed off when two surfaces scratch against each other without protective lubrication—in the joint. These wear particles are known to irritate the joint lining, producing pain and swelling. (This effect, however, is limited by the fact that the injected HA, without the addition of growth factors, may only last a day or two within the joint, though its effect can last for months. Exactly why is unknown.)
- **Permeability.** HA is able to penetrate deeply into cartilage, directly affecting the cells that support cartilage (chondro-cytes), as well as into the synovium (the joint lining).
- **Cell behavior.** HA suppresses the genetic expression of several inflammatory molecules, acting as an anti-inflammatory and reducing joint swelling. It also reduces the production of degradative enzymes from the cells that break down cartilage—a process that accelerates arthritis.

- **Scarring.** Scar formation and subsequent loss of motion is one of the most disabling aspects of any joint injury or surgical intervention. HA affects certain antibodies and cell receptors involved in cell adhesion, which reduces the formation of scar tissue after injury or surgery.
- **Collagen formation.** Excess collagen formation is another mechanism by which scar tissue forms after an injury. HA suppresses the gene expression for the specific types of collagen involved in the formation of scars but not those collagens involved in the formation of normal articular cartilage.
- **Antioxidants.** HA has been demonstrated to prevent chondrocyte cell death by promoting the expression of antioxidant enzymes.
- **Pain.** After an ACL rupture or any tissue tear in the joint, inflammatory molecules associated with pain (the COX-2 enzyme) are reduced by the application of HA. The activity of neurotransmitters that stimulate the pain receptors is also reduced.
- **Long-lasting effects.** Given that the bulk of injected HA is cleared from the joint in a few days, its biologic and clinical effects are most likely due to the penetration of the lubricant into the tissues and its effect on the underlying cells. There is a natural increase in the production of HA after injection and an improvement in the physical properties of the synovial fluid.

Some people do not respond to HA injections. HA is divided in the marketplace between low and high molecular-weight formulations.

It is not clear which combinations provide the best balance between the physical effects of mechanical lubrication (high weight/cross-linked) and the biologic effects (low weight) of cell stimulation. Our clinical experience is that the efficacy of HA injections can be improved by the addition of growth factors to the injections. In our clinic, we combine the stimulation/anabolic factors with the HA into a single injection.

Many Ways to Lube Our Joints

We know that HA injections into the joint can ease pain and relieve stiffness, but what are the other ways in which we can lube our joints?

First, nutrition matters. The natural supplements glucosamine and chondroitin are the building blocks of the joint-lining-cartilage matrix. Orally ingesting fifteen hundred to three thousand milligrams of glucosamine a day has proved to affect the joint chemistry in positive ways by increasing matrix production, decreasing degradative enzymes that break down cartilage, reducing inflammation, and increasing the lubricant hyaluronic acid.

Second, daily exercise increases blood flow to the joints, strengthens the surrounding muscles, and increases testosterone, pheromones, and adrenaline—all of which improve one's sense of well-being and mobility. Hydration with water—rather than with coffee, soft drinks, or alcohol—increases tissue elasticity. Dehydrated tissues are stiff, not stretchy.

Drinking beverages loaded with glucosamine and chondroitin sulfate stimulates lubrication in the cartilage and soft tissues, but drinking the natural joint lubricant hyaluronic acid (HA) does not work. HA is broken down in the stomach before reaching the bloodstream or the joints. At present, the only way to get these growth factors combined with hyaluronic acid into the joint is by injection. But like the vaccines that can now be given by needle-free vapor guns, these therapies may be delivered more easily in the future.

Cortisone: The End of an Era

Cortisone, a therapeutic drug used to fight ailments ranging from asthma to arthritis, is naturally produced by the adrenal gland in the body and influences the functioning of most of the body's systems. It was the athlete's best friend throughout the twentieth century. But in orthopaedics today, cortisone use has a significant downside.

Since the discovery of its antirheumatic properties in 1948 and its synthetic commercial production soon after, the drug has been injected into every variety of swollen joint, inflamed tendon, sore back, and aching body. The anti-inflammatory nature of the drug soothed pain and reduced swelling, and permitted the athlete to further injure themselves time and time again.

We now know that a cortisone injection interferes with the body's natural healing process, which works like this: When tissues are overused, overstretched, or torn, the cells of those tissues release factors that recruit blood vessels, stem cells, and healing factors. With that in-rush of fluid, the tissue temporarily swells. Over time, with the laying down of new collagen, the protein that makes up most of our body, the injured tissue heals. Some tissues heal normally; others heal with scar tissue that can often remodel into normal tissue over time.

Cortisone shuts down this cellular recruitment process by reducing swelling but also, unfortunately, by inhibiting healing. The result is that the weakened tissues stay in the weakened state for a longer period of time, sometimes exposing the athlete to repeat injury or permanent damage. This panacea drug has always had this hidden, harmful risk. If used too often or in the wrong place—such as the Achilles tendon—the tissues can completely rupture and never return to their full, uninjured state.

Tendonitis is a great example. It often starts at the elbow, for example, after a hard golf or tennis shot and becomes chronically sore due to microtears in the tissue that fail to heal. The tissue, over time, becomes chronically degenerative and sore. Cortisone sometimes helps but does nothing to repair the injury and often weakens it further.

Fortunately, the cortisone era is over. We have realized that the best response to tissue injury is to stimulate stronger heal-ing, to feed the cells that are trying to repair the injury, and to recruit more progenitor or stem cells to guide the complex healing process. This tissue stimulation is done by a combination of careful, early tissue mobilization. It is often performed by expert physical therapists, by early joint and tissue-controlled exercises that stimulate repair rather than irritate the injury, and by direct application of growth factors and sometimes stem cells.

There are, of course, times when healing won't occur and cortisone can be symptomatically helpful, but our job is to figure out how to promote healing in those tough situations as well as in the more straightforward overuse cases.

Since we now understand the injury-healing cycle well enough and have the tools to boost the system, we almost always use stimulation factors first. Hopefully it relegates shutting down the body's natural healing process to the twentieth century.

CHAPTER 7

SURGERY, RECOVERY, AND REBUILDING

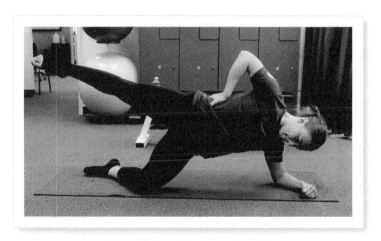

*Hannah D. • High-performance figure skater and
ankle articular cartilage repair patient*

Over the last decade, orthopaedic surgery has undergone a remarkable change. Surgeries such as total knee replacements have become outpatient procedures. What was once a week-long hospital stay—accompanied by terrible pain, narcotics, surgical drains, urinary catheters, intravenous medication pumps, passive motion machines, and significant complications—is now an outpatient procedure. Physical therapy is often started before surgery and continued before the patient leaves the surgical center, which is just an hour after entering the recovery room. How did this come about?

Several advances and changes in technique are responsible for the dramatic shortening of the surgical experience. (The exception is procedures for older people with significant health risks, who are still better off in a monitored hospital setting when undergoing any major surgery.)

First, prior to the operation, we focus on patient education. This includes preoperative physical therapy to maximize the range of motion of the joint and to introduce the patient to rehabilitation exercises and the use of cold compression therapy devices and crutches. (Cold compression devices, which circulate ice water through a pad around the surgical site, significantly reduce postoperative pain and swelling.) Of equal importance is a visit with the surgical nurse to review, in advance, the choice and use of nonnarcotic pain medications. These might include ketorolac (Toradol), aspirin, Tylenol, lidocaine patches, and possibly a "rescue" narcotic for breakout pain or sleep medication to be used if necessary.

Eliminating narcotics has been a primary factor in the reduction of complications. Narcotics not only make people nauseated; they decrease muscle function, cause urinary retention, and slow recovery. Having safe tools for pain reduction at home, and knowing how to use them, makes patients' first few nights after surgery far more pleasant than if they were in the hospital, awakened every few hours for monitoring of vital signs.

A few key changes have been made to surgical procedures as well. First, patient-specific cutting guides and customized implants, along with robotic or computer guidance, allow for smaller surgical incisions. This translates into less cutting of nearby tissue, more precise placement of implants, and faster surgery. A drug called tranexamic acid stops the bleeding locally, yet magically does not increase the risk of blood clots. This advance has eliminated the need for tourniquets, which produced significant post-op pain and muscle and nerve compromise.

Local anesthesia now plays a bigger role. We inject large volumes of diluted, Xylocaine-related drugs called ropivacaine or Marcaine in a pocket behind the knee capsule. These numbing compounds release slowly into the joint for twenty-four hours. The anesthesia team will add regional blocks in almost all cases, sometimes with long-acting slow-release lidocaine drug variants. Combined with cold compression, this strategy allows most of our knee-joint patients to leave the operating room pain-free—and stay that way—for twenty-four to thirty-six hours. A diligent schedule of additional nonnarcotic pain relievers makes the next few days quite manageable. Since the patients are in our physical therapy area each day for soft-tissue massage and guided exercises, any breakout pain can be controlled immediately.

Attenuated hospital visits benefit more than the patient. Cost savings to the medical establishment are also substantial. The current average hospital charge for a total knee replacement is $60,000.[27] Today, there are 719,000 knee replacements performed each year. Estimates suggest this will increase to 3.48 million total knees in 2030.[28] Moving to outpatient care can cut these costs by two-thirds, creating great savings for both patients and insurance companies. Getting patients into physical therapy sooner is also critical. Daily physical therapy mobilizes the joint, reduces the swelling that inhibits healing, and encourages well-body activities such as single-leg bicycling. Such exercise blows off the remaining anesthetics and stimulates well-being. Needless to say, there's a strong psychological benefit to starting the recovery program immediately, in an outpatient setting. Patients feel like athletes in training, not patients in rehab.

So the picture is much rosier. Artificial joint replacement has become considerably less painful, far quicker, and more accurate. When the best techniques are used, recovery times are faster than ever before. Moreover, we now have a clearer understanding of what post-recovery measures work, how to better handle pain, and what the patient needs to do to ensure a successful surgery as well as new insights into post-surgery diet, depression, and care. Let's deep dive into all of these so that you know what this orthopaedic surgical and recovery landscape now looks like.

---

[27] Samuel Greengard, "Understanding Knee Replacement Costs: What's on the Bill?" *Healthline*, updated April 13 2020, http://www.healthline.com/health/total-knee-replacement-surgery/understanding-costs.

[28] Steven Kurtz et al., "Projections of primary and revision hip and knee arthroplasty in the United States from 2005 to 2030," *Journal of Bone and Joint Surgery* 89 no. 4 (April 2007), https://www.ncbi.nlm.nih.gov/pubmed?term=17403800.

BECOMING A MORE EVOLVED PATIENT

Surgical procedures may have advanced in leaps and bounds, but patients, too, are evolving. It's not recognized that for a surgery to be truly successful, a patient must become a more active participant in controlling surgical outcomes. Here's how you can begin your journey as a more evolved patient:

Well before your surgery date. Exhaust all the alternatives to total knee replacement first. Depending on your exam, X-rays, and MRI, these alternatives may include physical therapy with gait, balance and muscle training, biologic joint replacement procedures with meniscus replacement, articular cartilage repair, or partial joint replacement if only one or two portions of the knee are worn out. Partial knee replacements work much better than in the past due to computer and robotic insertion techniques that have taken inaccuracy out of the procedure.

Envision a new you. Look at your procedure as an opportunity to become fitter, faster, and stronger than you have been in years. This is not usually possible when you are in pain, but it is a great goal to have once the discomfort is gone. Looking forward to "you, only better" makes the experience much less worrisome and turns it into a positive event in your life.

Before surgery. Line up a physical therapist, a trainer, a massage therapist, and a nutritionist. Yes, all of them, if possible. Use presurgery physical therapy and massage to increase range of motion and develop exercise routines focused on trunk and core strengthening.

See a nutritionist to help ensure that your dietary intake of protein is sufficient to respond to the stress of surgery. Protein matters. There is solid data that a low albumin level (protein level in the blood) correlates with increased infection during and after surgery. Also, optimizing your weight before and after surgery helps you preserve your new joint.

The night before your procedure, be entertained. Go out and see a movie, or watch a comedy series at home. Relax, laugh, and sleep well.

The day of surgery. Smile. Having a confident, calm, positive attitude affects you and your surgical team. Upbeat comments translate into happy outcomes. The advice of my nurse and surgical assistant, Ann Walgenbach, is to just "let it go" (as in the song). Be confident that you are in safe hands. You're going to have a really good nap, and in a few minutes, you'll have a new knee. If you are anxious, consider listening to a guided meditation or music (some surgery centers will allow you to listen in the operating room). If you are particularly anxious, talk to your surgical team about whether you can take a medication such as Valium in the morning with a sip of water.

After surgery. Set aside time to focus on physical therapy—the day after surgery and every day. A great physical therapist will help work on the entire body, restoring the ability of parts to work together. Take enough time off work to get into the physical therapy clinic as often as possible in the first six weeks. While some surgeons don't believe physical therapy helps, we are adamantly in the opposite camp.

Some physical therapists will focus on training and fitness, but others may not have the time or insurance permission to do so. Consider seeing a fitness trainer at a gym or hiring one to come to your home. It's often less expensive and feels less like medical treatment. Post-surgery, it is important to see yourself as an athlete in training rather than a patient in rehab. Focus on building muscle strength in your upper body, trunk, and core as well as the lower extremities. Bike and pool exercises cannot be overdone.

Book regular massages. A massage therapist can often augment the work the physical therapist does and keep your tissues flexible while your joint heals and your body retrains. Treat yourself as any pro athlete would; use all the tools of the fitness trade.

If you are thinking that only rich people or privately insured people can follow this advice, think again. Physical therapy is usually covered for at least a few sessions. Gym trainers and fitness classes can be found for less than twenty dollars an hour. Self-massage works too. Nutrition advice is widely available online. Focus on increasing protein and water intake, decreasing carbohydrates, and exercising more than you eat. Be more active, more aware, and more focused on your recovery, while working toward staying positive and visualizing the goal you're working toward—all of this helps in allowing you to get back on your feet and be better than you have been in years. Whether your sport is skiing or simply walking in the mall, our goal is to help you do these actively and without pain so that you can drop dead at age one hundred while enjoying your sport. To do that, seeing yourself as an athlete in training and treating yourself as the pros do is the trick.

Finding the Zen of Surgery

Calm, happy patients make calmer, happier surgeons. It adds up to better outcomes. Though it's hard to prove, the more the patient helps the surgeon relax, the better the surgeon perceives the patient and the job ahead. I know, having been both the surgeon and the patient.

As a surgeon, I see every patient as a unique challenge and every problem as an opportunity for improving my surgical technique and their outcome. An anxious patient—or worse, a distrustful patient— biases the decision-making process in surgery.

Let's take, as an example, a patient whose ligament is at least partially torn. Based on the patient's history, exam, and MRI, the surgeon decides whether to perform a primary repair (which has a higher chance of failing, but a better outcome if it works) or a full reconstruction (where the ligament is replaced by a new ligament, either from the patient's own knee or from a donor). This decision is based on a number of factors. Is the repair possible and likely to work? Is the patient willing to restrict their activities while the ligament heals? Did the patient understand the risks well enough before surgery, and will they be okay if it fails and requires another surgery?

While each of these decisions seems clear, there's another factor to consider. How patients present themselves in the pre-op holding room just before the surgery actually affects how the surgeon makes his or her decision. If a patient meets the surgeon with confidence and calm, it creates a certain mindset. A patient's smile and grace instill in the surgeon the confidence to do for the patient what they would do for themselves and approach the procedure with boldness and creativity.

If the patient is tense, wary, or unfriendly—or even if a family member or friend attending them is—the surgeon retreats to the safe zone of doing what is most likely to work rather than what might be a novel and potentially better approach.

As a patient who is also a surgeon, I understand that I probably induce a bit of over-caution in both the surgeon and the OR team. The natural intimidation of operating on one of your peers and knowing that your procedures will be reviewed by informed eyes makes the procedure that much more difficult. How to deal with this?

The answer—whether one is next to the operating table or on it —lies in the Zen of surgery. If both parties appear calm, display confidence and competence, and show a personal touch, the experience and outcome are more likely to be successful. As I tell my patients, "I can fix almost any complication, as long as your head is in a good space." When a patient has a positive attitude and approaches the procedure from a position of "Let's do this together," complications seem to occur less often.

So, the next time you find yourself heading into surgery, smile. Infuse the world around you with your grace. The whole operating room team will bestow their competence and creativity upon you.

VIP Patient? Choose Vanilla Care

Varying medical protocols because someone is extra special can lead to problems. If you are extra special, I suggest you request plain, vanilla care and expect the best outcome to occur. Here is why.

VIPs come in all forms: superstar athletes, politicians, CEOs, social media notables, rock stars. If they are humble and are treated at the level of excellence that we all expect, things go well. If they are arrogant, or if the staff is in awe, the problems begin early. Here are a few of the potential errors that you, the VIP, might make.

It starts with the first call to the office. If you are in a rush to get in immediately, you often fail to fill out all the forms necessary for us to understand your past medical background, allergies, or other risk factors for medical and surgical care.

You will push to be seen right away, even on a day that is not a normal patient exam day for us. If we acquiesce, the diagnostic testing team may not be available, and the full complement of physical therapists may already be booked out. Thus, you won't benefit from the PT assessment and instruction. We use physical therapists to help patients avoid surgery or to get the most out of any surgical procedure. The PTs often see issues the surgeon may not see, as well. This collaboration leads to the highest quality care. You risk missing out on that when you skip the full evaluation.

You may not book enough time for a pre-op conversation, the lengthy physical exam, and review of imaging studies, not to mention time for any additional MRIs or X-rays. Normal appointments with our clinic take from two to four hours.

Squeezing us in between your other obligations just doesn't cut it, assuming you want truly insightful diagnostic analysis.

Once scheduled for surgery, you forget the instructions on pain medications, blood clot prevention, and bowel management. You get constipated and woozy on unnecessary narcotics. You request extra opioids, and thanks to your extra doses of charm, you receive them, and the problems associated with opioids multiply. You sleep wearing a brace that you were supposed to take off. You can't remember how to use the ice machine, which is meant to keep your knee cold and reduces pain.

The surgical and rehab team do not get enough time to get to know you personally, so the little changes that we usually make to customize your surgery and rehab program get skipped. And you don't book enough days in physical therapy after surgery, forgetting that it takes months to fully heal. You forget that we are encouraging you to be an athlete in training, rather than a patient in rehab—a mindset that involves training your entire body while your injured joint is healing.

You jump on a plane to attend an "important" business meeting the week after surgery, which increases your blood clot risk, your swelling, and your stiffness.

Due to your busy schedule, you want physical therapy at home rather than in the clinic. While you are out of a trainer's sight, the little problems that pop up turn into big problems that may have been avoidable.

You accelerate the post-op protocols on your own due to the delusions of invincibility that made you a VIP in the first place. This acceleration sometimes works out great, and other times, it leads to procedure failure. But you would never acknowledge that it's your error.

The nursing team, meanwhile, has a hard time following up with you as you insist they go through your assistant to answer every question.

So even you—the VIP—are much better off being one of the very important patients in our practice, and not the standout. Plain vanilla is sometimes the perfect flavor.

Don't Die from the Hospital

Hospitals are wonderful places if you are very sick and need care. Top US hospitals have excelled in delivering leading-edge treatments and saving lives. But once that goal has been achieved, the rest of the care too often falls short. Hospitalization can be a pretty bad experience. Hospitals can be hotbeds of diseases, and mistakes in care can happen. So what can you do to ensure you have a successful visit to the hospital and minimize the risks of your stay?

First things first, in general, you need a protector watching over you at all times in the hospital. The excellent nurses and doctors are carrying too many responsibilities to get everything exactly right. One small error may mean that your lifetime is shortened.

Second, be vigilant from the moment you enter the premises. This is where the problems can start. If you are coming through the emergency room and your records are not on the hospital's electronic medical record system, the data you give may or may not be accurate. Your memory may fail you in the tension of the moment, and the diseases you have had in the past or the medicines to which you are allergic may be forgotten. The solution is to carry a copy of, or a link to, your complete medical record on your phone.

Bringing a smile into the hospital and maintaining it during every interaction with the staff will go a long way to improving your care. When you make others feel at ease and appreciated, they care for you with ease and appreciation. No matter how serious your condition, try to find the hopefulness and—better still—the humor in the situation. Additionally, the calmness and confidence you exude infuses the care team. Anxious, angry patients, unfortunately, get angry, anxious care. Your guardian also influences your care. Be sure he or she reflects your mission: to get healed and get out of there intact, without complications. Your personal team must help the hospital team deliver.

A doctor or nurse's evaluation may be the first real contact you have in the hospital. The time they take to assess you, the quality of their listening, and their exam may be high or low, fast or slow. Insist—or have your guardian insist—that you be completely undressed during this step. Let no part of you be left to chance.

The IV placed in your arm is often the first invasion of your body. This may be done with a highly sterile technique (the arm washed with alcohol and chlorhexidine, which has been shown to reduce contamination) or just a quick swipe with an alcohol swab. Insist on the more thorough wash.

The tests ordered for your condition may be the best ones, or maybe not. Be sure to have your primary care provider, who knows you, call in and speak to the doctor. Nothing beats a long-term patient/physician relationship. The great personal doctor you selected and stuck with, along with his or her deep knowledge of you and no other conflicting priorities, is the best medicine. If you don't have a primary care provider or you are in a system that doesn't assign you one doctor who knows you well, you may be out of luck in this regard.

Once admitted and treated, after surgery, the post-procedure stay in the hospital has been significantly shortened. This is mostly a good thing since too many bad things happen in hospitals. Still, you—or the guardian angel/nurse/friend/family member who has volunteered to stay with you—must insist on several things. First, the vital signs that are taken every few hours, all night long, guarantee a lack of sleep. They are often not necessary. Unfortunately, if the doctor checked the box for routine orders and did not think about it, your sleep is compromised. Just by asking the nurse to check with the doctor to see if you can have an uninterrupted night of sleep will usually solve the problem.

Second, insist on a private room. The data on shared rooms in hospitals is awful from an infection, sleeplessness, and quality of experience point of view. Bring in a pair of noise-canceling head-phones. As with being on an airplane, there is very little you need to hear most of the day in a hospital.

Third, if you are post-surgery, get the physical therapist and OT staff involved immediately. Even if you are bedridden, they can work on massaging your feet and exercising your arms within your doctor's limits. Hands-on therapy does a world of good for the body and the mind. Some hospitals allow outside massage therapists, physical therapists, and trainers to come in. If they do, hire them if you can.

Finally, order in great food. Food delivery from high-quality restaurants is available in every major city. Your nutrition counts. High-protein diets often help patients' recovery from injury and surgery. Check with your doctor, but eat well to live well.

Getting so sick or injured that you land in a hospital is bad luck. Getting well is an art form that requires all your imagination, engagement, and persistence. As a new, evolved patient, bring this skillset with you to the hospital so that you can leave with gratitude and the determination to not return.

ALIGNING EXPECTATIONS

We've covered what your surgical and rehab teams will (ideally) do to bring about successful results and what you can do to support their efforts. But what does "successful" mean? What do you expect to get from your surgical care? No one really asks this question, yet the answer determines your satisfaction. Surprisingly, the answers you receive from your surgeon, your physical therapist, your fitness trainer, and your coach may differ.

Let's look at the case of an injury to a high school football player. The athlete, a wide receiver, tears his ACL in the first game of the season, in his junior year. His expectation, if anyone asks, is to return to play by spring training and be back at his full potential by late summer, with his college recruiting opportunities unaffected.

The young man is treated by the team orthopaedic surgeon. He is given an ACL reconstruction that uses his own patellar tendon with bone from his patella and tibia. The surgery goes well, and his surgeon tells him and his parents that if all goes well in physical therapy, he will be cleared to return for the next season. His surgeon expects a "good" outcome.

He sees a physical therapist a few times a week for six weeks—the maximum his insurance will allow. The therapist knows this amount of intervention is not enough, but their hands are tied. The therapist works on his range of motion but tells him that after physical therapy, he will be on his own to regain strength, balance, proprioception, and all the components of fitness required by a successful football player.

Some of the player's buddies who have undergone the same surgery tell him about a trainer at their gym who seems smart about fitness. The trainer works with the player whenever he shows up, but school and other obligations get in the way. The trainer knows the kid won't make the team without a serious commitment.

The coach, who has been around for thirty years, knows the unfortunate truth: 30 percent of the ACL reconstructions in teenagers fail in the first two years. Harvesting the patellar tendon significantly weakens the front of the knee, and 50 percent of people with ACL reconstructions develop arthritis within ten years. The playing time in the pros after an ACL injury is only two to three years. The data for a college athlete who has experienced an ACL injury in high school is not known, but it probably isn't encouraging. The coach knows that the scouts will factor this in. He has also seen a lot of high school athletes drop their sport after ACL surgery and has observed others who return with a slight limp or favoring their surgical side. He tries hard to get more physical therapy for those athletes who are motivated, connecting them with trainers who will work with them daily and inspire them to return fitter than they were before they were injured. He has seen that athletes who buy in to this "better than ever" program actually do well in high school, college, and the pros.

So, if the surgeon knows the surgery is good but not perfect, the therapist knows that the time spent with the athlete is nowhere near enough, the trainer knows that it takes daily fitness coaching to excel, and the coach knows that the injury can be fatal to the athletic career—if all this is true—why do we persist with subpar solutions that lead to a low probability of success? Is it because this is the "standard of care" that the insurers will pay for? Perhaps. But how often do we ask the question, What are the expectations of everyone involved in my care, and what can I do to exceed historical outcomes?

This applies not only to ACL injuries. It is rare that significant musculoskeletal injuries requiring reconstructions with replacement tissues or devices ever return the joint to completely normal functionality. Yet the expectations of the injured patient are based on the hope that their medical and surgical care can restore them to a pre-injury state. The expectations of the doctors and therapists are that they will do their best, and the rest is up to the patient. The expectations of researchers in this field are that applications of growth factors—stem-derived cells combined with engineered and donor tissues—will make the outcomes significantly better.

Once expectations and therapies are aligned, doctors, therapists, and patients can work together to set achievable, superior goals. But if you don't ask—and *keep* asking—you will never know.

The fact is that a repaired joint injury is never again a pristine joint. Bone is the only tissue in the entire human body that regrows to a state that is indistinguishable from normal. All other tissues have a component of scar tissue, abnormal collagen fibers, and altered cellular distribution. Injuries and surgery, either overtly or subtly, change the athlete's attitude about their body. You, the injured athlete, have control over these five things:

1. how well you adhere to goals that help you achieve greater levels of performance and fitness than you experienced pre-treatment;

2. how well you train your mind and body to overcome deficits;

3. how well you use the resources available to assist you;

4. how well you choose and interact with your surgeon to be sure that he or she shares your goals and has the knowledge and tools to provide leading edge care; and

5. how well you and your physician use the evolving field of tissue replacement, growth factors, and progenitor/stem-cell therapies to accelerate healing and prevent the onset of arthritis.

Here Today, Gone Tomorrow

Not every medical "advance" ends up taking us forward. Take, as an example, the development of resorbable materials used to replace metals in joint repair surgery.

Metal has been used in patients since the time of Hippocrates (400 BCE) to repair broken bones and replace missing parts. The earliest metals included copper, tin, and lead, and often did not have the strength to last a lifetime. Over the centuries, surgical metals have improved. They have become stronger and leach fewer ions into the body. The vast majority do the job without causing complications, but since they remain inside the body, there is always a slight risk of problems developing.

Over the past thirty years, the use of absorbable or resorbable implant materials has grown. At first impression, it's an attractive idea: the body grows into the device, or it dissolves on its own as the body heals after the successful repair. Initially, absorbable synthetic materials, such as polylactides and collagen scaffolds, were the most commonly used materials to affix tissue. Sutures originally made of resorbable catgut became permanent with the introduction of cotton and silk materials and then evolved to resorbable threads made of lactide polymers.

One well-known application of resorbable material is a component of ACL reconstruction. Surgeons typically fixed the tissue with screws made of stainless steel, and then titanium. More recently, biodegradable screws made of lactides—often mixed with calcium phosphate—swept the marketplace.

The developers believed that as the body healed, these screws would be replaced by bone in the bony tunnels, making any future surgery easier. But as these screws were resorbed in the body, toxic materials were sometimes released, causing cavities and cysts in the bone. Follow-up X-rays showed tibias that looked like Swiss cheese.

What caused this to happen? Our bodies have evolved over millions of years to recognize and respond aggressively to foreign materials. Once materials are recognized as foreign, the body attacks with cells and enzymes that break down and chew up the invasive materials or wall them off with a protective layer of scar or bone. As the foreign materials are broken down by these systems, artificial components—which can have detrimental effects on the cells and surrounding tissues—are released.

Lactides, as mentioned earlier, are commonly used to make resorbable screws. But these screws release high concentrations of lactic acid in the tunnels where they press against the ligaments and bone. In this narrow space, the acid kills the responding cells, forming cysts in the bones. The acid also inhibits osteoblasts that build bone, preventing the body from filling in the defects. As a solution, permanent crystalline plastic materials called PEEK were developed to replace the resorbing screws. Though they worked well and were invisible on X-rays, they were hard to find and difficult to remove if the joint was reinjured.

The end result? In some cases, good old metal has returned as the material of choice in fixing bone to bone and sometimes even soft tissue to bone. The metal works without inciting the inflammation seen in resorbable materials. It's also easy to see on X-rays and straightforward to remove at surgery. Progress continues, however. There are now novel designs of sutures and anchors with cores of silk material that absorb salt water from the body, swelling and tightening the repair even after the surgeon leaves the table. These more biocompatible materials will evolve further to again replace metals and inflammatory materials in many applications. The lessons for those of us who have seen enough pendulums swing in medicine are that newer is sometimes better, but not always.

POST-SURGERY RECOVERY

You've come through your surgical procedure with flying colors. Now it's time to get back on your feet again as soon as possible. First on your to-do list: take care of your tissues.

What happens in the tissues when the body is injured? Damage occurs when you stretch tissue past its functional limit or traumatize it in some other way. We understand quite well how the body reacts to injury. When tissue tears or ruptures, bleeding occurs. A sequence of events then follows: tissue swelling, reabsorption of dead tissues, and remodeling with new collagen. The injury stimulates the body to recruit cells and blood vessels into the area so that eventually, healthy tissues replace the injured ones.

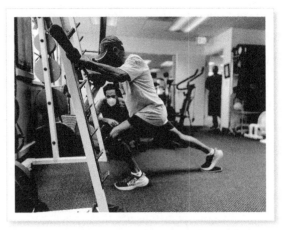

Lanny B. • Long-distance runner and partial knee
replacement & testosterone study patient

In some ways, the time immediately after surgery is no different from the moment after the first injury. You have been hit with an axe, otherwise known as a scalpel. No matter how delicately it was applied, the tissues were first surgically separated and held apart while the underlying injury was repaired. The body rushed a new blood supply to the incision. Pain fibers sent millions of signals to the brain (though the magic of anesthesia somehow blocked the memory of it), tissues swelled, muscles contracted, and all your injury protective mechanisms went into overdrive. The trick is to direct all of those responses into a healing rather than a recoiling response.

To do this effectively, you need to manage the pain. Suffering from pain after surgery is one of the most-feared experiences in medical care. Yet this fear is unnecessary because pain is largely preventable. No surgical outcome is improved by the patient having pain. Both you and the surgeon want to minimize discomfort so you can focus on your recovery exercises. Here's what you can do.

- **Talk to your doctors.** Before surgery, be sure to discuss the pain-relief strategies you and your doctor plan to deploy. Ask your doctor if you can take oral nonnarcotic pain medication such as Celebrex the night before and the morning of surgery. Ask your surgeon to deploy the newest long-acting local pain medications at the site of surgery before any incision is made. New versions of the traditional lidocaine numbing medications are bound to slow-releasing fat molecules and provide three days of anesthetic. They are so effective that many total joint replacement operations are now moving to outpatient centers as the patients can go home the same day. In addition, you can discuss with your anesthesiologist the use of regional blocks that also provide long-acting pain relief.
- **Get the right mix.** You want to find the combination of nonnarcotic plus narcotic medications that relieve post-op pain yet minimize the nausea normally associated with them. We use T&T first—Tylenol and Toradol—because they are great pain relievers without the narcotic downsides. When combined with ice, elevation, and soft-tissue massage, narcotics can often be avoided. With icing, newer sequential-compression ice machines, such as Game Ready, relieve pain by decreasing swelling with local cooling.
- **Use enough medication.** Many patients are scared of using too much medication. They then underdose and suffer needlessly. It is unlikely we will make you an addict after a couple of weeks of needed medications. However, it is likely you will be miserable if pain is not controlled.
- **Prepare mentally.** Remember the Buddhist advice that you can have pain but not suffer from it. This mental preparation

dramatically improves your ability to work with the symptoms and discomfort any surgical procedure has and yet not suffer from the underlying pain.

- **Use alternative pain-management methods if they work for you.** These can include acupuncture, electrical stimulation, and meditation. The wide variation in people's responses to these modalities is always surprising. When they work, they work without side effects.

- **Use alternative medications if they work for you.** The role of THC (tetrahydrocannabinol), CBD (cannabidiol), and other medical compounds extracted from cannabis is being evaluated in several studies. There probably is an important role for drugs that cause disengagement, mellowness, and euphoria in the postoperative time. Dosing and FDA-approved recommendations are not yet available, unfortunately.

Why R.I.C.E. Is Not Always Nice

For years, the traditional formula of R.I.C.E.—Rest, Ice, Compression, and Elevation—has been used for post-injury swelling. But this may not always be appropriate. Of course, we want to reduce swelling and stimulate cells to lay down their collagen, thereby strengthening the tissues. However, what we've accepted as "standard interventions" for those tasks are not necessarily the best ones.

Reducing swelling, for instance. We traditionally use ice, soft-tissue massage, and elevation to help reduce swelling. But that initial swelling is part of the body's healing response. Warmth is caused by vessels migrating to the site of the injury, and the massage can displace the tissues that are trying to heal. Elevation decreases the blood pressure to the site that needs increased perfusion. So, in a sense, each of those things is counterproductive to the healing process we are trying to stimulate.

"Wait," you say, "if swelling is good for us, why have we been taught to reduce it?"

Swelling isn't good for us all the time. It initially helps by recruiting healing factors that accelerate how quickly cells migrate to the site of injury. But swelling is also bad because it destructs and distends the tissues and distorts the anatomy. Fluid enzymes within the swollen fluid break down tissue as well as stimulate it.

Think of inflammation as appearing in two phases. Immediate swelling is required for tissue repair; it releases enzymes that break down tissue, along with anabolic factors and cells that rebuild tissue. But late swelling is almost always harmful, as those same enzymes have already done their job and now are attacking healthy tissue.

During the last few hundred years of medical science, we have figured out how to intervene with bold strokes for many problems. This is also true with anti-inflammatory drugs. If you hit something with an anti-inflammatory today, you hit ALL the tissues in the body. The entire patient gets that hammer of anti-inflammatories. To add to the complexity, we have limited ways of controlling what happens when you use both heat and elevation, ice and elevation, or an anti-inflammatory and ice. It's a complex dynamic. The next few years of trauma repair science will focus on understanding and managing these interactions.

The bottom line is that there is a wonderful and mysterious balance between when swelling is good and when swelling is bad. The question for doctors and patients is, What is the timing for swelling reduction, and what is the optimal way to do it? With advances in technology, we will get better at exposing the injured tissue to the optimal components of swelling at just the right time.

As of today, we counsel our patients post-surgery to use twenty minutes of ice compression, using machines such as Squid or Game Ready, every hour while awake—for swelling and pain control for the first few days, and then intermittently as needed for the next two weeks. We ask patients to elevate their leg above their heart when not exercising. Those that do that well, often turning around in bed and putting their feet high up against the wall for a few hours, often have much less swelling than those who ignore the advice and work all day with their legs down at their desk, or worse, go shopping. Manual physical therapy with an emphasis on effleurage—the technique of massaging fluid from distal to proximal, feet to hips, or hands to shoulders—practiced every day makes a huge difference. If a qualified physical therapist is not available, many athletic trainers and massage therapists can do the job well. Compression stockings worn when standing help reduce swelling and may help diminish the risk of blood clots. Novel wearable battery-powered compression pumps are quite effective as well.

The Opioid Crisis Solution

Weed. Almost 50 percent of the patients in my practice recently used marijuana to reduce their post-op pain. I didn't prescribe it; the word just seems to be out.

Postoperative pain is part of surgery. We do everything we can to minimize it. The available narcotic drugs are awful. They are addictive, produce constipation, nausea, and wooziness. Narcotics reduce the ability of the patients to participate in rehab exercises, slow their recovery, and are part of the cause of muscle atrophy. They are not even good pain relievers. Most work by making people feel dissociated from the pain, and not really interfering with the pain fibers. Despite the many measures we take to reduce pain, both presurgery and post-surgery, it's often not enough. Opioids such as Dilaudid, Percocet, OxyContin, and Vicodin are often prescribed, but the postoperative complications due to these drugs are too many to list.

Today, with the legalization of marijuana in California, many of our patients are self-medicating with various combinations of CBD and THC, the most well-known components of the marijuana plant. The local pot shops sell tinctures, edibles, and various other forms in a dizzying combination of THC-to-CBD ratios. The current buzz is that CBD is not psychoactive but reduces inflammation, and the indica version of marijuana plants helps with sleep and relaxation.

The reality of all botanical medications is that they contain a variety of other active components. Most likely, these work together —a synergy called "the entourage effect"—to be most potent. "For the relief of pain, there is no more useful medicine than Cannabis within our reach," wrote Sir John Russell Reynolds, physician to Queen Victoria, in 1859. Yet due to government restrictions, we are all at the very early stages of understanding the roles of the two main cannabinoid receptors, CB1 and CB2, found in the brain, and CB2 found all over the body, as well as the yet-to-be-found other receptors. Learning how each of these active ingredients works, both independently and together, is a work in progress.

Many of our patients are not waiting. They report to us a sense of well-being after using pot postoperatively. They use fewer opioids, often returning the bottles to the clinic unopened, and have no side effects from the home remedy. It is not just acute pain situations where cannabis is having a major impact. Chronic pain, which we used to treat with buckets full of narcotics, is also being impacted by the cannabis medical revolution.

I don't yet prescribe cannabis as it is not legal from a federal licensure point of view. But how can I not encourage it?

SURGICAL INFECTIONS

"Doctor, will I get an infection from surgery? If I do, then what?" This is a question your surgeon never wants to hear, much less have to answer. Why? Because no one knows the answer for sure.

Infections, fortunately, are uncommon in elective orthopaedic surgery. They happen in only 0.1 percent to 0.4 percent of cases,[29] and can usually be treated without long-term consequences. Sometimes, however, infection leads to disaster: the loss of the implant, or worse, the loss of a leg. For this reason, infection is feared by both doctor and patient. The randomness of infections, the cost, the loss of work time, and the risk to life and limb all drive a maniacal effort to prevent them.

As with much of medicine, there are many interrelated causes of infection. On the surgeon's side, these causes can be linked to errors in sterilization of equipment, breaks in surgical sterile technique, or failure to recognize unique risk factors the patient may have (such as an immune deficiency or simultaneous infection in another part of the body).

---

[29] Laura Prokuski, "Prophylactic antibiotics in orthpaedic surgery," *Journal of the American Academy of Orthopaedic Surgeons* 16 no. 5 (May 2008), https://journals.lww.com/jaaos/fulltext/2008/05 000/prophylactic_antibiotics_in_orthopaedic_surgery.7.aspx; Linda R. Greene, "Guide to the Elimination of Orthopedic Surgical Site Infections," *American Journal of Infection Control* 40 no. 4 (May 2010), DOI: 10.1016/j.ajic.2011.05.011.

All of these are avoidable. Checklists have popped up in operating rooms to raise the level of awareness about every single detail that might lead to an infection. Common behaviors of the past—such as too many people in the operating room or frequent opening and closing of the OR doors—have been virtually eliminated.

On the patient's side, there are the easy things to control and the impossible ones. Careful preoperative and postoperative washing of the skin with Chlorhexidine, a compound found in most antibacterial soaps, has proved to be the most effective skin preparation. Preoperative antibiotics timed just thirty minutes before surgery are more effective than antibiotics given long before or after surgery.

Huge variability exists in a patient's susceptibility to bacteria encountered in the operating room, which can never be perfectly sterile. Dust in the air, particles circulating through air-conditioning systems, and even small amounts of skin flakes from the surgical team's faces or eyebrows can carry viable organisms. We have often commented that a surgeon could spit into one patient's wound and the patient would never develop an infection, whereas a different person would grow a nasty bacterium despite sterilization procedures carried out as carefully as possible. How can that be?

The answer remains a mystery. Some people naturally host unique bacteria on their skin—so much so that a new field of forensic diagnosis of crime scenes focuses on which bacteria a criminal left behind. Some people can live with one organism all over their wounds, yet not tolerate another. With all the high-tech solutions we have to prevent infection, and with the best of practices and the healthiest of patients, an out-of-control growth of one specific bacterium can still blossom into infection. The future of preventive therapies may well lie in the testing of each individual for specific bacterial challenges, just as we now do for allergies. Once we know which bacteria a patient will not tolerate, targeted preventive steps may dramatically lower infection rates.

Fortunately, if identified and treated immediately, most infections (even deep ones around implants) can be eradicated with surgical washing of the wounds and organism-specific antibiotics. But even this is variable. Some patients will respond immediately, and others, not for weeks. Our advice to patients and their surgeons is to take all precautions, use the best techniques, identify the problems immediately, and treat each problem aggressively—like a cancer that could grow out of control. If this is done, only very few infections will become true disasters.

Infection is a rare possibility for all of us, but this fact should not prevent the right procedures from being performed for the right patients at the right time, all the time.

PHYSICAL THERAPY AND EXERCISE

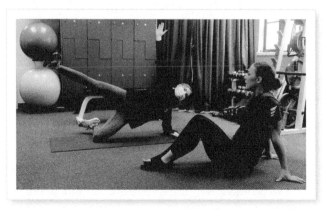

Athletic trainer Morgan from The Stone Clinic, carefully guiding the form of exercise and rehabilitation movements

Motion is life. Motion is also stimulus. After injury or surgery, scar tissue forms unless motion is applied. We want to get you moving as soon as possible.

When tissues are injured, a cascade of events occurs. These include inflammation and the release of chemical signals to recruit new cells. Some of these cells remove damaged tissue, while others form collagen: the fibrous material that makes up skin, bones, muscles, and all connective tissue.

At first, the eruption of the tissue repair process creates a tangled mess of collagen fibers. While normal tissues are made of a mixture of small and large collagen fibers, this new tissue contains only small-diameter fibers and has the biomechanical and structural properties of scar tissue. Over time, the body can either remodel this scar tissue into normal tissue (as it does with bone) or form the familiar scar tissue we often see with healed skin.

This remodeling process can be steered along more normal pathways using both chemical and physical factors. Motion is the most forceful of healing strategies.

Here is a typical example. When a football player's knee joint is hit from the side, the medial collateral ligament can rupture. In the past, the knee was placed into a cast or a fixed splint, and the ligament healed over a six-week time frame. But the physical properties and strength of the healed ligament were weak, leaving it—and the player—vulnerable to a repeat injury.

We have since learned that if motion is applied early in the healing process, the ligament heals with a more normal appearance. The motion has to be enough to provide stress, but not so much that it disrupts the healing fibers. This motion stimulates the repair cells to produce fibers that are oriented along the lines of stress. The motion-aligned fibers also have a more normal distribution of large and small diameters rather than the tangled variety of fibers formed when the knee is placed in a cast.

More than ligaments benefit from motion. The bearing surfaces of the joints are called articular cartilage. When injured, these surfaces do not heal on their own, and arthritis—the wearing down of injured cartilage—progresses. When the injury is repaired using techniques such as articular cartilage paste grafting, followed by the application of motion with the use of a continual passive motion machine, the healed cells of the articular cartilage look like normal cartilage tissue. Without the motion, only fibrous scar tissue forms.

The lesson that motion is critical for tissue repair applies widely in medicine and in life. Whether we are talking about physical trauma or mental injury, recovery from surgery, or adapting to pharmaceutical treatments, the advice of the past—when patients were told to "go home and rest in bed"—is rarely used today. Even head colds seem to improve with gentle exercise. The key is modulating the activity enough to stimulate repair, but not so much that it induces further injury.

How do you know exactly how much motion is enough and not too much? As physicians and physical therapists, we make educated guesses. We know impact exercises are often too much, and cycling is often just right. We wish the data were more specific to each tissue and each type of repair. The evaluation techniques of the future may involve extremely high-field, localized MRI machines that can focus on very small areas of tissue and provide real-time information on their healing status.

Physical therapy is the first step in getting in motion again. Remember those old lyrics, "The knee bone's connected to the thigh bone, the thigh bone's connected to the hip bone?" The song is actually a good anatomical reminder about the importance of seeing an injured or arthritic joint as part of your whole body and not something to be treated in isolation. If you are limping or favoring a joint, it's likely other parts of your body are off as well. The whole body is connected in one way or another.

The joined-up skeleton is the reason our team of on-site physical therapists and I put a great deal of emphasis on physical therapy: improving core strength, manually manipulating the joint itself, working on the soft tissue around it as well as working with the rest of the body, mobilizing the hip and the back, and helping to regain full range of motion and improved gait. Not every orthopaedic clinic has an on-site physical therapy program, but in our experience, soft-tissue manipulation makes a huge difference in how people heal, in large part by reducing swelling, inflammation, and scar tissue. You simply cannot manipulate your soft tissues as effectively as an excellent soft-tissue therapist. Soft-tissue manipulation works two ways: it directly mobilizes the collagen fibers that make up your tissues, and it stimulates the mechanoreceptors on the cells in the tissues. This helps them lay down new collagen repair tissue along the natural lines of stress, instead of forming disorganized scar tissue.

A smart physical therapist can look at a patient with an injury and figure out why they got injured, help the patient learn exercises and techniques to recover from the injury, and guide and motivate them to work to improve (without fear of pushing too hard). Most people are unaware of their posture, of how they walk, or how their feet hit the ground. They don't realize how loose or stiff their joints are or their back is. If you're hurt or in pain, a physical therapist can teach you about the mechanics of your gait and the mechanics of your sport, which is valuable information to help speed your recovery and protect you from further injury.

At my clinic, when we see people with a knee injury, the physical therapists teach them not only how to diminish the pain and recover from that knee injury, but how to train around the knee injury, so that if it requires a period of relative immobilization for the knee, we can train their hip joints, back joints, core muscles, and upper body. We can get them on a well-leg bicycle, where they spin with one leg and rest the injured joint. We can come up with all kinds of creative ways to help people train while they are in recovery.

In my view, patients who undergo surgical procedures and do not have a great physical therapy program before and after surgery, or who try to do the entire program on their own, will recover more slowly than those who go through a physical therapy program. They'll also tend not to have as complete a recovery and certainly won't learn as much from the experience.

What to Look for in a Physical Therapist

Choosing an excellent physical therapist can make all the difference to a patient's outcome. However, just as with any profession, the level of competence varies among physical therapists. In fact, the range of quality is distressingly wide. To help you find a good physical therapist, here's a guide to what we look for when hiring physical therapists, which includes outlining the skills we expect them to bring to the patient and to the doctor.

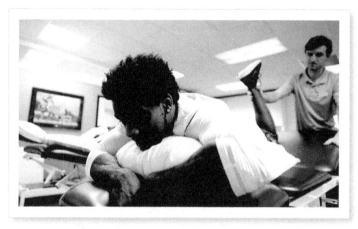

Tracy Porter • Super Bowl–winning cornerback and recipient of
Dr. Stone's biological knee reconstruction program, BioKnee,
receiving manual therapy from a StoneFit rehab trainer

First, a physical therapist must have great interpersonal skills and truly love caring for patients. We look for like-minded people to join our team whose primary goal in their professional life is to assist and inspire people to be better than they have ever been. To achieve this, each physical therapist must encompass the following.

- **Manual skills.** Every successful physical therapist uses their hands to mobilize, manipulate, produce motion, and improve function that cannot be accomplished by just stretching, strengthening, or other sorts of exercises. It is the knowledge and application of these skills that can set physical therapists apart. The use of hands mobilizes scar tissue in a fashion that leads to normal healing. Hands can sense areas of inflammation, pain, and motion restrictions. Hands must be both powerful and gentle.

- **Diagnostic skills.** As an orthopaedic surgeon, I learn from my physical therapists information that I would never know from my exam alone. The physical therapists spend more time with patients, hear more information than the patient might tell me, and see issues from a training perspective. When we discuss patients before they are treated, the questions the physical therapists ask illuminate subtle mechanical interactions that must be addressed to achieve a great outcome. After working with patients, the physical therapist's diagnostic skills often highlight contributing factors to the original cause of injury and help us design total body recovery and rehabilitation programs.

- **Communication skills.** Regular physical therapy appointments can only be satisfying for both parties if the information flow is smooth and informative. Also, case discussions with me and with the nursing team help us all keep connected to the patient throughout their recovery time.

- **Fitness training.** Physical therapy is more than just exercise to recover from an injury. Fitness training to avoid injury, during the recovery time and afterward, determines the likelihood of the patient achieving the "better than they were before they were injured" status. At our clinic, incorporating CrossFit and other fitness program principles has helped our elite athletes and our weekend warriors.

- **Continuing education.** There are a number of classes and courses that we require our physical therapists to complete during their career. Ongoing education from a variety of physical therapy education leaders is crucial to staying at the top of the field. The primary focus is to stay current on manual therapy treatment techniques and theory as well as the latest techniques in gait training, joint mobilization, orthotics, foot mechanics, and cervical and spinal mobilization skills.

Because our therapists have these skills, patients benefit physically, mentally, and spiritually, and my care of them is amplified to a level not possible without the team approach. The fact that we work together in the same space and discuss each patient, before and often after treatments, makes treatment efficient for patients and a great experience for all involved in helping them excel.

Once the doctor and the physical therapist have given the go-ahead, it's time to get the whole body strengthened in preparation for returning to your chosen forms of exercise. We encourage our patients to view their surgeries not as the reason they don't exercise, but as the reason they must. Still, it's unrealistic to jump right back into any given sport without first building up total body strength. The way we help our patients back to full capacity is with a program adapted from CrossFit, the fitness program started in Santa Barbara, California. Not only has CrossFit significantly influenced how fitness is defined and obtained today, but it has also made a substantial influence on how we rehabilitate patients from orthopaedic surgery.

As outlined in Chapter 2, the measurement of fitness in the CrossFit world involves assessments of ten abilities: strength, agility, balance, proprioception, cardiovascular/respiratory endurance, stamina, flexibility, power, coordination, and accuracy. Unfortunately, each of these physical skills is detrimentally impacted in most orthopaedic injuries, whether it is a knee, shoulder, ankle, or back injury. At the time of injury, the affected body part is partially disabled, but during treatment, the rest of the body is often also affected, especially if weight-bearing is prohibited.

What tends to happen, particularly in chronic injuries that lead to arthritis, is that the person favors a joint, limits their motion, and/ or compensates by using other body parts, and their overall fitness declines. To address this, doctors have often prescribed physical therapy for the injured joints. Yet therapy usually focuses only on the site of injury and traditionally ends when that particular part of the body is at least partially healed. It's not designed to get a person back to total body fitness and strength.

That's why, in 1995, we made some changes to how we went about helping injured people get back to full fitness. We recognized that recovery from injury was not sufficient to protect the person from further injury. We hired an early CrossFit leader, Eva Twardokens, to come and teach our physical therapy team the CrossFit techniques of efficient training. We modified their standard CrossFit program to suit an injured patient and the rehabilitation environment and developed a total body recovery program with the goal of returning people to a state "better" than they were before they were injured. We defined better as "fitter, faster, and stronger," and as I've said, we encouraged our patients to see themselves as athletes in training and not patients in rehab.

The outcome of this shift has been that patients now see that their recovery from injury is a lifelong activity. By using their injury as an incentive to develop an efficient fitness program, they achieve a better outcome, and we have the sense of accomplishment that comes from not just helping a patient heal but from helping them improve their lives.

SPORTS INJURY DEPRESSION

You ski fast. You make one small error. You get back on the tails of your skis, but one ski skids out to the side. That's when you hear a pop, and you get a nauseating feeling in your stomach.

Your binding hasn't released; it's your knee that has given way. Your ACL—the key stabilizer of the knee—has ruptured as your shin bone is locked in your ski boot. Your ACL moved forward while your thigh bone, or femur, moved backwards.

After your fall, you try to get up, but when you put pressure on the ski, your knee buckles. Intuitively you know what you have done, though you hope it isn't so.

The ski patrol arrives, checks you out, loads you into the toboggan, and slides you down to the mountain base clinic. There, you encounter four other people with the same story. A brief exam by the all-knowing medical staff, a recommendation to see your orthopaedic surgeon when you get home, and an ice bag for your knee are your souvenirs, marking the early end of your vacation.

There is a morbid frenetic excitement about the whole process. You realize that your ski season is over, and your plans for the spring are up in the air. You make multiple phone calls to see the top doctor, the one you have heard has the best results. Finally, the exam confirms the diagnosis. The X-rays show your healthy bones, and the MRI shows the ruptured ligament. You schedule the surgery, meet with the physical therapists, and reorganize your life and work.

Finally, the surgery happens. All goes well. You begin your rehab, but a couple of weeks later, you hit the skids. You've had it. You are sick of the soreness, the dressings, the ice machines, the knee braces, and the physical therapist appointments. You just want your life back.

There's a name for this malaise. You have officially acquired "ACL depression syndrome." A recent study documented that 40 percent of people who undergo ACL surgery experience clinically diagnosable depression. Life disruptions are a drag, especially when they put the brakes on your active lifestyle.

Of course, sports injury depression is not just confined to those with ACL ruptures. Any major injury can cause our mental wheels to spin out. Perseveration—a recycling through the mind of thoughts that won't go away—traps you in the pain or anger of a past event. It can be hard to break free.

Sports injury depression may not seem to be in the same league as PTSD, suicidal ideation, or other severe depressive disorders. But it is far more common. We have all encountered an unexpected injury that derails us. The sudden calamity first produces anger, and then sorrow, and the long recovery from surgery induces another type of anguish. But chronic injuries can leave you with pain of the worst type as it seems your life will never be as good again.

In the pharmaceutical world, anti-depressants are often prescribed for this spiral, with widely varying results. In the sports world, these drugs decrease performance. However, since most injured athletes were not depressed before they were hurt, they don't see themselves as needing or wanting a "psychiatric" drug treatment.

In the experimental world combining both science and recreation, the use of hallucinogens is teaching us interesting lessons. When Timothy Leary lectured in the late 1960s that a single LSD trip led to permanent improvement in some people's outlook on life, he was right. Current studies are trying to understand the phenomenon of therapeutic, professionally guided "trips." Results suggest that these therapies have the potential of curing PTSD and severe depression.

Once a person sees himself or herself floating in space, free of the rigid attachment to the trauma that holds them down, they recognize the person they could be, rather than the angry, depressed person they are. This experience of joy may clear the cobwebs or actually rewire the brain. It can be convincing enough to change the course of a person's life.

After sports trauma or surgery, we seek the same release. We coach our patients to see themselves as athletes in training, not as patients in rehab. If the injured can view their injury as an excuse to train more creatively and work around their injury while that part of the body heals, and if they can use the gift of downtime to rethink their approach and reduce the likelihood of future injuries, then they have the possibility of returning from their injury in better shape than they were before they were hurt. This requires letting go of anger about the injury, or about any previously failed surgeries, or about the person who may have caused the injury. It requires letting go of perseveration and envisioning a new, positive goal.

The tools we use to help athletes get to this point include coaching with hands-on physical therapy, where the touch and experience of a skillful therapist dramatically builds confidence while mobilizing stiff tissues. Daily sweat workouts are creatively designed to protect the injured part of the body while raising the heart rate. Pilates, pool exercise, upper-body weight lifting—we recommend them all. Muscle building releases pheromones, testosterone, adrenaline, and dopamine, which enter the bloodstream and reset the competitive athletic spirit. Combining a vision of who you can become with this level of coaching is a tremendously effective healing strategy.

Sports injury depression is endemic to all athletes who begin as driven, healthy, fit, and life-loving people. In a moment, they become victims of a sports injury, facing an uncertain future. Those who buy into the importance of an ambitious exercise program succeed in warding off the depression, or at least in shortening its length and intensity.

HEALING DIET

Low carb, low fat, low calories—"low" is the common denominator of nearly every diet fad.

The harm is done when it is low protein. While there are varying statements on how much protein a person needs each day, my observation is that those levels are far too low when you are injured or sick. (And they are probably too low to keep you from getting injured and sick.)

People are influenced by sensational online and print media. The touting of new diets by movie stars and supplement manufacturers masquerades as science. On top of that, scientists at our government institutions use poor-quality studies to create nutritional pyramids that guide American food choices and diets. The combination of marketing and low reliability, when mixed with the opportunity for profit, has led to harmful diet recommendations. Vegetarians and vegans may adopt meatless diets for other reasons, of course—as a lifestyle choice due to moral convictions, for example. But the meat they forego must be replaced with significant amounts of other proteins in order to avoid illness and injury.

For healthy individuals, the margin for error when following diets that eliminate certain food groups is reasonably large so people do not become too sick too fast. Yet I see many injured athletes, weekend warriors, and people with arthritis who wonder why they don't heal as fast as they used to. One reason for this is their low protein intake.

An even more dramatic correlation exists between low blood albumin (a marker for protein load) and infection. Put simply, if your dietary intake of protein is low, your blood albumin level is low, and your risk of infection after a surgical procedure or with an open wound is high. Anyone who tells you that a low-protein diet is a good idea simply does not see what I see.

When a bone is fractured or a limb is immobilized, muscle atrophy can be measured after as little as eight hours and continues until motion and weight-bearing are restarted. The loss of muscle exposes the limb to further damage. Regaining that muscle requires training. The benefits of training depend on protein availability more than any other factor.

Here is what you need to know. Complete or quality protein is protein that has all the essential amino acids required for health. Lean protein sources, such as skinless chicken or turkey, 90 percent or leaner ground beef, low-fat or nonfat dairy, seafood, soy products, pork loin, and eggs are ideal. Incomplete proteins, such as beans, oatmeal, barley, corn, nuts, and seeds are missing some of the essential amino acids and must be combined with other foods.

For good health maintenance, the range of recommendations for protein intake is as follows: 0.8 to 1.5 gm/kg of body weight (17–21 percent) of total calories. (To convert to metric, first divide your weight in pounds by 2.2. Then multiply by the protein recommendation.) For example, a 220-pound person weighs 100 kg, and therefore should consume 80 to 150 grams of protein a day for health maintenance alone. For sick or injured people trying to build muscle, the recommendation increases to 2gm/kg a day. (Note: other health issues must be taken into account before introducing dramatic increases in protein intake. Always consult your physician before making these changes.)

Look at yourself. If you are injured and want to repair your tissues, what do you want to repair and rebuild them with? Do you want to be mostly fat? Mostly carbohydrates? Or protein? Eat mostly what you want to be, and feed the systems you need to restore health.

HEALING TOUCH

We all love touch. So why are people most in need of it the most often denied it? Old people and injured people often lie in their beds or live in rehabilitation environments: places where touch is rare.

Things can be even worse if the patient is sick. Everyone keeps their distance as if cancer or heart disease will jump across the room and afflict the visitor. The awkward hospital gown, wires attached everywhere, and beeping machine monitors make the patient feel like a specimen in a laboratory, while the families react with fear and faint gratitude that they are not the ones in this imprisoned state. Here is how to change that.

- If you have an old person in your life, touch them. Hold their hand whenever you can. Talk to them while massaging their neck, their feet, their fingers. Don't let your voice be their only connection with you.
- If you know someone who is injured or sick, observe what happens in the hospital or nursing home, or even in their own home. Nurses come in with clipboards (or now, computers), and the only form of touch is a thermometer stuck into their patient's ear. The doctors make their rounds standing at the side or foot of the bed, possibly with a stethoscope pressed to their patient's chest. The orderlies,

food delivery people, and everyone else drifts in and out with no physical contact at all. Even the physical therapists may forget their most basic training. While they may get the patient up and walking with crutches, they avoid the manual soft-tissue massage that separates great physical therapists from the rest.

- For the injured young or old, visiting a physical therapist who spends most of their time with hands-on manipulation of the injured tissues—combined with guided rehabilitation exercise—leads to more rapid recovery than any "modality" of ultrasound, laser, hot packs, or ice could ever achieve.

"Tactile queuing" is used to help a person focus on a body part they may be ignoring. Tapping the quadriceps while the patient contracts it awakens the brain-body connection. Deeply massaging the legs can mobilize pooling fluids back to the central core and reawaken the lymphatic system. Head rubs lower stress, and affection, and any form of touching—while looking the person in the eyes with warmth and love—restores their sense of humanity.

The reason casts have been largely abandoned in our practice is that they prevent touch to the injured part. So why treat the elderly, sick, and injured as if they are wearing a "virtual cast" when their skin is so desperate for contact with yours? Among the many missing things in caregiving, the lack of touch is the easiest to remedy. Whether it is for love, affection, therapy, or strengthening, the touch from a family member or professional is a magical—and healing—gift.

ONE AND DONE IS NOT ENOUGH

A top skier breaks her leg. A doctor fixes it, gives her narcotics, and sends her home. She's told to come back in two weeks for a checkup and have the rod taken out in a year. The doctor moves on to the next patient. What is wrong with this picture?

It's not the narcotics. Yes, those drugs stink, but unfortunately, they are the best we have for pain medication today. What is wrong is the absence of all the other information the athlete deserves to hear.

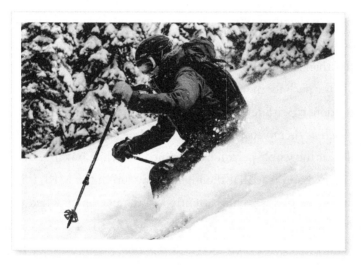

Jenn Hudak • X Games half-pipe gold medalist, winning eight months after ACL reconstruction with articular cartilage and meniscus repairs

This situation happened recently at the World Pro Ski Tour. A skier launched over a jump in the qualifying races, landed badly, and broke her tibia. She received excellent surgical care from the orthopaedic surgeon at the local hospital, where a rod was placed into her tibia. She returned to the ski hill the next day to watch the race finals. She and her parents were taking in the shock of her injury and its impact on her ski racing career. They had no information and no guidance.

Here is what she should have been told: "Bad luck that you broke your tibia. All athletes get injuries. The best athletes use their injury as an excuse to come back to their sport fitter, faster, and stronger than they were before they were injured. Here are some suggestions to help you heal." And then she should have been talked through each of the steps we've covered in this chapter: pain management, healthy exercise on a timeline, a good high-protein diet, the use of a physical therapist to massage her soft issue, a trainer to build her fitness program, especially with a focus on returning her to her sport better than she was before.

In the push for more efficient medicine, by less-trained healthcare practitioners, with fewer possibilities for engaging ancillary personnel such as therapists and trainers, the time and ability to diagnose and treat the whole person has declined. So while it is true that you are injured and true that the injury shows up in the MRI, it is also true that no one is paying attention to the person attached to the injury spot.

This is not good enough. As orthopaedic surgeons, it's no longer good enough for us to just do our job and leave athletes—or any patient—to their own devices. The treatment plan should not just focus on healing the injured site but also tap the resources of physical therapy, fitness training, and medical guidance to enhance all of your body. I teach our doctors-in-training this approach. Each and every time they see a tweaked body part, they must take full stock of the human attached to the injury. Treat them as a wonderful performance unit that responds to tender loving care, meticulous repair, and total body assessment, and offer training and fitness improvements as a lifelong gift.

Equally important is understanding the patient's personality and outlook. If the patient is an athlete, for instance, as our skier is, then they have the ability and the desire to train hard and to endure pain to reach a physical goal. Engaging that drive in their recovery process determines both their future healing and athletic success. Ignoring it leads to depression. As surgeons, we have that power to direct our patient's focus, and to harness their strengths. To do so effectively, we must cater our treatment plans to the person. We must understand their mindset and personal crutches, for the mind game of injury recovery is different for each person. Finding the path that works for each athlete is part of the fun and satisfaction of being a sports orthopaedic surgeon, but that takes an understanding of the patient, an ability to engage at a very personal level, clear communication, and an openness to guide them through the process.

PART III

MEDICINE TODAY AND TOMORROW

CHAPTER 8

ENHANCING A CURRENT MEDICAL PRACTICE

A medical degree confers on a doctor a responsibility to care for patients. That should not be all we aspire to. Physicians in every discipline are scientists by training, and thus have the tools to probe the medical knowledge base and test new possibilities. Pushing boundaries can bring about discoveries that enable us to provide better care for patients.

As I've pointed out throughout this book, what we in the medical profession think we know today is probably not accurate. If we are practicing medicine the same way next year as we are practicing it this year, we clearly haven't taken opportunities to learn. This is the principle on which I have built my practice and research career —with a healthy skepticism of both "accepted" knowledge and "standard-of-care" practices. Insistence on established protocols and evidence-based medicine sounds like a good thing. Yet most people are unaware that the evidence is often not that well-founded, and the standards are sometimes based on economic factors rather than quality metrics.

In this chapter, we'll explore where medicine is now: what's missing in medical training, mindset, and approach, and how the current system works, what its flaws are, and how we could move forward to perfect them. In many ways, this chapter is for medical professionals and my peers, but it's equally valuable for anybody—athlete, sportsperson, those just beginning their fitness journey, those continuing it, or those dealing with the effects of aging on their body. Understanding a physician's perceptions and attitude—as well as the constraints of the healthcare system in which they're functioning—helps patients recognize the kind of care they will receive and choose that care (and their physician) more carefully. Perhaps if we were all more aware and better informed, we could put our heads together to fix the current flaws in the medical field, plug the existing gaps, and reach for that brighter future.

CREATIVITY, CONFIDENCE, AND COMMUNICATION

Most of the information I learned in medical school is now outdated. Most of what's "tried and true" is not really all that good. For the most common surgical procedures in orthopaedics, for example—which include total knee replacement, ACL reconstruction, rotator cuff repair, and meniscectomy—the failure rate varies from 15 to 30 percent. If we in our profession succeed only three out of four times, we must acknowledge that the "state of the art" in orthopaedic practice is still in the formative stages.

So what is missing in medical training and practice? One of the building blocks of world-class medical care is creativity. Innovation is part of what differentiates standard care from superlative care. It is taking what is known—what is presented by each patient—and combining or inventing the best ways to solve their problems. It is assuming that every tool and every procedure can be improved.

Starting in medical school, we should train physicians to be creative thinkers, show them the benefits of working both collaboratively and independently, and give them the confidence to question the status quo. Unfortunately, developing these qualities is not a common area of focus of any program. A student's four medical school years are crammed with massive doses of information requiring rote memory. On top of that, students must learn the evaluation skills of the physical and mental exam. The clinical rotations endured by medical students are often structured with punishingly long hours—time often spent performing menial tasks at the beck and call of more senior residents. Residents-in-training are commonly used by attending physicians as servants to treat patients in the middle of the night, or as clones to absorb what the attending wants to teach. Many attending physicians, of course, are inspiring teachers and role models, and the best residencies produce well-trained, wonderful doctors. But can they innovate?

After five to eight years of training, most residents then spend another year or two in fellowship training programs. This is an opportunity to be mentored by someone with exceptional skills. Clearly, the residency didn't prepare them to function in the real world, and this final stage is required to learn the art of medicine and surgery.

Most residents do it—must do it—to get a good job and to really learn a specialty. And most such fellowships follow the model of cloning the professor.

If we want creative doctors, is this the way to get them? The system doesn't change, because the people in it value basic competence more than creativity. And healthcare systems, hospital chains, and the public don't place a high value on the difference.

Creativity *can* be taught. Engineering schools and biodesign programs have mastered the "brainstorming" session—a forum in which all ideas have value, and each can be presented in ways that stimulate solutions to unsolved problems. In fact, creativity training—from the way we approach problems to the way we solve them—has been integrated into almost every field *except* medicine.

To accelerate the creative aspect of education, training, and practice, a deep and systematic change must occur. Students must be recruited for their ability to think and educated in problem-solving and innovation. Residencies must go beyond the medical needs of today's patients and model future practice, including work with robotics, artificial intelligence, genetic engineering, and 3D modeling. Insurance companies and hospitals must provide incentives and reward those who push forward the envelope of medicine.

There's another quality that serves a physician well, in tandem with creativity: confidence. In this context, confidence is a synonym for ego, and while most would say that ego is not lacking in the medical profession, or at least the surgical specialties, I would maintain that a healthy ego is worth nurturing. I suspect that all highly ambitious, driven, success-oriented people have outsized egos. High levels of self-confidence permit you to believe in what you are doing, to make split-second decisions without self-doubt, to push the boundaries, and to absolutely believe in yourself. So let's strip the term "big ego" of its pejorative connotations and link it to the potential power for greater good.

Of course, there is a downside of having a supercharged ego. Toes can get stepped on, and team members may not always get the credit they deserve. Hardheadedness sometimes creates tone deafness to other ideas or flags of caution. The big ego is not always right.

In my line of work, a big ego is not an excuse for a lack of empathy, especially when it comes to dealing with patients. There's a world of difference between confidence and arrogance. If you believe that most of what we know is not true, that everything we see and touch we can make better, that there is so much we can contribute to this world, that the more you contribute the better you feel, and that there is no end to learning and applying those lessons, then you must develop the confidence and courage to push your ideas to fruition.

So should we train medical students to have big egos? Is it even teachable? My wife and I tried in a subtle way with our kids. We told them that if every day they did four things—educate themselves, be good people, contribute to the world, and have fun—they would thrive. It actually takes an ego to live every day by these goals. Yours can be a quiet, conservative, subtle, big ego, or it could be a louder, gregarious, big ego. Either way, it takes confidence to see what could be better and guts to make it so.

Balancing self-confidence with humility and compassion is essential. Fortunately, if you have people you love around you or have wisely empowered your staff, colleagues, friends, or teammates to interject, interview, and speak up, then a misdirected ego can be nipped in the bud. That takes teamwork. And teamwork is the key to big egos becoming big successes.

A study led by a team at the Harvard School of Public Health is currently examining teamwork and communication in cardiac surgery operating rooms and is finding that the biggest egos only sometimes make the best surgeons, but the best communicators are always the best surgeons. Great leaders are able to take good skills and make them shine nearly every time, where poor leaders fail without backup support. Most interestingly, the study is demonstrating that interventions with the poor communicators lead to improvements, even at the extremely high-ego level of top heart surgeons.

Learning how to express ideas, how to give and take direction, and how to be part of a team are intertwined with developing the ego as part of a student's total skillset. When an athletic coach says, "There is no 'I' in team," that indicates that they don't get it. The 'I' is the leadership provided by those with self-confidence—those who understand that teams need to be led, and leadership is as much about communication as it is about action.

How to Survive Medical Training

F or medical students, years of school and resident training can be abusive. (Probably not much more than training for other high-pressure fields, but still tough.) Rising doctors must learn to perform in competitive, high-pressure, high-stakes learning environments, at the low end of a strict pecking order, with an ongoing sleep deficit. And they receive criticism—lots of it.

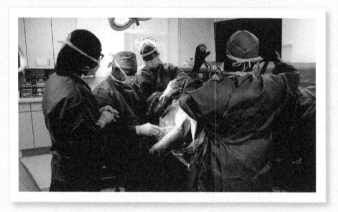

Dr. Stone training new doctors

There is a trick to swimming, not sinking, in a sea of criticism. It's a strategy that can in fact be applied to any learning or working situation. It consists of just two words: "Yes, and…"

First, though, some context on medical training. It is a tremendous honor and a privilege to be trained as a doctor. With this training comes the responsibility of caring for patients. This means, in part, placing the patient first, above all other

considerations, even if that means being there for them in the
middle of the night or in the midst of a disaster. The ability to act
alone—or to be part of, or in charge of, a team during any number
of crises—defines a critical part of a doctor's skillset. Gaining
those skills takes years and requires melding with a system.

The military figured this out a long time ago. To become a
soldier, everyone has to go through basic training. It isn't as much
about learning to shoot a gun as it is learning to take orders.
It's about learning how to be screamed at for no good reason and
still say, "Yes sir!" It is learning how to subjugate one's own
personality while playing a role.

Medical education, especially for surgeons, starts with
treating the person who is the most junior member of a surgical
team as an idiot. Residents, just a few years older, have responsibility for patients' lives, often while the senior surgeon is at home
in bed. Without years of experience under their belts, residents
are terrified of screwing up, losing face among their peers,
harming the patient, and being knocked out of the program.
They take out this insecurity on the first-year residents and on the
medical students below them. Many young doctors-in-training
push everyone below them mercilessly, hoping not to fail themselves. Where the military drill sergeant doesn't want his troops
to get their asses shot off, the young doctor-in-training has his
or her own bottom in the crosshairs.

For the medical student, the key to survival lies in Tina Fey's
wisdom about improvisational acting. In improv, if one person
says, "It's hot in here!" and the other replies, "No it's not," the

act thumps to a stop. But if the response is "Yes, and maybe we shouldn't be standing in the pizza oven!" the improv goes on.

For the medical student, or anyone facing withering scrutiny, saying "Yes, and…" is the key.

"You idiot!" the senior resident says. "You should have known that diagnosis!"

"Yes," replies the student. "And tonight I will study it and all its variations."

Saying "Yes, and…" elevates a student's stock far above the one who says, "No, I never thought of it," or, worse, "Don't blame me; I'm tired from being up all night."

Medical superiors need to have confidence in their students. They need to know that future doctors have the spirit to persist, to be ready and alert in the middle of the night if need be, and to have a good attitude when things are going badly. They need to know that their students don't take themselves so seriously that they must defend their honor against an onslaught of harsh criticism. This holds true in any field, both in the spheres in which you are a leader and those in which you are a student. "Yes, and…" is how you inculcate this confidence in your medical superiors. It is how you show you are ready to face whatever the world of medicine holds.

It is easy to say there shouldn't be abuse in medical training or even in the training of soldiers. But this is not realistic, nor would it make for dependable soldiers or surgeons.

Indeed, once you rise through the ranks from first-year medical student to resident and beyond, you do not need to become an abusive leader yourself. If you can become a kinder, wiser, and more competent human by leading well and learning from the examples (positive and negative) of your own leaders, while still ensuring you train those under you properly and prepare them for the rigors of this profession, then you will contribute to your field and enrich yourself. For now, just remember to say: "Yes, and…"

COLLABORATION IN MEDICAL CARE

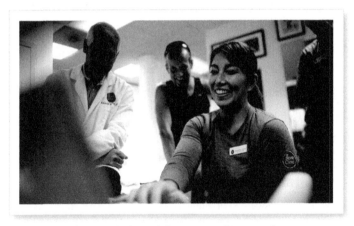

Dr. Stone and physical therapist working together on optimizing their patient's recovery strategy

The oft-heard expression that two brains are better than one seems logical, yet teamwork is discouraged in most of medicine. Insurance companies discourage assistants in surgery, consultations among peers, and collaboration between providers of similar skills, despite the fact that two brains dramatically increase the quality of care in so many cases.

Recently, a patient in our clinic complained of calf pain without clear trauma. In the seventh decade of life, blood clots are worrisome, and this possible diagnosis can jump to mind—especially in this particular case because the patient had an underlying blood disorder. Late Friday afternoon, after he'd experienced several hours of discomfort, I began to organize an ER visit for him to obtain an ultrasound test that would confirm the diagnosis. Before doing so, I discussed his case with my nurse practitioner of twenty-three years. She suggested a little quinine and waiting a few more hours, suspecting that this highly athletic patient was probably under-reporting his activities that day. Sure enough, the simple trick worked, and the patient was saved an unnecessary trip to the ER.

We have seen this in everyday surgical cases. Routine or common procedures are approached with greater insight if two people who know the patient are thinking together about potential related issues and conceiving new and better ways to solve the patient's particular problems. It takes years of experience and working together to be able to push each other clinically, surgically, technically, and creatively. Instead of pushing out routine care, nothing is routine because each case represents a new opportunity to collaborate on the art and science of medicine.

Two brains can also vastly improve diagnostic studies. In our practice, every MRI is read by the orthopaedic surgeon, the supervising musculoskeletal radiologist, and the radiology fellows-in-training. We share an annotated grid of the images each day and discuss the interesting cases and any differences in diagnostic interpretations. It doesn't matter that the radiologist is in Los Angeles and our clinic is in San Francisco. The technology for global collaboration is available with the click of a mouse. I get better with every discussion, and my patients benefit with every collaboration.

The interplay of brain power that two or more driven, curious people bring to the table is more likely to result in innovation. Nurses can play an invaluable role in this creative interchange. One of my nurses is my surgical assistant. My other nurse is the patient assistant in my office. Though insurance companies don't seem to realize it, both nurses matter to the patient a great deal.

My current surgical nurse has been my first assistant for over twenty-four years. She sees every patient before surgery, operates on them with me, and follows up with them after surgery—often for years after the procedure. Because she knows their specific issues, because she listens with different ears than I do, because she is there to guard them and help me, she provides an extra level of expertise and protection that every patient deserves. No matter how great a surgeon may be, every patient, every problem, and every day has unique issues. Having more than one person pay attention and think about these issues substantially improves the quality and consistency of care.

Surgical nurses have a unique role that allows them to bring up issues and point out problems at each phase of surgery. Their skill with instruments, tissue preparation, and positioning the patient continues to increase each year. The nurses also interface with the rest of the operating room staff in ways that build community and team dynamics. This dramatically decreases the stress and errors that come from miscommunication.

The office nurse plays a similar role. By interviewing patients before the surgeon sees them, a more complete picture of their problems, symptoms, and goals is obtained. The bond between the nurse and the patient often provides assurance that their issues are being heard. By double-checking the patient's dressings and medications after surgery, the office nurse diminishes the common office-based errors that can lead to poor outcomes. The patient is confident that their medical record will be complete and that the care given will be intuitive and sensitive to their specific issues. Follow-up phone calls, post-op care, and ongoing concern all expand the quality of care.

The nursing team elevates the "standard" of care to exceptional care. And, if things go wrong, the nurses are often first to know, to respond, and to initiate corrective actions. Without their ears, eyes, and hearts, the injuries and diseases that patients suffer from are seen with far fewer dimensions. When practiced as a team, medicine and surgery are an elegant display of caring and competence in the service of mankind. If we empower, fund, incent, encourage, facilitate, and foster collaboration with every problem, and with every patient, the world will be a healthier place.

The New Doctor Disease

A new doctor, fresh out of a top residency and fellowship, wants all the right things at the wrong time. She wants to be busy with lots of patients, and if she is a surgeon, she wants to be operating every day. In fact, it is better *not* to be busy, and instead to think long and hard about each patient: listening, pausing, recommending nonoperative treatments, and being patient. Doctors learn the most from the patients they take the time to truly listen to and care for with extreme attention and lovingness. They learn nothing from those they have little time for.

A new doctor wants to market himself. He wants to tell the world how well-trained he is, how up to date he is with the literature, and how knowledgeable he is about the latest techniques and tools. What he should really do is read more than he speaks, listen more than he argues, and apply the accepted techniques, while ever so slowly introducing novel approaches. He should stay under the radar, find and cultivate the wisest mentors, stand behind the pillars of the community, and gain their trust for several years before challenging and eventually leading them.

The new doctor wants to computerize, modernize, electronic medical "recordize," and robotize every aspect of medical care. What she doesn't realize is that most of the current digital data is not compatible with any other system, can't be moved to a new hospital, and is subject to viruses, malware, and corrupted programs. Mostly likely, twenty years from now, all her computerized records will be unreadable, inaccessible, and useless. She must take note of the growing trend of a computer humming between every doctor and their patient, further distancing the doctor from learning the subtleties of the patient's needs and the subtleties of medicine, and she must find a way to overcome this.

The new doctor wants security while making money, independence while having a job, and freedom to practice while contracted with insurance companies. What he doesn't realize is that the security of working for someone else can evaporate in the first downsizing. The independence once visualized in medical practice is lost when taking a paycheck, and the freedom to practice is crushed when contracting with the lowest-cost bidders—i.e., the health plans. The socialization of medicine is a choice a doctor makes when they choose not to work independently.

The new doctor wants to lead her field. She understands that performing research, presenting papers, writing books, and lecturing are the paths to stardom. She doesn't understand how to do this while also practicing full time and meeting the financial and personal demands of a new practice and maybe a family. What she really needs to do is accept that to be both a fabulous doctor and a researcher, one must commit full time to both, integrating the research directly into the practice and setting the practice up to permit the research. It is all possible, and definitely worth it, though the sacrifices are usually financial and personal for many years.

New doctors want to be all they can be on Day One. The reality is that each decision on how to become the superstar affects the likelihood of getting there. Patience, exquisite care of each patient, quiet tactical maneuvering, and phenomenally hard work are all necessary ingredients. Keeping a low profile early on, under the guidance of a wise mentor, is by far the best way to start out.

STUDYING OUTCOMES

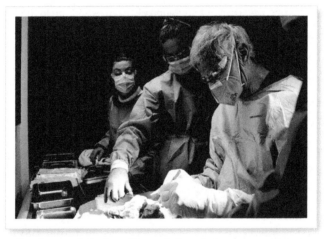

Dr. Stone and the Stone Research Foundation team conducting an experiment to optimize Dr. Stone's cartilage regeneration surgical procedure: the articular cartilage paste graft

I believe that no doctor should do anything to or put anything into a patient without knowing or studying the long-term outcome. Seems logical, doesn't it? Yet, most doctors do not know the outcomes of their interventions. In fact, most of the data they need to do this is not available. Fortunately, this may be about to change—due to a combination of new outcome tools, social media, and the ability to mine enormous data sets from disparate inputs.

First, the unknown "facts." Only a tiny percentage of all published articles in the medical literature are based on Level I studies. Level I means that the studies are done well enough, with proper controls and appropriate blinding, so that the conclusions are highly likely to be accurate (though not necessarily correct). The reliability of the other 90 percent of studies varies widely as most of these are based on the clinical experience of the reporting doctor, biased data, or study designs that are not always completely robust.

Here are the effects of a lack of broad-based outcome data in several medical spheres, and what the future may hold.

Surgical Procedures

Minimizing surgical and hospitalization time has been a welcome, cost-effective trend in both medicine and surgery. What's not to like? Gone are the days when patients routinely spent days in the hospital after delivering babies, undergoing heart surgery, or having joint replacement. Hospitals saved on extended care and had low return or readmission rates to hospitals. The lower the cost, the better, and if the patient doesn't come back, they must be cured. Right?

Wrong. What is lost in this equation is an assessment of the quality of care. Hospitals are now basically acute-care facilities, sending patients who need longer stays to secondary facilities instead. Rehab and physical therapy visits have been cut to the bone.

What's not to like are the results: a lack of them. The quality of medical care is now measured as the "cure." If a patient gets a total knee replacement and does not come back, the surgeon and hospital get an "A" grade. But what about the patient who lives with pain and doesn't complain? Or the patient whose knee doesn't get back to full motion? Or the patient whose knee is loose and mildly unstable? Or the patient who continues to limp? Worse still, what about the patient whose knee replacement fails after the one-year "final" assessment?

The point is that outcome measures that accurately demonstrate the quality of surgical care are neither standardized nor required, and the data is simply not being collected in the vast majority of cases. This is in an era where we quantify everything about ourselves with Fitbits, food scales, and smartphones. So why do we not collect this crucial data on hospitalization outcomes?

There are several answers. First, it is not required, partly because data collection was difficult in the past. In addition, surgeons are not trained well or compensated for collecting outcome measures. The insurance companies, meanwhile, have only short-term goals, so the costs of any failures are someone else's problems.

Fortunately, because the long-term success of any surgical procedure is in everyone's best interest, solutions are at hand. Tools for collecting and storing outcome statistics are now widely available and are becoming easier and cheaper for both doctors and patients to use. Since all patients now have smartphones and almost no one changes their cell phone numbers, it's possible to create an app or a text messaging tool that reaches out to every patient—monthly at first, then annually—to follow up and collect validated outcome measurements.

In the past, the wide variety of hard-copy patient records and electronic medical records did not cross-communicate with each other. This was a barrier to any kind of global medical record analysis. New clinical outcomes software, which mines various data inputs from a wide variety of medical records, is now available through companies like LynxCare. These permit the creation of enormous data lakes, which can be fished for the pearls that physicians need to truly understand their patients' outcomes.

By effectively crowdsourcing the outcomes of all procedures, we will have a far better idea how well our healthcare system is working.

Medical Devices

Despite lack of data and analysis on surgical outcomes, a patient might still assume that the effectiveness of the device a surgeon may be planning to implant in their body has been well studied. Unfortunately, they'd most likely be wrong. There is no required reporting on nearly any of the medical devices used in the United States once the implant has been approved by the FDA, and most procedures do not even require FDA approval. The approval protocols for devices are based on small safety trials, and usually on one or two efficacy trials reported from a relatively small (usually less than a few hundred) number of patients.

Only a small number of doctors participate in wide clinical trials or device registries that track the outcomes of implants they use, such as artificial joints, vessel stents, and meshes for hernias. In fact, there are no national registries of orthopaedic surgical implants used in America. Shocking? That means that when a doctor implants a total knee or a hip prosthesis, there is no professional body tracking whether or not those implants fail—not at the federal, state, or local level. There isn't even a company registry. The only way most doctors know if a device fails is if patients come back to them. If a patient moves away or is angry about their outcome, the doctor may never know.

This applies not just to implants. There is no registry or required post-market approval (meaning after the FDA gives its initial blessing) for drugs, braces, breathing devices, or just about anything doctors place into or on patients. We rely solely on reports to the doctor, and then hopefully the doctor reporting to the FDA.

Now, it might be argued that the rigorous initial FDA-approval process makes all products highly likely to be safe and effective. It's true that this process is arduous and expensive—so much so that few new products are actually being introduced, which is problematic. The process now is estimated to take an average of four-and-a-half years for a new device to complete pilot and pivotal clinical phases, with average costs of $30 million for low- to moderate-risk devices and a whopping $91 million for higher-risk devices. For new drugs, the costs are in the hundreds of millions of dollars.

So what is the solution? What could improve the safety, lower the cost, and speed the time to commercial use of medical devices in the United States? The answer lies in a nonintuitive combination of relaxing the rules for approving medical devices while strengthening the requirement to report any problems.

We could start with a new way of approving medical devices. It would go like this: A company completes all the safety testing required and then conducts a Phase I clinical trial in a small number of patients. This would be required to prove safety, not efficacy. After the initial safety trial, the FDA could permit sales while simultaneously requiring all manufacturers to do a "post-market approval study." All doctors who implant a device would then be required to place an app on a patient's smartphone. The app would permit the doctor and the patient to monitor all outcomes, using standardized, validated outcome questionnaires. The data would be posted publicly, and all physicians, scientists, and manufacturers would be able to see the results as they unfold over months, years, and even decades after implantation.

By crowdsourcing the outcomes of medical devices, the safety and efficacy of these devices could be revealed, studied, and potentially improved over time. Complications would be spotted early, and problem devices could be removed. With this system, companies would be free of the burden of decades of expensive studies to prove efficacy in a relatively small clinical trial. They could sell and create revenue immediately, and most importantly, doctors and patients would actually *know* which new devices work and which don't. By gradually extending this model to a comprehensive, web-based national medical products reporting program for devices currently on the market, we could then build a complete living data bank that would provide the basis for informed decisions around every medical device in use.

Therapies

Last, how well do we know the outcomes of tried-and-true therapies? Once again, not well enough. Here are some examples of widely recommended remedies that have not proven to be as straightforward or effective as we once believed.

Ibuprofen and anti-inflammatories. Inflammation is the normal response to injury. As we've covered in previous chapters, anti-inflammatory drugs inhibit prostaglandins, the inflammation mediators in all tissues, and so if you take anti-inflammatory drugs, you actually inhibit this healing process.

Moreover, while these drugs are potent pain relievers and reduce inflammation, reports of their negative effects are growing. Recently, ibuprofen has been linked to reducing testosterone production in men, causing infertility. All prostaglandin inhibitors—meaning all anti-inflammatory drugs—likely have the same effect. This is unfortunate because when I think about the things I want my injured and healing patients to have, increased testosterone is one of them. Testosterone builds muscle and enhances well-being. Inflammation reduction is an important part of therapy for many chronic diseases such as inflammatory arthritis and cardiovascular disease (where inflammation in the walls of blood vessels may be a key contributor to abnormal clot formation and heart attacks). Yet the side effects of the drugs we are using to reduce inflammation may, in some cases, be worse than the disease.

Ice. We use cold therapy after surgery to reduce swelling and pain. It is highly effective and reduces the need for pain medications. Yet all healing tissues require *increased* blood flow. Ice reduces blood flow. So where is the trade-off? Should we be cycling heat with cold? When is one better than the other? This remains unknown.

Cortisone. We know that cortisone powerfully shuts down inflammation by inhibiting cell metabolism. It restricts cells' ability to recruit new cells to the site of inflammation and tissue repair. We also know that cortisone causes long-term damage to cartilage, weakens tendons, and inhibits healing, yet it remains the number-one injection ordered by physicians for painful joints. This is changing, however, with the introduction of stem cells.

Stem cells. Stem-cell-derived self-repair cells are potent growth factor production engines. Unlike cortisone, they appear to do no harm. The factors they release are anti-inflammatory, antimicrobial, anabolic, and "professorial" in that they teach other cells what to do at the site of an injury. There are various types of stem cells in the body; some are more specialized than others. Each injury profile is unique. The blood and fluid released in a newly torn ACL is very different from the blood and fluids in a joint with chronic arthritis. Today, we inject cells—most probably progenitor cells—and combinations of growth factors into joints without knowing which combinations are ideal for which tissues. Clearly, we can get more targeted in our therapies.

Calcium, vitamin D, and bone. For decades, we have recommended that our patients use calcium and vitamin D supplements to prevent hip fractures (everyone becomes more osteoporotic as they age, women faster than men). Yet a review of randomized clinical trials involving fifty-one thousand patients fifty years and older showed no significant positive association of calcium and/or vitamin D treatment compared to placebo—regardless of dose, gender, fracture history, dietary calcium intake, or baseline vitamin D concentration.[30]

So if some of these time-tested therapies—with megabillion dollars invested—are rife with uncertainty and even possible harm, what are we to do? Once again, we can look to crowdsourcing as a means of collecting data. Unprecedented access to patients (via their smartphones) enables us to seize the opportunity to track and assess all therapies that patients undergo.

Imagine if every patient were given the opportunity to use a cell phone app to participate in a study for any therapy they are being administered. The app would ask the patient to enter data on the therapy's effectiveness on a regular basis. By adding their patients' information into outcome trials, every doctor would now be a researcher. The number of participants in clinical trials and patient outcomes

---

[30] Jia-Guo Zhao, Xian-Tie Zeng, Jia Wang, and Lin Liu, "Association between calcium or vitamin D supplementation and fracture incidence in community-dwelling older adults: a systematic review and meta-analysis," *JAMA* 318 no. 24 (2017): 2466–2482, https://doi.org/10.1001/jama.2017.19344.

could number in the tens of millions rather than just a few thousand. Though this platform does not yet exist, we're working on it.

Hopefully, in the near future, instead of just saying, "All my patients do well," physicians will be able to state, "Here is the outcome data from my practice, and reports from all the surgeons around the world implanting this device, and aggregated efficacy data from millions of patients who have used these therapies." We may all be pleasantly surprised by what these spotlights reveal—or at least informed by it. This would truly advance the art and science of medicine.

"NEW AND COOL AND NOT FOR YOU"

Traditionally, conservative care meant nonoperative care: a person injured their knee or shoulder, and the doctor said, "Let's try conservative care first and see if you get better." These days, though, conservative care often means that the insurance company has only authorized physical therapy or medications, with the aim of delaying a full workup or surgical repair as long as possible. But conservative care may not be in the patients' best interest. Let's take my favorite subject, a knee injury. The data shows that if a patient twists their knee, hears a pop, and the knee swells, there is a 90 percent chance that a significant injury to the meniscus, articular cartilage, or ligaments has occurred. Current understanding of these tissues is that they are crucial to knee function, rarely heal on their own, and are best treated with surgical repair as soon as is practical.

In the case of the meniscus cartilage, when a patient hears a pop and the knee is swollen, this means a significant portion of the tissue has been torn. This won't heal on its own. Nonoperative care, such as physical therapy, means the torn tissues are exposed to repetitive motion, which, in this instance, further damages the tissue beyond the ability of the surgeon to repair it. Unrepaired meniscus tears lead to arthritis. Not very conservative.

In the case of ligaments such as the ACL, the longer the knee is left unstable, the more the secondary restraints and the ligaments on the side of the knee become stretched, and the higher the chance of a secondary injury to the supporting structures, such as the meniscus. This leads to a worse result when surgery is eventually performed, even more so if the patient is young.

The same is true for the articular cartilage, the bearing surface of the joint. Acute damage that leads to knee swelling never heals. Articular cartilage has no nerve supply (it is aneural), and so the damage may not initially be painful, but if left unrepaired, the lesions expand into early arthritis and persistent pain.

In this twenty-first century, the ability to make an extremely accurate diagnosis of joint injuries lies in the combination of obtaining a careful history (i.e., talking to the patient about exactly how the damage occurred), an experienced examiner, accurate X-rays, and a high-field, high-quality MRI. It is pennywise and pound foolish to skimp on these resources after significant joint injuries since it is far cheaper and much more efficient to fix injuries sooner rather than later. I predict the cost of an MRI will be driven down so low that in the near future, most acute joint injuries will be scanned without hesitation. Hopefully, the knowledge will become widespread that early repair is far better for the patient than false conservative care. Efforts to reduce health insurance costs are also having a dramatic impact on utilization of state-of-the-art devices and techniques. The number of patients allowed coverage for one of the new and improved implants now available is declining rapidly. The most significant change is that "out-of-network benefits" are being reduced to almost nothing—despite the language on an expensive healthcare plan. "New and cool and not for you"—not what the patient wants to hear, but increasingly true.

Since health insurance plans are so costly, most employers now buy the lowest-cost coverage for their employees. This means these employees can only go to doctors who accept the lowest fees, and these doctors can only use devices that are "approved" (i.e., cheap) for treatment. Most of the new, cool, and hopefully better products are not reimbursed, or the hospital will not add them to the formulary. This means out-of-network surgery centers or hospitals will not get reimbursed if they are used.

If a patient buys a more expensive insurance plan, believing it will empower them to go to other doctors and get what those doctors determine is best for treatment, the patient is often mistaken. The out-of-network benefit coverage they buy today has hidden caps. At an outpatient surgery center, for instance, most plans now have a cap of $300 to $400 per day. That might cover a few more minutes in an operating room, at best.

True private insurance plans without caps are now rare. While healthcare costs are being reduced overall, today's doctors-in-training are exposed only to the limited techniques and devices allowed under current plans. How are they going to expand their knowledge and develop into superstars of medical care?

The pendulum of controlling healthcare costs has swung too far. Anthem BlueCross now lists almost all but the most basic therapies as follows: "Cannot be approved. Needs more data." Even when controlled clinical trials and meta-analysis show the efficacy of new tools and techniques, the reviews are unwavering: "Not enough studies to approve…"

This can be said about nearly everything in medicine and surgery, which is why we have come to trust our doctors' judgment and why when something serious occurs, we seek out the best doctors in their field. But many of those doctors are now operating with one hand tied behind their backs. In the past, doctors charged patients what we thought was a reasonable fee for the care given. Those who could afford to, paid for it, or their insurance did. For those who could not pay, we found creative ways to negotiate with our hospitals. Fortunately, there were enough patients who could pay the full fee so the development and use of novel techniques was both possible and expected.

If patients are actually paying full fare for their care, they expect their doctors to have access to and experience with the best tools, the best implants, and the best devices for their bodies. Generic drugs might be okay, but generic knee surgery is not, and generic implants are often simply out of date.

Today, healthcare quality and training are being reduced to the lowest common denominator. This may be a good thing when we are trying to protect the entire population with at least basic care. But it has a chilling effect on the development of new techniques and on the training of doctors. The solution? Get rid of the Medicare-type rules that forbid voluntary overcharges. Permit patients to pay and doctors to charge above the minimum-set fees. Those who can afford it will pay, and the demand for top-level care will drive innovation. It is time to let doctors be doctors, before there aren't any creative ones left.

FIVE LESSONS
MY FATHER TAUGHT ME

We've explored the current state of the medical field, its major limitations, and possible solutions. We've also touched on what good doctors need in terms of perspective, mindset, and personal qualities to excel as leaders and healers.

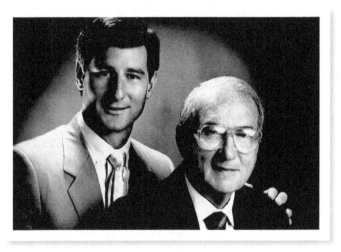

Drs. Kevin and Jacob Stone

I want to leave you now with five lessons my father taught me. He was an internal medicine physician in solo practice for thirty-five years in Providence, Rhode Island. A man of few words—yet recognized as a brilliant diagnostician—he passed on a few pearls that I have always found deeply valuable. They were offered in the context of the medical field, but I've found that they apply to almost all areas of life, and all professions.

- **Overlook it.** So many of the insults, errors, and odd things people do should simply be overlooked. Commenting on them or doing anything to try to change them is mostly unnecessary and only expands the problem.
- **Listen carefully.** The patient almost always knows their own diagnosis. Patients will tell you what is wrong if you ask enough questions and listen carefully. Being a good diagnostician means being well informed, smart, intuitive, compassionate, and patient. If you let the information come to you, it will. You don't need to do every test or engage every consultant. You need to listen and think.
- **Quiet is best.** The louder you are, the harder it is to hear. Hold your peace between comments, let people speak, and let silence occur. Let others take meetings in the directions they want to go. My father believed that this applies to most business and medical settings as well as interpersonal encounters.
- **It will be better by the time you are married.** Almost all of our aches, pains, and complaints as children were met with, "Don't worry; it will be better by the time you are married." The message was patience. Most things heal on their own. Some take a lot longer than you would ever expect, while others resolve overnight. But the confidence that things will get better, according to my dad, is what matters most.
- **It is good enough.** Leave some on the table for the other guy. Don't get the last nickel. Don't be seen as aggressive when grateful is good enough. Be satisfied with what you've done, and you will be happier. Unfortunately, the drive for excellence often overwhelms this advice.

It's difficult to say how many of us put into practice the best of the lessons our fathers teach us. We could view so much of this counsel now as "old school," and many of us would be brash enough to believe that we could do better. In an age where we measure time as the nanoseconds between clicks, where does patience come in? When do we practice listening? When are we quiet? And why do we often "forget" to apply these lessons in the moments of stress?

I urge you to ask yourself these questions and interrogate your answers. If we are to truly build a better and brighter future, we must build it on the wisdom of the past. As I look at my personal success at adopting my dad's lessons—and my failure to adopt others—I wonder why so much of the wisdom of the ages is lost in practice. Why do some, and not others, of these childhood lessons become ingrained into our personalities? Why do we discard so many of them as "outdated?" And what would you like to pass on to your children, and how would you ensure they practice it?

We hope that our immediate response to any challenge will reflect our best possible selves. When we can do this across the board, we become the truly better people our fathers wished us to be.

CHAPTER 9

WHERE WE'RE HEADING

I t is a heady time in the world of human empowerment. We are seeing technologies that can alter our genetic code, augment our brainpower, enhance our physique, and extend our lives. Our goals as physicians are no longer limited to healing injuries and curing disease. The question "Can you make me better than I have ever been?" has moved from fantasy to near reality.

In my part of the medical science space, we are not overly concerned with life extension. We are focused on living life to its fullest—and "full" now has new meaning. Building superhumans is becoming part of our everyday medicine. This chapter focuses on what you, as a patient, can expect to experience in your future healthcare (some of it in the near future) and some of the implications.

DISEASE CARE VS. HEALTHCARE

In this modern moment in the trajectory of healthcare, doctors still can't tell you what is about to happen to you, because we don't know. We are still reacting to, rather than preventing, illness and injury. We make diagnoses of diseases after they affect you and treat injuries after you suffer from them.

But what if a significant portion of our work was focused on testing you before you got sick or injured? We might develop exquisite predictive tools and great preventive treatments. All of medicine—and life—would be changed. "Healthcare" would mean just that—not the disease care we currently practice. Here's how it is going to work, in five of its early stages.

Advanced in-patient profiling. Multiple body scanning devices will obtain all your standing and volume measurements and correlate them with various orthopaedic disease states. A dynamic gait lab will capture your movements. A spit test or swab will produce a full human genome sequence, which will get better at telling us which diseases are likely to pop up, which therapeutic drugs you will best respond to, and which diets are likely to be most effective.

Predictive proteins. Many diseases and most cancers release identifying proteins prior to the disease becoming clinically recognizable. They have to start somewhere, and they all start small. An expanding number of these biomarker proteins are being found each week. What we don't know is, how often does your body kill off the cancer (or ward off a cold) before the symptoms hit you? One day, when you and your doctor are alerted to the possible coming storm, you will take preventive action. This will usher in a whole new era in which we can define which disease precursors need to be addressed and eliminate diseases before they eliminate us. We see predictive diagnosis now with arthritis: joint cartilage health can now be measured with novel MRI techniques, and subtle changes of both aging and injury can be subject to early intervention.

Predictive errors. Many sports injuries and work-related traumas start with mental errors. A momentary loss of focus, a "mental error," a poor decision—all can be precursors to the injury. But focus and attention to detail are now measurable, both by brain wave recordings and eye motions. The quantified health devices of today will morph into tomorrow's skin patches and eyeglasses—wearables that won't merely record data but intervene, much as a pacemaker does for the heart. You will thus be warned of an upcoming error—though heeding the warning may or may not be up to you.

For serious athletes, the interfaces will be even more sophisticated. Coaches will store your propensity data, monitoring your response and timing in a vast array of possible sports encounters. By wearing a virtual reality headset before you play, you will train while visualizing these various scenarios, improving your performance while lowering injury rates. And not just before, but during play. NFL helmets are now fitted with all kinds of communication devices. The Google Glass of the future helmet will provide data on the most likely moves of the opponent and the success odds of each of your potential countermoves, based on real-time information.

Arthritis. While not as dramatic as cancer or as sudden as a heart attack, arthritis is still a devastating disease. The markers for arthritis exist within the joints and within your genes. Currently, the tools for measuring these markers are needle aspiration, X-rays, MRIs, and genetic sequencing. Before injuries occur, the genetic markers reveal propensities to develop arthritis. Choosing jobs and sports that diminish impact will be wise for an arthritis candidate. After injuries occur, but well before arthritis sets in, replacing the damaged tissues (missing meniscus cartilage in the knee, for example) or regrowing the articular cartilage will stop the disease's progression. The key is intervention, either at the time of injury or even before, using biologic joint replacement therapies.

Aging. Much of aging is self-induced disease. Yes, the clock goes by, but how healthy, fit, and calm we are helps determine how old we look and feel. While the mirror and the staircase may have warned us in the past, the newly ubiquitous "Internet of Things"— the extension of connectivity into everyday devices—will take over, reminding us how often we have opened the refrigerator door and what we've ingested. More than just how many steps we took today, the next Fitbit will record balance, coordination, strength, agility, and flexibility, along with other markers of fitness. The levels of smoke and air pollutants we inhale will trigger changes in the air quality in our homes and cars, ramping up filtering systems and providing fresher air. Our daily Aging Impact Scores will be totaled, reported, and adjusted. Our stress levels, excitement, and depression stages will be predicted by a cocktail of blood tests, brainwave recordings, and our activity on social media. Interventions—suggested actions to change our destructive paths—will occur about as often as they do today, when we reach for a mood lifter, be it a cup of coffee or a chocolate bar.

ROBOTICS

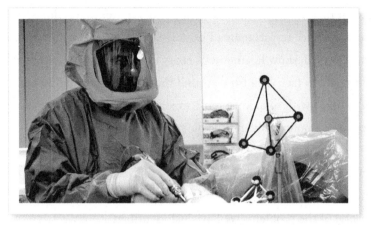

Dr. Stone performing robotic knee replacement surgery

Total knee replacement has been a godsend for many people with severe bone-on-bone arthritis. Many of my patients are skiing, hiking, and playing sports on replaced knees at levels they have not done in years, or even decades.

So, thinking about the hundreds of knees I have replaced with total artificial components over the decades, why am I holding my breath? Because no matter how accurate I was in placing the new knees, I was limited by the accuracy of the saws and manual guides that were available to me. Even slight inaccuracies led to abnormal wear and early failure.

No matter how well I cemented in the components of the new knees, I was limited by the survival of the cement. Over time, the cement inevitably breaks down. So the cement-bone interface was the weak link, especially for my patients who wanted to return to a high level of athletic performance.

No matter how well-designed the implants might have been, the inability to manipulate the implants virtually on a model of the knee meant that the ligaments often stretched out over time. Almost all of the total knee replacements I examine, whether or not I performed them myself, show ligamentous laxity or looseness of the knee after ten years. In fact, data from around the world states that 50 percent of patients with total knee replacements have pain at ten years. This becomes a potentially unsolvable problem.

So in march the robots. Unlike the computer-generated, custom knee implants and cutting guides that have become popular over the last ten years, the surgical robot provides a real-time solution for several of the problems we have just identified.

And it is going to get much better. The current robots still depend on a tremendous amount of surgeon judgment and are not interactive. Future versions will be more professorial, telling the surgeon the outcomes of doing option A or option B, proposing solutions for difficult revision cases, and highlighting errors as they happen so that the patient can leave the operating room benefiting from the best human–robot interaction.

While I am still biased toward replacing injured knee tissues biologically, with new meniscus cartilage and paste grafted articular cartilage, those patients with true bone-on-bone, worn-out knees now have a potentially longer-term bionic option.

Other, nonsurgical, uses of robotics are now coming to the fore with the development of brain-body connections. Contract a muscle, and the artificial limb moves; this technology was once a dream for those who have lost limbs. The interfaces between the motor nerves and prosthetic devices have rapidly improved, permitting power-assisted extremities. Next to come are the "think it and move it" interfaces. Restrictions imposed by human inaccuracy in hand movements or by time delays (between a command and its execution) will be removed.

ARTIFICIAL INTELLIGENCE

AI is already present in many spheres of our lives. Despite its tremendous potential for medical applications, it's surprising how little we've turned to artificial intelligence for help with managing healthcare. For example, could AI end the electronic medical record nightmare?

Medicine has been, and should continue to be, an oral science. People talk to doctors about their problems. Doctors listen and ask questions. Doctors tell the patient's story to other doctors to share information and gain new ideas. Doctors and nurses talk about a patient's progress. They talk to social workers and physical therapists and all sorts of experts who can help solve the patient's problems and improve their healthcare.

The electronic medical record has killed this oral science. Doctors now hunt and peck for information to share. Nurses stare at screens, taking half an hour to enter data, something that used to take three minutes. As far as I can see, everyone in healthcare hates the new quantified medical record except the insurance companies. There are hundreds of editorials by doctors documenting the fact that they can only see two-thirds of the patients they used to see when they must spend chunks of their days entering data.

Apple's Siri, IBM's Watson, and their relatives could solve this. For example:

"Siri, I would like to admit Ms. Jones to the hospital for her knee replacement."

"Sure, Dr. Stone, shall I use your pre-op order set?"

"Yes."

"Tell me the medications she is on."

After I speak the medications' names, Siri might ask, "Okay, let's be sure to let her cardiologist know to adjust her blood thinners a few days before surgery. And by the way, the medication she is on has been recalled and this alternative is recommended."

You can see how this could go. Artificial intelligence has long offered an improvement for these highly formulaic situations and could prompt doctors to be better at their jobs. Medical staff would never have to waste precious time looking through a dozen menus and screens of unrelated information to get to the piece they need. Nurses could dictate their findings as they made their rounds and ask Siri (or her equivalent) to notify doctors if something is amiss—if, say, a wound were not looking right. Patients could tell Siri their medical history before coming in for an office visit, and the doctor could review it with them in person and fill in the shading.

The point is, we can all have conversations. We just can't simultaneously listen, talk, think, and type efficiently. An AI assistant can both listen and add information we may not have learned in medical school—making both the patient and the doctor smarter.

Even big insurance companies might love this scenario as more accurate medical records replace cut-and-paste versions of preexisting records. Not to mention that the bot in the room could prompt doctors to consider less expensive alternatives to drugs, dressings, or therapies. When doctors have the knowledge base of supercomputers just a voice prompt away, diagnoses become more accurate and treatment more efficient.

As you might imagine, there is also an important role to play for

AI surgical assistants. I encounter little surprises in every surgical procedure. Every person is different, and each tissue has its own characteristics—from the obvious tear patterns to the hidden degeneration within the tissue's collagen structure. To my mind, there are no "routine" or "standardized" cases. Each procedure has its own beauty and intrigue. Each can be performed better than the last. Thanks to AI, there is a world of data out there that can instantly respond to my curiosity and influence my decision-making in the operating room.

The source of patients' surgical differences may be in their sports habits. Are they a pro athlete or an out-of-shape desk jockey? How much are they going to push the limits of a repair? Will they follow the postoperative rehabilitation program? Have they been repaired before and reinjured? The tissue differences can be obvious muscle sizes, the shape of the bones, the angle of the joints, the blood supply to the torn fragments, and/or the unique locations of the ligament insertions.

The medical database version of IBM's Watson—and similar knowledge repositories from Google, Apple, and even Amazon—are now available at the tip of my tongue. These tools are called "voice agents." They listen passively and are available to answer any question I may have. I might ask for a reminder of a patient's surgical history, for the data on a specific type of meniscus tear, or for a suggestion on how to remove a broken screw that resists the techniques I have used before.

While much of the information is accessible before I enter the operating room, the surprises I encounter in surgery are still significant. Why? Because there are wide variations in each patient's tissues, where they insert, how they interact, and how they are injured. No two people are exactly alike, yet the similarities are what permit us to aggregate this data into our voice agents' AI.

Before, surgeons usually had to go it alone. Today, we are empowered with the world's knowledge of each case, each technique's outcome, and with the many surgical variations that have been tried. While my head may hold a career's worth of knowledge, and my hands are skilled by practice, I was but one individual. I am alone no more.

AI will soon play an important role in interpreting medical diagnostic images. AI-enabled systems that interpret radiologic studies are advancing to the point where they often match the best radiologists in the world, and they are getting better every day. From CT scans to MRIs, angiograms to Doppler studies, the data captured is digital, and digital data can be read by machines.

Radiologists traditionally sit in dark rooms studying diagnostic images. A resulting report is then given to the practicing physician, who merges the objective digital image interpretations with the more subjective clinical presentation and exam. Often there is more information read by the radiologists than is relevant to the physician and patient. At other times, important information is missed. In a knee MRI, for example, there may be degeneration of a meniscus tissue reported, but this finding has no importance to a patient with bone-on-bone arthritis in need of a joint replacement.

As with genome interpretations, where there is data overload and the possibility of over-diagnosing problems, patients have generally not had direct access to their radiology images or reports. Coalescing this data can take days, if not weeks.

This may soon change due to several parallel advances. AI bots will no longer be interpreting only isolated radiologic scans. Due to the wide availability of electronic medical records, a patient's entire medical history will be available to these bots. In combination with data-mining programs, all of the diagnostic information in a person's medical record will be correlated with any symptom, exam finding, or lab result. With the advance of do-it-yourself image uploading systems, any patient may be able to send their images not only to their doctor but to a cloud-based radiologic interpretation station as well.

Here's an example of where we are heading with the first stages of this system. Let's say a woman injures her knee while skiing in a remote part of Alaska. She gets an exam, X-ray, and MRI done by a local physician in a mountain clinic. The doctor enters this information into an electronic medical record and provides the patient with a web link. The patient uploads the links or the images directly using a cloud-based radiology storage system like Purview.

The patient's own physician, who subscribes to the future "Global Medical AI" network, is notified of the injury and provided with the AI bot–produced report overread by a supervising networked radiologist. This report combines all of the medical information with human and computer software interpretations. It not only diagnoses a torn cruciate ligament (ACL) but also highlights some important genomic information previously submitted to the doctor and patient: Due to a specific genomic pattern, a blood clot in the leg is 10 percent more likely to form during the post-injury period. Since the AI bot has also reviewed the entire pharmacy records available for this patient (in addition to their credit card purchases of over-the-counter drugs), it is clear that the patient has been consuming high doses of NSAIDs. These NSAIDs, the bot notes, might increase the bleeding risk if the patient were to be placed on anticoagulants before being taken off the other drugs. In addition, the evaluation of the patient's recent tweets indicates a new level of depression that may require extra psychological support during the postoperative healing phase.

So, before the skiing patient has even left the remote mountain town, the level of medical insight about their underlying conditions, lifestyle choices, and potential risks exceeds most of what is known today, yet very few extra resources were consumed.

Several recent events are making this future possible. First, general acceptance and recognition of the lack of privacy in medical and consumer information is growing. Electronic medical records are improving by sharing information about patients, no matter where they are being treated. On the positive side, this permits the doctor to know a great deal about the patient. All of their credit card or Apple Pay–like purchases are recorded, and that information is mined to paint a general picture of the cardholder. When combined with analysis of a patient's Facebook and Twitter feeds, Instagram pictures, and other social media findings, a highly detailed portrait of the patient emerges.

In addition, because they are self-learning, AI bots and data-mining technologies are improving more rapidly than humans ever will. They are not intimidated by vast amounts of data and can quickly correlate disparate information sources. Genetic information able to predict disease or highlight risks is rapidly improving. Today, we are researching a sliver of this information as it relates to injury and arthritis. While we still do not have a handle on exactly how certain conditions predicted by the genetic code are expressed or suppressed, such patterns will be more predictive after billions of people have been sequenced.

Patient access to direct medical resources—through medical data uploading services, along with data mining their own healthcare data—will democratize medical diagnoses. This will not reduce the physician's role. It will empower doctors with potent interpretation tools, making them far better diagnosticians. And it will free patients from the tyranny of socialized medical care systems and insurance companies that, in their effort to drive down costs and improve profits for their executives and shareholders, have robbed millions of patients of the best that medicine can offer.

Does all this mining and synthesis of personal information make you squeamish? I believe it is time to embrace the belief that at least in medicine, "all things digital are public." And if they are going to be, we might as well all benefit from this transparency by mobilizing the best minds to keep us healthy, even if those minds are not human.

All Things Digital Are Public
(and Mark Zuckerberg's Lost Moment)

Privacy used to exist only to the degree that one did not share one's information. That standard is now breached on a daily basis. Every time you drive over a bridge that photographs your license plate, walk down a street where face recognition technology records your every step, use your credit card, make a digital phone call, or send a message, you are recording for posterity your actions, locations, and even emotions. We live in a digital world, and all things digital are public.

Forget about privacy. Accept the public nature of all things digital, because it is now indisputable. Once a piece of data is digitized, there is no government agency, no corporation, no software, no server, no encryption, and no blockchain known to modern science that is not vulnerable, penetrable, and hackable. If it is digital, it can be opened, shared, and modified in every way possible.

When you accept this fact, your world changes. HIPAA—the Health Insurance Portability and Accountability Act, designed to ensure medical privacy—is revealed as the expensive and useless encumbrance that it is. The password jumble we all create and forget is removed. You live your life knowing privacy exists only in the analog world.

This realization has tremendous benefits and unfortunate side effects. On the beneficial side, we are compelled to communicate honestly. We know our audience is larger than our intention, our words are permanent, and what we say will help some and hurt others.

All moments captured are public. We see this when we take a photograph with a smartphone; it almost instantly becomes a shared image. (Social media companies' servers store your images, even if you have deleted them on your own devices.) Once you accept that the person you hugged, the bar you danced on, or your child's first steps are visible by the world community, you begin to act as though you are part of the ocean of life rather than an isolated puddle. All aspects of recorded human life digitally influence all others and hopefully increase the maturity of the species.

On the negative side, secrecy is nearly impossible. It is a tremendous effort to take important communication offline. It may no longer even be possible since cameras and the potential for voice capture are ubiquitous. Few conversations occur outside the proximity of a cell phone, computer, or video cam. All of these can be set up to spy on our conversations. (Even Zuckerberg can't hide and has tape covering his smartphone camera lens). Our current loss of privacy is stunning to many people, though it has been years since true privacy was possible.

In medicine, patients used to think their medical records belonged to them. Now they realize that every record is mined for health data. This data is used by insurers to limit costs, by pharmacies and drug companies to target advertising, by hospitals to limit their expense exposure, and by employers to cut insurance costs. The only person who has a hard time accessing a person's medical record is a doctor outside of your health plan from whom you want a second opinion. Your diseases, ailments, and neuroses are far from private.

So does all this help or hurt our health? It could be that once we embrace our truly public lives, we may lift ourselves out of the silos we thought we lived in and act as the communities we really are. We may actually make better-informed decisions when all of the data is crowdsourced. Our entrancement with smartphones, Fitbits, and other intelligent devices may show us, at last, that we're truly interdependent. (Isn't that why this media is called "social?")

Which brings us to Mark Zuckerberg. When he went to Washington, DC in April of 2018 to testify before the joint Senate Judiciary and Commerce Committees, he had a wonderful opportunity to educate the US Congress about the public nature of digital life, but he missed it.

The absurdity of the otherwise elegant presentation that Zuckerberg gave to Congress rests in his statement that you own your own information and can choose who to share it with, and that you can opt out of the various data sales schemes Facebook uses to make money. In fact, you can't. This isn't all Facebook's fault; they may indeed mean well and be sincere in their efforts to give you at least the semblance of control over what you post. But the moment you take a digital picture and store it on Facebook, other social media outlets, Google, Apple, Amazon, or any cloud server, you have transferred that information to a hackable site. The world's hackers strip images for nefarious uses—so that as you text your best friend, your worst enemy can monitor your keystrokes and know your thoughts before your friend ever gets the message.

More than our social interactions are at risk of invasion. The contrived, convoluted HIPAA (Health Insurance Portability and Accountability Act)—a set of rules that supposedly guards our medical information—is a joke on the human privacy condition. Every digital medical record is designed to be shared among the vast array of medical professionals who need to see your information and the insurance companies who pay out for your care. They, the hospitals, and even some employers then sell that information (supposedly stripped of your name) to drug and medical supply companies. Yet once diabetes is put in your medical record, you start getting ads for diabetes medications. How anonymous is that?

And the invasion goes even deeper into our psyches. Our moods are quantified by the words and emojis we put into our texts, by the smiles and frowns in our photos, and by the websites we visit. Our psychological profiles are examined and quantified. We are then targeted by Cambridge Analytica (for example) with ads that are based on these factors. We can also be scrutinized by prospective employers or potential dates. Our thoughts are no longer our own—never mind our posts.

What about our souls? If the soul is the reflection of our moral, ethical, and spiritual being, is it not being exposed by our simple, everyday choices? What we say, who we associate with, what we believe in, even what we confess—all are becoming commoditized.

Once we understand that all things digital are public, we can craft a new sensibility around what privacy means— or if it still has meaning at all. It's even possible that complete transparency will transform our world into a better place. Zuckerberg could have taught Congress that we suddenly live in a new world—a world that they, and even you, have not yet come to grips with. Legislation? Legislate what? Our dreams? Guess what! With some of the new brain wave recorders and artificial intelligence interpreters, even our dreams will soon be up for sale.

VIRTUAL REALITY

Virtual reality is about to hit the inflection point. Soon, nearly everyone will have a VR device or use one regularly. The well of content is rising, and the cost is dropping; only the execution of the various applications is limiting exponential growth. The experience of almost every educational interaction—whether teacher to student, coach to athlete, or doctor to patient—can be vastly improved by this new tool.

Here are a few examples. Through VR, patients can preoperatively experience the surgical center, the recovery process, and their rehabilitation exercises. Not only can instruction on postoperative gait training and range of motion be given, but the patient can actually do the exercises under the virtual guidance of the physical therapist. When combined with wireless activity trackers (e.g., Fitbit), evaluation of the patient's outcome—let's say, range of motion after a total knee replacement—can be actively demonstrated, scored, and reported without the patient leaving home. Problems can then be red-flagged to the doctors' office, activating early interventions. Truly valid outcome scores for surgeons and implants will then be possible. Patients will compare their post-procedural progress to that of their surgeon's previous patients, and they can even check their scores against a national database of patients who are in similar physical therapy recovery processes. All of this data will be measured and collected in virtual-reality physical therapy sessions, then uploaded or accessed on your smartphone, which will be connected to a VR headset.

Surgeon training films and videos have traditionally been visual; now they will become tactile. Feedback devices that increase and decrease resistance (depending on the density of the virtual tissue) will provide the "touch" training long missing in the teaching of new doctors (or in teaching old doctors new tricks). Not only will a potential surgeon's dexterity be trained and measured, but the skillsets needed to respond to crises in the operating room, such as a sudden vessel rupture or heart attack, can be practiced in the virtual body as well. The "See one, do one, teach one" homily of the old days becomes "See a hundred, and practice until your scores match the top 10 percent—then do one on a live patient."

The benefits will stretch far beyond medicine. EMTs, emergency responders, and firefighters will go in and out of every conceivable disaster scenario, following the training manuals and guidelines set down by their specialties, long before donning a uniform.

Sports teams are also increasing their use of virtual reality training. Imagine if professional football prospects are given not just a 150-page playbook to memorize preseason but a VR headset with which they can practice the team's signature plays in real time. Then imagine each week's opponents added to the virtual game with their likely formations and responses. It makes Madden NFL Fantasy Football seem dated and our fantasy future look fabulous.

NEXT GENERATION BIOLOGIC TISSUE

Many athletes hurt themselves while pushing themselves, seeking greater athletic glory at the expense of their bodies. They train through the pain, ignoring the warning signs of injury. They stop only when they can't go on. And we glorify this irrationality, admire those who push past the perceived limits of human performance and reward them with shiny medals, ridiculously large sums of money, and fame that often ruins them in the end. This cycle will not stop. It has occurred since the dawn of competition.

My job is to restore the injured. When I do it well, they return to the glorious destructive process of pushing themselves and seeking greater athletic glory at the expense of their bodies. When the injuries become cumulative, we reset goals, modify the activities, and find satisfaction in lowered standards. The average age of the irreparably injured is being lowered every year. My hope is that our continuing research into and development of regenerative medicine techniques will lead to more than just pain relief. However, our treatment tools— and patients' abilities to use them—sometimes fall short. In what I call the "anabolic era of orthopaedics," we use the body's own response to injury (e.g., rushing blood with stem cells and growth factors to the site) as a model for how we should treat tissue damage.

We now augment almost all tissue injuries with a cocktail of cells and growth factors. We bathe donor tissues in these same compounds, and we stimulate new blood supplies to heal tissues previously thought to be untreatable. The next step is to refine these treatments by identifying which specific growth factors are needed and applying them in a selective manner. An ACL-injured knee clearly has a different biochemical profile than an arthritic knee. We will soon have a much clearer picture of how to augment the healing process.

Our goal is the true restoration of the original materials: the meniscus, the cartilage, and the ligaments that have been so abused. Our aspirations are not in vain. Over the last twenty-five years, my research and the work of my peers has led to novel ways to repair, regrow, and regenerate tissues that were previously thought to be unsalvageable.

Our efforts have expanded into the remodeling of animal tissue for use in people whose own tissues have been used up. The dream is that by using younger and stronger tissue (usually from pigs), the injured person might return as good or even better than they were before their injury. This fantasy has become a reality. Pig ligaments passed a wide clinical trial in Europe and South Africa as ACL replacements and pig tissues eventually will be approved for use for all of the other musculoskeletal tissues of the body.

Our next step will be to use pig organs, such as kidneys, liver, pancreas, and heart tissues, by stripping them of the antigens that cause rejection and repopulating them with the human patients' own stem cells. This tissue engineering process may solve the current scarcity of young, healthy donor tissue for people with end-stage diseases. This work is in its infancy, but the horizon is not far away.

Our bodies once knew how to regenerate tissues. We did it in utero, but then shut off the genes that drive organ growth. Salamanders, on the other hand, never shut off those genes. They can regrow their lost tails throughout life. Sea cucumbers can regenerate organs. Starfish can grow new arms. One approach to solving the human repair problem may lie in the removal of the gene inhibitors that prevent our own limb regeneration.

Only by working on these tissue regeneration solutions can I justify encouraging my patients not only to rehabilitate, but also to get back into the game. I maintain the hope that one day soon we will be able to truly solve their self-inflicted, societally encouraged injuries.

Of Pigs, Ligaments,
and Tendons of the Future

Imagine that in the future, you badly tore a ligament or a tendon, and it was beyond repair. Imagine again that instead of replacing the tissue by taking tissue from your body, the surgeon could replace it with something stronger yet still biologic; something your body would remodel into being all you. For some, that future is now.

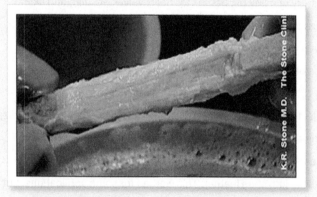

A pig ligament for surgical implantation after undergoing the Z-Process, a technique invented by Dr. Stone that humanizes animal tissue for transplantation

In 2016, a patient in Poland had his ACL replaced with a Z-Lig, an off-the-shelf scaffold device made from a pig ligament. It was the first commercial use of this device and the culmination of many years of work, which my team and I began over two decades ago with early-stage development and pilot trials. The Z-Lig was subsequently developed by Aperion Biologics and was cleared for marketing and distribution in the European Union and other markets that recognize the CE certification mark (indicating conformity with health standards for products sold within the EU).

Why pigs? Pigs grow to over four hundred pounds in just six months. Some porcine tissues are stronger than human tissues due to their thickness, yet they have the same collagen organization as humans. In evolutionary terms, we say the collagen is quite "conserved," meaning that it matches ours. There is a long history of using pig tissues for heart valves, insulin, and skin. Pigs are plentiful, and the unused medical parts can be eaten. Even many Muslim and Orthodox Jewish authorities allow the use of pig tissues for medical necessity.

The problem with using any animal tissue is immunologic rejection. Specific carbohydrates on animal tissues are recognized when transplanted into humans. In the past, the body blocked these immunologic red flags by aldehyde fixation, turning the tissues into shoe leather. This worked for some applications, but not where the tissues had to be both flexible and able to be remodeled, as is the case with ligaments and tendons.

The new solution is to strip away the carbohydrates with a specific enzyme, thereby humanizing them. This solution, called the Z-Process, was successfully tested in a randomized prospective double-blind trial in Europe and approved for use. The Polish patient became the first patient outside of the trial to receive the graft. Patients in Italy and South Africa followed. A pivotal trial in the US was planned as well. Unfortunately, underfunding caused the commercial entity, Aperion Biologics, to fail. Stay tuned for further commercialization progress.

Ligaments and tendons of the future will be stronger than those they replace. Torn ACLs and PCLs, rotator cuffs of the shoulder, collateral ligaments of the elbow, and tendons in the hands and feet, when ruptured, will all be replaced by stronger, younger, and healthier tissues from pigs. And these pig tissues may be preloaded with stem cells and growth factors from the injured patient.

Fixing broken people with the goal of making them better than they have been in years is a dream come true for surgeons around the world. If the patients do their part, our goal of helping people become fitter, faster, and stronger will be realized more often than not.

LONGEVITY AIN'T WHAT IT'S CRACKED UP TO BE

The longevity movement is pushing science to explore the possibilities of keeping people alive well past one hundred. Recent conferences on radical life extension explore "hacking" various body systems to stop the aging process, diminish genetic telomere changes, and defeat death. The upside to this research is the identification of life-shortening behaviors, foods, and chemicals that should be avoided or eliminated. In addition, the habits of a healthy lifestyle—via nutrition, exercise, and stress reduction techniques—can be quantified and taught.

The downside to radical life extension is that it might partially work. That changes the appeal considerably. Who wants to be 150 years old if half of your body's systems work and half do not? The likelihood of medical science solving the related issues of cardiac weakening, brain deterioration, joint destruction, muscular atrophy, dental decay, and taste reduction, are so low as to be scary.

Who wants to outlive all of one's friends and family? Who is going to fund your life past one hundred years old? What healthcare system can afford a society that includes thousands—or millions—of super-aged people? What's the point of living past the age when you can contribute effectively? Are the perspectives of very, very old people really relevant to youthful societies they may inhabit but hold little in common with?

What about the orthopaedic challenges? Life past one hundred is a life lived on fragile bones, weak muscles, arthritic joints, and often with significant pain. While we are working hard to prevent and repair these problems, reversing the aging process would create a mismatch between age and musculoskeletal function. This will require equally ageless mental, cardiac, and sensory systems to utilize our new, mythic, god-like physiques. One is really wishing for a freezing of time—for the eternal body and mind of a 25-year-old—rather than wanting to be a 125-year-old stud.

So let's amuse ourselves with the radical life extension discussions. We'll take the best of the anti-aging advice to heart and focus the majority of our precious resources on healthcare rather than disease care.

Remember that living well now is far better than living overlong and that our great-great-grandchildren really don't want to support us.

BIODYNAMIC HEALTH

From Bordeaux, France, to Sonoma, California, the vineyards of prominent winemakers are foregoing pesticides, tractors, and modern farming techniques in favor of a method called biodynamic farming.

Biodynamic farming goes beyond "organic" standards. It is a technique of agriculture where plants, insects, and farm animals are purposely comingled to optimize the growth of the crops without the use of chemicals, pesticides, or nonnatural fertilizers. While some proclaim a spiritual connection, the practical reality is the balancing of organic materials from multiple sources to optimize the quality of the crops.

Controlling pests by balancing competing large and small living things is exactly what humans did before industrial "modernization." There is now a significant push in medicine, orthopaedics, and other specialties to do this same balancing by harnessing the power of viable microbes, viruses, and organisms to promote health and cure disease. Here are a few of the most recent examples.

In orthopaedics, sports and arthritis injuries are being treated with blood derivative injections containing growth factors and stem cells to stimulate healing rather than using cortisone and pharmaceutical anti-inflammatories that sometimes inhibit healing. Natural sugars, such as glucosamine, are being combined with gelling factors and injected into joints to promote cartilage repair. Even a few homeo-pathic compounds that were once thought to have no measurable amounts of therapeutic agents are now being shown to have some possible effect by the presence of low-level antigens that instigate a healing response.

In gastrointestinal disorders, such as infectious C. difficile colitis disease, a practice called fecal microbiota transplant (FMT), or just fecal transplant, takes stool from healthy family members, concentrates it into a pill, and gives it to the patient with the bowel disorder. FMT has cured a once-incurable disease. Many other GI diseases, in which the natural microbes of the body have been overwhelmed by an unfriendly variant, may also fall to probiotic therapies since they may be susceptible to a competing microbial infusion—the most prominent being colitis, food allergies, gluten insensitivity, and many so-called autoimmune disorders. Each of these may be interpreted as a misbalancing of viable organisms within us.

Viruses are now being harnessed to use their invasive powers to deliver foreign proteins to cancers that then are recognizable by the immune system and destroyed. The most recent successful use involved injecting the partially inactivated poliovirus into a previously incurable brain tumor, a glioblastoma, to induce the tumor's destruction. Even carbohydrates from pigs are being used to label cancers as foreign, again exposing them to destruction by normally circulating antibodies.

The biodynamic health era is upon us again. Working with nature and natural compounds permits the interactive dance of living things. It's a dance developed over millions of years of evolution, which may be applied to the many disorders that humans, animals, and plants experience. By avoiding selective pharmaceuticals manufactured in the lab that focus on one target, and by using all the components existing in nature, we benefit in extraordinary ways.

In the case of biodynamic wine, we get to drink the results.

BRAIN NUTRITION

Multiple times each day, we reach for an "altering" substance. It may be an upper: a piece of chocolate, an espresso, a Coke, a candy bar. After a day of stressful work, we may switch to a downer: a cocktail, a beer, or a marijuana joint (now legal in at least eight states). All of these are brain supplements, neural nutrition, or attitude modifiers. Where do you think this constant up-and-down, unscientific brain modulation is leading?

The state of happiness in America is not very highly ranked. Most people seem to be stressed, overworked, emotionally frazzled, angry, and sometimes even violent. To counteract these traits, we seek stress reduction through yoga, meditation, and sports activities which— while sometimes competitive—leave us in a happier place. We also turn to reading, arts appreciation, and shared group interactions. A surprising number of people have spent years seeking solace in psychotherapy, in retreats designed to calm the brain, and in counseling of all sorts. All these strategies attempt to put us in control of our out-of-control mental states. Mindfulness is the goal. Yet the paths to get there are filled with anxious efforts.

The most common brain modification activities surround the foods we put in our bodies. Those foods have been corrupted for decades by the sugar industry's realization that while a little sugar is good, a lot is addictive. Worse than the nicotine lobby, the sugar lobby entered our lives through our children's cereals and has stayed there in our soft drinks. The negative health effects from conditions like diabetes and obesity dwarf all other self-induced illnesses.

Yet paralleling the sugar industry's effort, our government waged a "War on Drugs" that effectively crushed experimentation on mind-altering substances. Research on MDMA, LSD, mescaline, Ketamine, and marijuana was suppressed. The development of thousands of other compounds that could helpfully affect our brain receptors never got any funding.

This is changing. Marijuana, proven not to be a gateway to the use of other drugs, is opening the path to research on mind expansion in a variety of ways. Scientists have discovered defined receptors—cannabinoids being just a single example—that can be stimulated to provide pain relief without addiction. Other receptors may help release creative energies, open blocked memory passages (both for people with healthy brains and those with dementia), intensify mathematical acumen, unleash musical skills, empower empathy, suppress violent thoughts, cure depression, provide satiety to inhibit overeating, and trigger a thousand other useful traits yet to be identified.

Our days of living in fear that the use of "drugs" is always a crutch, and leads inevitably to addiction, are fading fast. We are all using drugs or supplements in the form of sugar, chocolate, or caffeine uppers and alcohol-based downers. Yet we have been held back from access to effective, targeted interventions that could streamline our paths to happiness, productivity, and peacefulness.

Throughout Silicon Valley and the Bay Area, many professionals are experimenting with micro-doses of various drugs, including LSD, to enhance their work performance. This is a lousy way to develop the body of scientific research we need to measure the brain's receptivity to targeted therapies. Instead, I suggest we fund massive amounts of brain nutrition research, and cure what ails us in the most productive, safe, and scientific ways. I look forward to my daily glass of brain juice and hope everyone toasts to a happy life with theirs.

GENE EDITING

From my point of view, the diseases that afflict my patients—arthritis in particular—may be partially eradicated in the remarkably near future because the action mechanisms of these diseases can be determined from the patient's genetic code. Then the expression of the disease can be prevented by early gene manipulation, and the disease's clinical manifestations blunted by therapeutic interventions.

Today, we are interfering in the expression of the genetic code in a variety of ways. Most simply, we give over-the-counter supplements that affect the telopeptides: terminals of the genetic code that enhance certain functions and suppress others. Nutrition counseling will move from focusing on weight to focusing on specific, genetically directed cellular activity. We are modifying the genetic activities of our injured patients (with various injections and medications) to treat, augment, and prevent a number of diseases. Our genetic map is no longer a sacred, unalterable chart of biological destiny but rather an alphabet with which we can write new stories.

The first known experiment using the CRISPR gene editing technique with live human embryos was conducted in China in November 2018. The joy of seeing babies born with potential immunity to the HIV/AIDS virus was, unfortunately, dulled by a chorus of critics. What was not said is that the potential for good is unlimited and that the first real success will launch a thousand ships carrying weapons capable of killing off the diseases of old.

Yes, the genetics experiment carried out in China raises many questions. Yes, it could have been done with more transparency, more consent, and more protections. No, it does not represent the dawn of unnatural selection, leading to super races that will dominate the world, but it *does* open up the possibility that every disease with genetic origins is now a fair target.

There are diseases, and there are proclivities. The diseases of arthritis (osteo, psoriatic, and rheumatoid), while varying widely in their clinical presentations and mechanisms of joint destruction, may have common pathways in genetic alterations. Obesity, diabetes, and hemophilia have already been shown to have associated genetic patterns and susceptibility to target interventions. The possibility that diseases like arthritis could be eliminated before birth opens up vast potential for increased human performance, health, and happiness.

The proclivity of one person to develop a syndrome or a late-in-life manifestation of a systemic weakness presents another set of challenges to the human species. We are on our way to understanding how and why conditions such as cardiovascular disease, loss of hearing and eyesight, and sensitivity to sunlight that develops into skin cancer are predictable from certain genetic patterns and inheritance. Knowing who has these proclivities, and when these afflictions will occur, may not be far away. Changing the epigenetics—the proteins and messengers that deliver both the bad news effects of the genetic patterns or the good suppression of unwanted genetic expressions— could lead to an increase in human longevity only dreamed of a few years ago.

All of this depends on safe alterations of the genetic makeup of humans. In fact, we do this kind of genetic suppression and stimulation every day. When you take a simple supplement like glucosamine, it upregulates the cellular machinery that produces hyaluronic acid, the lubricant in joints. This effect then diminishes stiffness, a complaint of many arthritic patients. The effect of this supplement works largely through its effects on the patient's genes. Upregulation and downregulation occur millions of times per day, sometimes intentionally, sometimes beneficially, but not randomly. What you do and what you eat makes you who you are.

You are constantly genetically modifying yourself—and your loved ones as well. Your interactions with them, the transfer of your microbiome by a handshake or a kiss, has real genetic ramifications. The more we understand these mechanisms, the more intentional we will be in our transference. Soon your doctor will give you drugs and surgical interventions that are specific for your receptivity to these therapies based on your genetic patterns and that may alter your epigenetic expressions to make these more successful.

So when a doctor and researcher attempt to suppress a fatal disease like HIV/AIDS as the first step to eventually curing a thousand diseases, speak up. While you may suggest refinements to their process and even engage in ethical explorations, remember to celebrate the phenomenal achievement that may lead us to a healthier population. Our ability to survive our planetary pollution, our disease-spreading behaviors, and even our nuclear misadventures depends on our ability to evolve faster than natural evolution alone permits.

NANO COMMUNICATION

How low does communication go? Will we one day be able to understand and influence communication at the atomic level?

Humans, fish, and other animals talk to each other, even if they don't always listen. We all know that bees talk. They communicate where the best forage is and when it's time to swarm, and they even collaborate to commit regicide and raise a new queen. We've also learned that plants communicate about their surroundings, a subject most elegantly written about in Michael Pollan's bestselling book, *The Botany of Desire.*

Surprisingly, we have learned that even bacteria talk, a phenomenon called quorum sensing. A group of bacteria can recruit others of its kind to join them, raising their level of potency to cause an active infection. They can also lie dormant and awaken together at just the right time for them, and often the wrong time for a patient.

Viruses clearly talk. They infect healthy cells and inject their DNA into nuclei to turn them into killers. HIV is the best (and worst) example of this genetic conversation.

Even smaller units of life talk. Enzymes signal to effect protein activation and feedback controls. The regulation of entire cascades of biomechanical processes depends on complex communication systems that might last fractions of a second or days at a time.

We now know that all of these inputs can affect our genetic makeup and its expression. Our genes change with drugs, stimuli, and an infinite number of other forces. They then produce a phenomenal variety of chemical markers, all from a genetic language containing only four letters: A, T, C, G. What happens when we learn how to add letters to the four that now constitute our human genome? This synthetic biologic syntax is already in the testing stage. The human dictionary is about to expand exponentially.

What if we can learn to listen, understand, and respond to genetic communications? Could we have a genetic Fitbit and language translator? And as gene editing techniques like CRISPR Cas-9 continue to become less expensive and more available, could we engage in a daily conversation with our personal genetic dictionary? When George Jetson came home and walked through his doorway scanner, could he have chosen which version of him would say, "Hi, Honey, I'm home!"?

Don't be so quick to laugh this off. We already take medications that change our protein constitution. We touch, kiss, make love, and share microbiomes in thousands of ways each day. In our current practice of orthopaedics, we inject stem cells and growth factors from healthy donors into injured patients. This is turning out to be the most potent, effective therapy we have ever seen. We believe that the stem cells in these preparations communicate with each other, recruiting other stem and progenitor cells to the site of injury or arthritis. Once there, they instruct injured tissues, inducing them to heal.

We are actively engaged in the transmission of cellular and gene-altering vectors and studying what happens on the level of cellular communication. What we need is a tool to help us interpret this language on a much smaller, even atomic, scale. For now, it's mostly Greek to us.

IMMORTALITY

The Singularity—the merger of machines and humans in a dawning era of nonbiological intelligence—is a hot topic in the Bay Area. The algorithms of deep mathematics, combined with neural networks and high-speed processing, permit human systems' monitoring to a high degree. A robot programmed with the right information could potentially act as a "mirror" of ourselves, responding in real time, just as we would, to all kinds of inputs, both social and biological. Here's how this is developing.

Today we text nonstop. This messaging tool has all but replaced email, faxes, phone calls, and the ancient "snail mail" letter. These messages, when analyzed, reflect our business, social activities, and our family lives. They can serve as windows into our moods, our fears, and our desires.

Consider the enormous number of selfies people take each day, and each of the personal fitness devices we wear, sleep-monitoring apps we open, and all of our other self-measuring tools. Based on these mechanisms, a bot, troll, or computer agent can monitor our lives and replicate much of it by approximating, with increasing skill, our actions. After a while, it can deduce exactly how we would respond to many of life's inputs and even predict how our lives will progress. With Photoshop-like "aging" tools already available, our online profiles can "naturally" age 20, 50, or even 150 years.

Our thoughts can now make artificial hands move. They can be transmitted through neural networks and activate various control mechanisms. Soon, they'll be good enough to fly an airplane. The humanoid robots that embody this technology will move and may even act better than we do. They can already write poetry, create original paintings, and dance ballets.

Given time, this is likely to evolve beyond merely actionable thoughts. By mapping our neural networks as they respond to emotional and moral issues, a window opens onto consciousness itself. By reading the Fitbit of your soul, of your spirituality, of your creativity, a bot may ultimately bring a "human" quality to its decisions.

Once this is fully realized, we will gain a sort of digital immortality. In the same way your Facebook page lives on after your death, your bot may live on—counseling your children as you would, and their children—with its point of view evolving just as yours would as new information enters your decision-making process.

So while we have emphasized physical fitness in this book so far, we recognize that your mental fitness, along with your social and emotional intelligence, needs as much training as your body does. Not only do you want to play until you are one hundred years old, but you also want your immortal bot to reflect the best mindset forever.

Who is going to create these monitoring agents, and what ethical rules will the bots be governed by? What does "human" mean if a time comes when algorithms can evolve our mental and spiritual beings as well, or better, than we can? What would you do or say if you knew your words and actions would be immortal? In some ways, they already are. So, there's another reason to think about what you say and do before you do it.

TOP FIVE REASONS TO AVOID SPACE TRAVEL

I've presented a variety of ways the future will make us superhumans (at least, from today's perspective). I'll leave you with one invaluable piece of health advice for the day after tomorrow: Stick close to home. Planet Earth, that is.

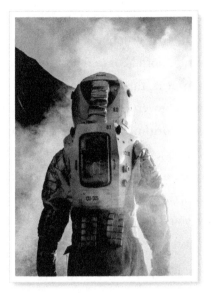

The reality of living on another planet

The list of bodily systems that don't work properly grows with every examination of astronauts who spend prolonged time in space. Here are the top five hazards for would-be space explorers.

1. Effects of Gravity

Lack of gravitational force is deadly to humans. Starting at the top, the cerebrospinal fluid does not circulate properly in low-gravity states, causing brain swelling and cerebral motor dysfunction. While loss of balance may be obvious, all types of proprioception are affected—some perhaps permanently. Changes in the brains of astronauts, as noted by MRIs, suggest premature aging, and the trips so far have been relatively short.

Normally, our body's fluids are pulled down by gravity, and our systems adjust. In low gravity, the fluids redistribute. Faces, eyes, and brains all swell, overloading the cardiovascular system. Cardiac atrophy, with weakening heart muscle activity, will eventually disable all humans in space.

Bone formation depends on resistance exercise. Because it simply is not possible to exercise enough while in space, loss of bone mineral essentially ages astronauts by decades and makes fragility fractures a huge risk. Bone loss accelerates from 3 percent cortical loss per year to 1 percent per month. Most astronauts take up to three years to recover from a simple four-month visit in space. The osteoclast cells that break down bone are ramped up more than the bone-forming cells, leading to an overload of calcium in the system.

Long-haul astronauts experience a decreased production of red blood cells. Inner ear and blood pressure are so disturbed that all astronauts develop nausea for varying periods of time. A single episode of vomiting in a space suit can be fatal.

2. Effects of Radiation

Radiation exposure is ten times higher in low orbit than it is on land. As insulating lead is too heavy for spacecraft, astronauts receive toxic doses of radiation every second. The damage to the retina, the thyroid, and the brain, along with the body's most sensitive tissues, is permanent. Any residence in space would require massive shielding of housing and mobile units, along with clothing—making colonists of Mars or the moon relatively stationary. Unanticipated solar flares produce fatal radiation doses in minutes, even through the walls of spacecraft. In one measured solar storm, the surface level of radiation on the planet Mars doubled.

Human eyes are particularly sensitive, and a higher incidence of radiation-induced cataracts in astronauts has been noted. Alzheimer's and other degenerative brain diseases are accelerated in the astronauts who have traveled into space so far. The immune system is weakened with chromosomal changes in the white blood cells (lymphocytes), and T cell function is reduced.

No fetus could ever come to term healthily in such a low-gravity, high-radiation environment. Most likely, they would be deformed upon delivery or stillborn, due to exposure to radiation in the womb.

3. Depression

Fresh air is not only key to physical health; it's also critical for mental health. People who are confined indoors with no exposure to fresh air (e.g., prisoners) display depression and multiple other health issues. While indoor gardens may provide the simulated scent and humidity of outdoor nature, they are a poor substitute for the real thing. In space, foods do not taste the same, and at the same time, our sense of taste is reduced. Smells freed from gravity permeate the shared living space, diminishing the quality of life. Combined with claustrophobia, lack of biodiversity, lack of privacy, no family, and reduced opportunities for social, romantic, or sexual engagement, extended time in space is a prescription for mental disease.

Spacefarers' complete reliance on a complex maze of critical engineering and life-support equipment, all supplied by the lowest bidder (if from public sources), or by private contractors with varying experience and little accountability, leads to a constant underlying fear of a fatal technical failure. There is a no-return policy once in space, even for Amazon Prime.

Aside from personal depression, there are other mental health dangers, such as the lack of a police force with the ability to resist one man gone mad. Even if you could imprison someone for a crime in space, how could the colony spare the resources for even one unproductive member? There will be no provisions to support the mentally ill, the sick, or the incarcerated.

4. Infection

Microbes and viruses become more virulent in space, possibly leading to food poisoning, antibiotic resistance, and hard-to-treat infections. A likely confluence of microbiomes—interacting without medical services, a hospital environment, or advanced testing facilities to control and treat infectious agents—risks complete colony wipeout from a single antibiotic-resistant organism.

5. Lack of Healthcare

The high likelihood of cancer formation from radiation, blood pressure elevations from lack of gravity, and the stress of living in confined quarters will all lead to complex health challenges in an environment where only basic emergency care is available. Astronaut crews will not have the range of medical experts, CT, MRI, or other tools necessary for accurate diagnoses. Nor will they have the surgical facilities for critical healthcare. The expected lifespan of extraterrestrial inhabitants will be shockingly short. And the reproduction of human babies would be nearly impossible due to radiation-damaged DNA.

On Earth, we spend relatively little energy surviving in our atmosphere, leaving most of our efforts for productivity or recreation. In space, even if a small colony could survive, they could not innovate, manufacture, or farm at scale unless massive innovations in living quarters and health maintenance were achieved.

So, by all means, let's leap forward toward a future filled with new technologies that can make us more superhuman, that can repair our bodies and eliminate our diseases, and that offer us a plethora of opportunities to live fully while we are alive. But when it comes to our future as a species, my wish for all my readers is that they look around; let us invest in the earth and save this planet while we can.

FINAL CHAPTER

I often ask people what they look for in a doctor. The most common answers are friendliness, availability, caring, and thoroughness. These are all wonderful traits, but they are not what I look for. I want the best brains and with it, extensive knowledge of the field. I want curiosity and the power to look beyond the routine. I want courage and the ability to act on what the doctor sees. Yes, of course, the other traits are nice, but they won't determine if I live or die, or if I can return to my life with the ability to become better than I was before.

I hope this book has prompted you to think about each of the issues that hold you back from recovering from injury or overcoming arthritis. I hope that you now seek a level of care that helps you see yourself as an athlete in training and not a patient in rehab and returns you fitter, faster, and stronger than you have been in years. May you play until you are age one hundred, and may your brains, soul, and character live forever.

If you have questions or need help, I invite you to reach out to me. I can be reached by email at info@stoneclinic.com, or you can schedule a complimentary medical consult at www.stoneclinic.com/consult.

APPENDIX A

INSIGHTS ON SKI BINDINGS

Most ski bindings have not changed in thirty years. When bindings comply with international safety standards, they do a brilliant job of reducing tibia fractures. However, these fractures account for only 3 percent of all skiing injuries, while ACL damage has risen to one in five of all skiing injuries. Surprisingly, bindings are not designed to protect the ACL while skiing. Over time, skis have changed in both shape and length, so why haven't bindings evolved to offer protection for the ACL?

There are several issues with current ski bindings. First, capturing both the toe and the heel is a recipe for disaster—with the heel capture being the primary problem. The forces experienced by the leg and then the ACL (which, in part, holds the femur to the tibia) vary widely, depending on hundreds of factors. These include snow conditions, the body of the skier, the length of the tibia, the flexibility of the ski, the flexibility of the boot, the relationship between the ski, foot, and knee…the list goes on. Boot fit and boot buckling also contribute significantly to the transfer of loads between the ski and the tibia.

The ski, acting as a lever, leads to the tibia fracture problem, but it is the length of the tibia itself that affects the ACL problem. When a ski slips sideways, then catches while the heel is captured, the ACL sees abnormally high forces at the top of the tibia, leading to rupture. (Note that while the heel is captured by the snow in skiing, it can also be captured in soccer and football by heel cleats and in basketball and handball by the high friction between modern athletic footwear soles and the playing surfaces of well-kept gym floors.)

The challenge with ski bindings is to find just the right amount of control—an amount that keeps the skier attached to the ski when desired (retention control) and avoids prerelease, and yet releases the boot just before an injury occurs. To do this effectively, the binding design must decouple release forces from retention forces and decouple certain retention forces from each other.

For racers and steep terrain skiers, releasing at the wrong time is believed to produce as many severe injuries as not releasing—though there is no hard data to support this belief. For recreational skiers, failure to release during a fall is the most frequently stated cause of injury (though skiing injuries that involve "no release" are evenly distributed across skier types). Most ACL injuries are incurred before "falling," so the skier's report of what happened to their knee is often unreliable.

In the meantime, the ski binding industry continues to make what are called "two-mode bindings," which release laterally at the toe and vertically at the heel. Some also have a multidirectional toe release. These ACL-unfriendly designs continue to dominate the marketplace and, consequently, fill the orthopaedic surgeon's office.

Currently, no binding on the market addresses ACL injury mitigation. Despite suggestive marketing names, recent alternative designs have not made a dent in ACL injury rates. What is needed are ski bindings that release in the presence of certain levels of downward and lateral forces at the heel (mostly) and certain levels of upward and lateral forces at the toe. Most importantly, the retention mechanisms and release controls need to be independently incorporated into the same binding mechanism.

INSIGHTS ON SKI BOOTS

Ski boots haven't changed much in twenty years. Stiff and stiffer cuffs, rounded Italian-molded toe shapes, heavy polyurethane plastics with cold, hard buckles—this pretty much describes most of the downhill boots on the market. This is about to radically change. While not nearly as radical as needed, boots over the last ten years have featured wider toe boxes and wider lasts. In many cases, the rear cuff heights have been lowered a bit to accommodate less tip pressure needed with tighter radius sidecut skis.

Skis have evolved. The old narrow, straight shapes are now curvy with waists narrower than tails and tips that permit anyone to turn after just a few lessons. The cambered bottoms have given way to rockers that ride forward and backward on the snow, cruise through crud, and float on the powder. The technology for actually making the skis has gone high-tech, with carbon fibers laid between novel materials that produce a range of ski responses tailored to each snow condition. Yet the casts that skiers put on their feet, which extend across their ankles up to mid-calf, lock in most people's ankles so effectively that the skis they're clamping onto may never be used to their full potential.

This is how we got here and where we are going. Ski racing captured our imaginations with ABC's *Wide World of Sports* glorifying the courageous, good-looking athletes who flung themselves down icy racecourses, mostly in European mountains. The speeds they were achieving kept rising, and to manage those steep hills, the skiers had to be locked into a rigid connection between their boots, their bindings, and their skis. This technique required a forward stance, deeply bent knees, and the ability to put pressure on the front of a long, straight, metal-edged racing ski. Only tremendous musculature, combined with fearlessness and skill, could control this stiff construct.

No one appears to have told the rest of the skiing public that they were not facing the same challenges as their idols on the race slopes. Though racing boots make no sense for recreational skiers, boot companies invested heavily in molds made for thick polyurethane, a heavy material that could be stiffened to meet a variety of skier abilities. Marketers made clear that "real" skiers skied with stiff, heavy, toe- and shin-crushing boots.

We now realize that the new ski shapes make skiing so easy that stiff, heavy boots make less sense than ever. Our ankles can now be used to turn the skis. This means the softer the forward flex, the more the skier feels the ski. Importantly, with dorsal flexion, the skier is able to manipulate her center of gravity more readily to maintain pressure over the arch and metatarsals as opposed to the heels. This can only occur, however, with new materials. It is not stiffness the skier wants, but reactivity. How fast does the boot return to its optimal shape after being flexed? It turns out that if the polyurethane is replaced with specialized nylons, such as Grilamid or thin carbon fiber skeletons, the ski boot can be made 75 percent lighter. It remains stiff in lateral positions but super reactive in forward and back motions. All of a sudden, the skier becomes a dancer, with quick, light motions driving their skis anywhere on the slopes.

With these high-tech materials come new boot shapes. When skiers flex forward through the ankle, they first apply pressure on the ski at the first metatarsal, or great toe. To allow that pressure to be applied optimally, the toe box needs to be widened—more like a Birkenstock than a pointed shoe. The arch, meanwhile, needs to engage with the forward pressure, then spring back when released. In the old boots, the heavily clamped-down buckles that locked the foot to a raised boot bed eliminated this anatomic interplay and distanced the skier from the ski. In newer designs, the fit, flexibility, and reactivity are designed to permit the skier to rely on their feet, not just on their egos.

So try these new boots out. Once you go soft, flexible, and reactive, you will never go back.

THE POWDER CURE

"There are only so many moguls in any given knee," said Warren Miller, the famous ski filmmaker. I use his observation for many patients who love skiing but have arthritic knees. Skiing is actually pretty kind to the knee joints as long as you don't fall and if you don't ski hard bumps all day long. Skiing powder uses all the body's muscles and improves balance and coordination without impact. I sometimes write prescriptions that say, "Must ski powder." Every knee, it seems, can miraculously ski or board on a fresh powder day.

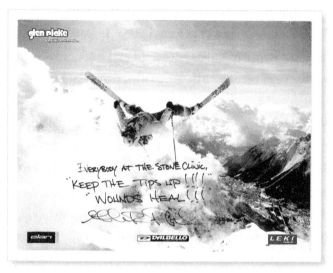

Glenn Plake • Hall of Fame skier and longtime Stone Clinic rehab patient

If you have arthritis in your knees, and it is too late to replace the cartilage or resurface the bones before the ski season, there are three things you can do: start on glucosamine for its joint lubrication properties; visit your doctor for joint lubrication injections; and work with a physical therapist to maximize your range of motion.

Here's why powder is helpful for arthritic knees. The bones of the knee joints are covered with a smooth layer called hyaline cartilage. This surface is made up of collagen, a protein fiber, and a matrix of charged sugar molecules that attract water. There are a few specialized cells within the matrix called chondrocytes. The surface has a boundary layer of lubricants called hyaluronate and lubricin. Together, these remarkable materials have a slickness five times smoother than ice on ice.

This beautiful construct can withstand skiing or running for a lifetime. It rarely wears out—unless there is a specific injury to it, to the meniscus fibrous shock absorber that protects it, or to the underlying bone.

In very general terms, there are four types of arthritis that can damage the joint surface. "Wear and tear" arthritis is really the name of a disease that occurs only after injury. Osteoarthritis, on the other hand, may be caused by an underlying genetic condition or possibly by an as yet unidentified infectious disease. Inflammatory arthritis commonly involves the reaction between the lining cells of the joint and circulating antibodies that damage the cartilage surface. Infectious arthritis is characterized by the damage done by enzymes released by bacteria during such infections.

Absent these diseases, what happens when the cartilage gets damaged is that the scarce cells within the cartilage matrix are not activated adequately to instigate a repair process. Just as a bulged-out area on a tire eventually leads to a failure of the surface and a flat, the damaged area of the joint surface fails to properly absorb the forces of walking or sports. The "flat tire" in arthritis produces bone spurs that form underneath the cartilage surface and at the edges of the bone, eventually deforming the knee joint. When worn severely enough, the knee misshapes into varus (or bowed leg) on the inside or valgus (knock-knee) on the outside.

The solution is to repair these injuries as soon as they occur by stimulating a healing process in the damaged articular cartilage (articular cartilage paste grafting is our preferred method) and by repairing, regenerating, or replacing the damaged meniscus shock absorber as soon as it is injured.

Once arthritis is present, a range of effective treatments—including cartilage replacement—can be offered. All therapies, however, work better in people who remain active. Activity stimulates muscle development, improves blood flow to the joints, increases a sense of well-being, and increases free testosterone, pheromones, and adrenaline.

So the message for my skiers with arthritis is, ski the powder. The smooth, nonimpact runs will bring smiles to your face and happiness to your knees.

ACKNOWLEDGMENTS

Inspiration, motivation, and creativity unrestrained needs editors, lovers, friends, and family to modulate words into palatable morsels. For this I have a cornucopia of wise people to thank…First, my wife, Susan, and daughters, Jennifer and Juliana, whose constant amusement at my antics and input to my thoughts make life beyond meaningful. This book is a note to them.

Tashan Mehta, Katherine Harmon, Colleen Shelley, Sharon Bobrow, and Jeff Greenwald have edited my verbiage to make sense and my grammar to please all of our second-grade teachers and rear-seat drivers. Continuous thanks to them.

Kat Salsman brought anatomy to life with her beautiful illustrations.

Christine Mason and Ann Walgenbach added the stimulus and the softness to make my impulses productive and not negative, kind and not so often critical. I only wish I could be as nice as Ann.

May this book be a gift to all and an inspiration to become fitter, faster, and stronger than you thought you could be.

Made in the USA
Las Vegas, NV
16 December 2021